ADVANCED DIGESTIVE ENDOSCOPY: ERCP

ADVANCED DIGESTIVE ENDOSCOPY: ERCP

EDITED BY

PETER B. COTTON

AND

JOSEPH LEUNG

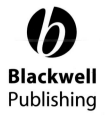

Blackwell
Publishing

Contents

List of contributors

BERGMAN, JACQUES J.G.H.M., *Department of Gastroenterology and Hepatology, Academic Medical Center Amsterdam, Meibergdreef 9, 1105 AZ Amsterdam, The Netherlands*

CHUNG, SYDNEY, *Department of Surgery, Prince of Wales Hospital, The Chinese University of Hong Kong, Shatin, NT, Hong Kong*

COTTON, PETER B., *Medical University of South Carolina, PO Box 250327, Ste 210 CSB, 96 Jonathan Lucas St, Charleston, SC 29425, USA*

FOGEL, EVAN L., *Indiana University Medical Center, 550 N. University Drive, Suite 4100, Indianapolis, IN 46202, USA*

FREEMAN, MARTIN L., *Hennepin County Medical Center, GI Division, 701 Park Avenue, Minneapolis, MN 55415, USA*

GUELRUD, MOISES, *New England Medical Center, 750 Washington Street, Booth 213, Boston, MA 02111, USA*

HOWELL, DOUGLAS A., *Portland Endoscopy Center, 1200 Congress Street #300, Portland, ME 04102, USA*

LEE, JOHN G., *University of California Irvine, Division of Gastroenterology, 101 The City Drive, Bldg 53, Rm 113, Orange, CA 92817, USA*

LEHMAN, GLEN, *Indiana University Medical Center, 550 N. University Blvd, Rm 4100, Indianapolis, IN 46202, USA*

LEUNG, JOSEPH, *Division of GI UC Davis, 4150 V Street, Ste 3500, PSSB, Sacramento, CA 95817, USA*

MCHENRY, LEE, *Indiana University Medical Center, 550 N. University Drive, Suite 4100, Indianapolis, IN 46202, USA*

NG, ENDERS K.W., *Upper GI Division, Department of Surgery, The Chinese University of Hong Kong, Hong Kong*

PARASHER, GULSHAN, *Division of Gastroenterology and Hepatology, University of New Mexico, Albuquerque NM87131-0001, New Mexico*

SHERMAN, STUART, *Indiana University Medical Center, 550 N. University Drive, Suite 4100, Indianapolis, IN 46202, USA*

Preface

There was a time, long ago, when endoscopy was a small off-shoot of gastroenterology, and when most of what budding endoscopists needed to know could be covered in a slim book. Thus *Practical Gastrointestinal Endoscopy* was conceived by Christopher Williams and myself over 25 years ago, and had a successful run through four editions. The field has expanded enormously over that time. The number and variety of procedures, and the relevant scientific literature, have proliferated, and there is now a hierarchy within endoscopy. There are 'standard' procedures which most clinical gastroenterologists master during their training. These constitute routine upper endoscopy and colonoscopy, with their common therapeutic aspects, which may be needed at work every day (and some nights). Then there are recognized 'advanced' procedures, such as ERCP and EUS, and the more adventurous therapeutic aspects of upper endoscopy and colonoscopy, such as fundoplication, EMR, and tumor ablation. These are practiced by only a small percentage of endoscopists, who need more focused and intensive training. In addition, for a few of the leaders, there is much to be learned in related fields, such as unit design, management, teaching, and quality improvement. It is clear that no one person (or two) can speak or write about all of this territory with any authority. Advice and instruction are best given by acknowledged experts in each specific area.

My publishing journey reflects these changes. Thus, the latest (5th) Edition of *Practical Gastrointestinal Endoscopy*, sub-titled 'The Fundamentals', published in 2003, is devoted solely to the basic facts which all trainees need in their first year or two. It is accompanied by 2 practical CDRoms, one devoted to each 'end'. We removed all of the 'advanced stuff', such as ERCP, teaching methods, and unit management.

We then sought to serve the needs of the established endoscopists, and of those learning more advanced aspects, with a new series called 'Advanced Digestive Endoscopy'. Reflecting the acceleration of our world, we saw this primarily as a virtual 'ebook', presented electronically for speed of posting and for easy updating. This is now evolving on the comprehensive Blackwell Publishing website www.gastrohep.com. It has 5 separate sections:—Endoscopic Practice and Safety, Upper Endoscopy, Colonoscopy, ERCP, and EUS. I was delighted to be joined in this endeavor by new partners; Joseph Leung, Joseph Sung, Jerry Waye, and Rob Hawes. Between us we have persuaded over 40 distinguished colleagues from all over the world to make contributions.

Despite the multiple benefits of electronic publishing, there is still a demand for print books. Jerry Waye's book on Colonoscopy, co-edited with Doug Rex and Christopher Williams, is already in print (the ebook version consists of a selection of those chapters).

Here we present the print version of ERCP. I am enormously grateful to Joseph Leung and to the 12 other contributors who have labored long and hard to bring it to fruition. The fact that most of the authors are based in the USA should not be misinterpreted, for the expertise and methods of ERCP are now truly international. The electronic version will continue, and will be updated every year or so. We welcome your criticism and suggestions for improvement.

Joseph and I offer our sincere thanks to our families for their support and forbearance, and to our colleagues and trainees who have taught us so much, not least how much we still have to learn.

Peter B Cotton MD FRCP FRCS February 2005
Digestive Disease Center, Medical University of
South Carolina, Charleston, USA

CHAPTER 1

ERCP Overview—A 30-Year Perspective

PETER B. COTTON

Historical background

Endoscopic cannulation of the papilla of Vater was first reported in 1968 [1]. However, it was really put on the map shortly afterwards by several Japanese groups, working with instrument manufacturers to develop appropriate long side-viewing instruments [2–5]. The technique (initially called ECPG—endoscopic cholangiopancreatography—in Japan) spread throughout Europe in the early 1970s [6–13]. Early efforts were much helped by a multinational workshop at the European Congress in Paris in 1972, organized by the Olympus company. ERCP rapidly became established worldwide as a valuable diagnostic technique, although doubts were expressed in the USA about its feasibility and role [14], and the potential for serious complications soon became clear [15–18]. ERCP was given a tremendous boost by the development of its therapeutic applications, notably biliary sphincterotomy in the mid-1970s [19–21] and biliary stenting 5 years later [22,23].

It is difficult for most gastroenterologists today to imagine the diagnostic and therapeutic situation 30 years ago. There were no scans. Biliary obstruction was diagnosed and treated surgically, with substantial operative mortality. Nonoperative documentation of biliary pathology by ERCP was a huge step forward. Likewise, ERCP was an amazing development in pancreatic investigation at a time when the only available test was laparotomy. The ability to 'see into' the pancreas, and to collect pure pancreatic juice [24], seemed like a miracle. We assumed that ERCP would have a dramatic impact on chronic pancreatitis and pancreatic cancer. Sadly, these expectations are not yet realized, but endoscopic management of biliary obstruction was clearly a major clinical advance, especially in the sick and elderly. The period of 15 or so years from the mid-1970s really constituted a 'golden age' for ERCP. Despite significant risks [25], it was obvious to everyone that ERCP management of duct stones and tumors was easier, cheaper, and safer than available surgical alternatives. Large series were published, including some randomized trials [26–31]. Percutaneous transhepatic cholangiography (PTC) and its drainage applications were also developed during this time, but were used (with the exception of a few units) only when ERCP failed or was not available. The 'combined procedure'—endoscopic cannulation over a guidewire placed at PTC [32,33]—became popular for a while, but was needed less as both endoscopic and interventional techniques improved.

The changing world of pancreatico-biliary medicine

The situation has changed in many ways during the last two decades. ERCP has evolved significantly, but so have many other relevant techniques.

The impact of scanning radiology

Imaging modalities for the biliary tree and pancreas have proliferated. High quality ultrasound, computed tomography, endoscopic ultrasonography, and MR scanning (with MRCP) have greatly facilitated the non-invasive evaluation of patients with known and suspected biliary and pancreatic disease. As a result, the proportion of ERCP examinations now performed purely for diagnostic purposes has diminished significantly. However, it remains a very accurate diagnostic tool, and continues to shed important light in selected cases where all of the non-invasive tests have been inconclusive.

Extending the indications for therapeutic ERCP

The second major change has been the attempt of ERCP practitioners to extend their therapeutic territory from standard biliary procedures into more complex areas such as pancreatitis and suspected sphincter of Oddi dysfunction. The value of ERCP in these contexts remains controversial [34].

Improvements in surgery

The third major change is the substantial and progressive reduction in risk associated with conventional surgery (due to excellent perioperative and anesthesia care), and the increasing use of less invasive laparoscopic techniques [35]. It is no longer correct to assume that ERCP is always safer than surgery. Sadly, serious complications of ERCP (especially pancreatitis and perforation) continue to occur, especially during speculative procedures performed by inexperienced practitioners, often using the needle-knife for lack of standard expertise [36].

Risk reduction

These facts are forcing the ERCP community to search for ways to reduce the risks. Important examples of this preoccupation are the focus on refining indications [34], prospective studies of predictors of adverse outcomes [37], and attempts to remove stones from the bile duct without sphincterotomy [38], at least in younger patients with relatively small stones and normal sized ducts.

Patient empowerment

Another important driver in this field is the increased participation of patients in decisions about their care. Patients are rightly demanding the data on the potential benefits, risks, and limitations of ERCP, and the same data about the alternatives. Report cards are one response [39].

Current focus

The focus in the early twenty-first century is on careful evaluation of what ERCP can offer (in comparison with available alternatives), and on attempts to improve the overall quality of ERCP practice [40]. Equally important is the increasing focus on who should be trained, and to what level of expertise. How many ERCPists are really needed? (See Chapter 2.)

These issues are important in all clinical contexts, but come into clearest focus where ERCP is still considered somewhat speculative, e.g. in the management of chronic pancreatitis and of possible sphincter of Oddi dysfunction [34].

Benefits and risks

Evaluation of ERCP is a complex topic [41,42]. Its role is very much dependent on the clinical context (Table 1.1), and colleagues contributing to this resource provide guidance about the current state of practice in their main topic areas. This discussion focuses on the general difficulties in defining the role and value of ERCP [41]. Figure 1.1 attempts to illustrate all the elements of the 'intervention equation'. There is much talk about 'outcomes studies', but 'outcomes' cannot be assessed without detailed knowledge of the precise 'incomes'. Thus, a patient with certain demographics, disease type, size, and severity causing a specific level of symptoms, disability, and life disruption is offered an ERCP intervention, by a certain individual with a particular experience and skill level, with certain expected, planned, burdens (i.e. pain, distress, disruption, and costs). All of these metrics need clear and agreed definitions if we are to make any sense of the evaluation. The conjunction of the patient and that intervention results in the 'outcomes' (Fig. 1.1). Ultimately, we are most interested in the clinical outcome (reduced burden of symptoms and disease), but there are many factors along the way, including the technical results (influenced by the 'degree of difficulty'), and the occurrence of unplanned events (or complications), which add to the actual burden.

Table 1.1 Clinical contexts for possible ERCP use.

Biliary
- Jaundice
- Abnormal LFTs
- Suspected/known duct stone

Pancreatitis
- Chronic
- Acute gallstone related
- Idiopathic recurrent
- Complicated

Pain
- Chronic
- Acute intermittent (includes postcholecystectomy)
- Early postsurgical

Imaging findings (papilla, pancreas, biliary)

Stent service

Other

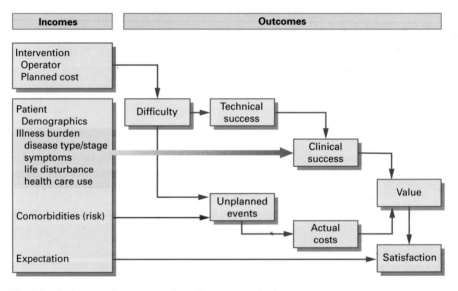

Fig. 1.1 The intervention process: data elements required.

Unplanned events

The word 'complication' is emotive, raising issues of medical error and legal liability. We prefer to discuss 'unplanned events', since they are best described simply as deviations from the plan which had been agreed with the patient. The phrase 'adverse events' has been used too, but not all unplanned events are negative. A patient with suspected cancer may be delighted to wake up from a procedure with an unexpected cure (sphincterotomy and stone removal). All unplanned events should be documented in a standard format, as an aid to efforts at quality improvement. Some are relatively trivial, such as transient hypotension or self-limited bleeding. At what level of severity do they become 'complications'? An influential consensus conference [43] set the threshold at the need for hospital admission, and defined levels of severity by the length of stay, as well as the need for surgery or intensive care. Details of complications, and their avoidance and management, are addressed in Chapter 13.

Clinical success and value

Clinical success may sometimes be relatively obvious, e.g. removal of a stone or relief of jaundice with a stent. However, in many cases (e.g. chronic pancreatitis, sphincter dysfunction), the judgement can be made only after long periods of follow-up. This greatly complicates evaluation studies in just the clinical circumstances where the knowledge is needed most. Patient satisfaction is another important parameter. It is determined partly by the clinical results (and how that compares with the patient's expectation), but also by patients' perception of the process (accessibility, courtesy, etc.). The cost (burden) of the intervention is obviously a key consideration. This consists of the planned burden, plus the result of any unplanned events. The ratio between the clinical impact (benefit) and the burden (cost) determines the 'value' of the procedure in that individual patient (Fig. 1.1). Attempts to provide definitions for all of these metrics are advancing slowly. Their incorporation in endoscopy reporting databases will allow ongoing useful outcomes evaluations to guide further decisions. If the same or similar metrics are also used by those performing alternative interventions such as surgery, we will obtain a clearer idea of the relative roles of these different procedures [44]. In some cases randomization will be necessary to make a final judgement. However, the issue of 'operator dependence' will always exist. A randomized trial of two techniques performed by experts may not be the best guide to the choice of intervention in everyday community practice.

The future

The trends which we have outlined are likely to continue and to accelerate in the coming years. Quality is the big issue. That means making sure that we are doing the right things, and doing them right. It has been clear for a long time (but is only now becoming generally accepted) that ERCP is a procedure that should be undertaken only by a minority of gastroenterologists. The amount of training and continuing dedication in practice needed to attain and maintain high levels of competence, and to improve, means that the procedures should be focused in relatively few hands. The increasing variety and safety of alternative procedures, and the vigilance of our customers, will drive that agenda. The other imperative is to pursue the research studies necessary to improve current methods, and to evaluate all of them rigorously. This is best performed in collaboration with colleagues in surgery and radiology to establish the best methods for approaching patients with known or suspected biliary and pancreatic disease. The dynamics between specialists will change with time, which is one excellent reason for organizing care to be patient-focused, rather than in traditional technical silos. Multidisciplinary organizations, like our Digestive Disease Center, attempt to provide that perspective and a platform for the unbiased research and education that aim to improve the quality of service [45].

References

1 McCune WS, Shorb PE, Moscovitz H. Endoscopic cannulation of the ampulla of Vater: a preliminary report. *Ann Surg* 1968; 167: 752–6.
2 Oi I, Takemoto T, Kondo T. Fiberduodenoscope: direct observations of the papilla of Vater. *Endoscopy* 1969; 1: 101–3.
3 Ogoshi K, Tobita Y, Hara Y. Endoscopic observation of the duodenum and pancreatocholedochography using duodenofiberscope under direct vision. *Gastrointest Endosc* 1970; 12: 83–96.
4 Takagi K, Ideda S, Nakagawa Y, Sakaguchi N, Takahashi T, Kumakura K *et al.* Retrograde pancreatography and cholangiography by fiber-duodenoscope. *Gastroenterology* 1970; 59: 445–52.
5 Kasugai T, Kuno N, Aoki I, Kizu M, Kobayashi S. Fiberduodenoscopy: analysis of 353 examinations. *Gastrointest Endosc* 1971; 18: 9–16.
6 Classen M, Koch H, Fruhmorgen P, Grabner W, Demling L. Results of retrograde pancreaticography. *Acta Gastroenterologica Japonica* 1972; 7: 131–6.
7 Cotton PB. Progress report: cannulation of the papilla of Vater by endoscopy and retrograde cholangiopancreatography (ERCP). *Gut* 1972; 13: 1014–25.
8 Cotton PB, Salmon PR, Blumgart LH, Burwood RJ, Davies GT, Lawrie BW *et al.* Cannulation of papilla of Vater via fiber-duodenoscope: assessment of retrograde cholangiopancreatography in 60 patients. *Lancet* 1972; 1: 53–8.
9 Gulbis A, Cremer M, Engelholm L. La cholangiographie et la wirsungographic endoscopiques. *Acta Endoscopica Radiocinematogr* 1972; 2: 78–80.
10 Heully F, Gaucher P, Laurent J, Vicari F, Fays J, Bigard M-A, Jenpierre R. La duodenoscopie et la catheterisme de voies biliares et pancreatiques. *Nouv Presse Med* 1972; 1: 313–18.
11 Safrany L, Tari J, Barna L, Torok I. Endoscopic retrograde cholangiography: experience of 168 examinations. *Gastrointest Endosc* 1973; 19: 163–8.
12 Liguory C, Gouero H, Chavy A, Coffin JC, Huguier M. Endoscopic retrograde cholangiopancreatography. *Br J Surg* 1974; 61: 359–62.
13 Cotton PB. ERCP. *Gut* 1977; 18: 316–41.
14 Morrissey JF. To cannulate or not to cannulate [Editorial]. *Gastroenterology* 1972; 63: 351–2.
15 Blackwood WD, Vennes JA, Silvis SE. Post-endoscopy pancreatitis and hyperamylasuria. *Gastrointest Endosc* 1973; 20: 56–8.
16 Classen M, Demling L. Hazards of endoscopic retrograde cholangio-pancreaticography (ERCP). *Acta Hepatogastroenterol (Stutt)* 1975; 22: 1–3.
17 Nebel OT, Silvis SE, Rogers G, Sugawa C, Mandelstam P. Complications associated with endoscopic retrograde cholangio-pancreatography: results of the 1974 A/S/G/E survey. *Gastrointest Endosc* 1975; 22: 34–6.

18 Bilbao MK, Dotter CT, Lee TG, Katon RM. Complications of endoscopic retrograde cholangiopancreatography (ERCP): a study of 10 000 cases. *Gastroenterology* 1976; 70: 314–20.

19 Classen M, Demling L. Endoskopische sphinkterotomie der papilla Vateri und steinextraktion aus dem ductus choledochus. *Dtsch Med Wochenschr* 1974; 99: 496–7.

20 Kawai K, Akasaka Y, Murakami K, Tada M, Kohill Y, Nakajima M. Endoscopic sphincterotomy of the ampulla of Vater. *Gastrointest Endosc* 1974; 20: 148–51.

21 Cotton PB, Chapman M, Whiteside CG, LeQuesne LP. Duodenoscopic papillotomy and gallstone removal. *Br J Surg* 1976; 63: 709–14.

22 Soehendra N, Reijnders-Frederix V. Palliative bile duct drainage: a new endoscopic method of introducing a transpapillary drain. *Endoscopy* 1980; 12: 8–11.

23 Laurence BH, Cotton PB. Decompression of malignant biliary obstruction by duodenoscope intubation of the bile duct. *Br Med J* 1980; I: 522–3.

24 Robberrecht P, Cremer M, Vandermers A, Vandermers-Piret M-C, Cotton PB, de Neef P *et al.* Pancreatic secretion of total protein and three hydrolases collected in healthy subjects via duodenoscopic cannulation: effects of secretin, pancreozymin and caerulein. *Gastroenterology* 1975; 69: 374–9.

25 Byrne P, Leung JWC, Cotton PB. Retroperitoneal perforation during duodenoscopic sphincterotomy. *Radiology* 1984; 150: 383–4.

26 Vaira D, Ainley C, Williams S, Caines S, Salmon P, Russell C *et al.* Endoscopic sphincterotomy in 1000 consecutive patients. *Lancet* 1989; 2: 431–4.

27 Cotton PB. Endoscopic management of bile duct stones (apples and oranges). *Gut* 1984; 25: 587–97.

28 Leung JWC, Emery R, Cotton PB, Russell RCG, Vallon AG, Mason RR. Management of malignant obstructive jaundice at The Middlesex Hospital. *Br J Surg* 1983; 70: 584–6.

29 Cotton PB. Endoscopic methods for relief of malignant obstructive jaundice. *World J Surg* 1984; 8: 854–61.

30 Speer AG, Cotton PB, Russell RCG, Mason RR, Hatfield ARW, Leung JWC *et al.* Randomized trial of endoscopic versus percutaneous stent insertion in malignant obstructive jaundice. *Lancet* 1987; 2: 57–62.

31 Smith AC, Dowsett JF, Russell RCG, Hatfield ARW, Cotton PB. Randomised trial of endoscopic stenting versus surgical bypass in malignant low bile duct obstruction. *Lancet* 1994; 344: 1655–60.

32 Shorvon PJ, Cotton PB, Mason RR, Siegel HJ, Hatfield ARW. Percutaneous transhepatic assistance for duodenoscopic sphincterotomy. *Gut* 1985; 26: 1373–6.

33 Dowsett JF, Vaira D, Hatfield AR, Cairns SR, Polydorou A, Frost R *et al.* Endoscopic biliary therapy using the combined percutaneous and endoscopic technique. *Gastroenterology* 1989; 96: 1180–6.

34 Cohen S, Bacon BR, Berlin JA, Fleischer D, Hecht GA, Loehrer PJ *et al.* NIH State of the Science Conference Statement: ERCP for diagnosis and therapy. *Gastrointest Endosc* 2002; 56: 803–9.

35 Cotton PB, Chung SC, Davis WZ, Gibson RM, Ransohoff DF, Strasberg SM. Issues in cholecystectomy and management of duct stones. *Am J Gastroenterol* 1994; 89: S169–76.

36 Cotton PB. ERCP is most dangerous for people who need it least. *Gastrointest Endosc* 2001; 54: 535–6.

37 Freeman ML, DiSario JA, Nelson DB, Fennerty MB, Lee JG, Bjorkman DJ *et al.* Risk factors for post-ERCP pancreatitis: a prospective, multicenter study. *Gastrointest Endosc* 2001; 54: 425–34.

38 Huibregtse K. Endoscopic balloon dilation for removal of bile duct stones: special indications only. *Endoscopy* 2001; 33 (7): 620–2.

39 Cotton PB. How many times have you done this procedure, Doctor? *Am J Gastroenterol* 2002; 97: 522–3.

40 Quality and Outcome Assessment in Gastrointestinal Endoscopy. *Gastrointest Endosc* 2000; 52: 827–30.

41 Cotton PB. Income and outcome metrics for objective evaluation of ERCP and alternative methods. *Gastrointest Endosc* 2002; 56 (Suppl. 6): S283–90.

42 Cotton PB. Therapeutic gastrointestinal endoscopy: problems in proving efficacy. *N Engl J Med* 1992; 326: 1626–8.

43 Cotton PB, Lehman G, Vennes J, Geenen JE, Russell RCG, Meyers WC *et al.* Endoscopic sphincterotomy complications and their management: an attempt at consensus. *Gastrointest Endosc* 1991; 37: 383–93.

44 Cotton PB. Randomization is not the (only) answer: a plea for structured objective evaluation of endoscopic therapy. *Endoscopy* 2000; 32: 402–5.

45 Cotton PB. Fading boundary between gastroenterology and surgery. *J Gastroenterol Hepatol* 2000; 15: G34–7.

CHAPTER 2

ERCP Training, Competence, and Assessment

PETER B. COTTON

ERCP is challenging, and not for all gastroenterologists

ERCP is the most challenging endoscopic procedure performed regularly by gastroenterologists. It is often difficult technically, and may fail. Optimal practice requires considerable manual dexterity, a broad knowledge of pancreatic and biliary diseases, and familiarity with the many alternative diagnostic and therapeutic approaches. Furthermore, it carries substantial risks, even in the hands of experts [1,2].

ERCP has been seen also as rather glamorous, so that most gastroenterology trainees have aspired to master the techniques, and to practice them independently. Many factors make that inappropriate. Firstly, it has become obvious (as detailed below) that attaining competence takes far more training and experience than previously appreciated. This is time consuming, and also detracts from time needed to study other specialist fields of gastroenterology and hepatology. Secondly, the increasing refinement and availability of imaging techniques such as CT scanning, MRCP, and EUS have rendered diagnostic ERCP to be (almost) obsolete [1]. This means that any endoscopist offering ERCP must be geared up to provide therapy for the likely problem. Thirdly, it is now clear that less experienced practitioners have more failures, and also have more complications. Fourthly, many ERCP endoscopists have been trained (albeit not all very well) in the last two decades, and very few more are needed each year to maintain the ranks. Finally, consumer empowerment will be an important driver. Patients are beginning to understand that not all endoscopists are alike, and are seeking out experienced practitioners when they need more aggressive procedures.

All of these facts mandate that only a few people should be trained, and that they should be trained well. This is far from a new idea, having been stated clearly and repeatedly over the years by many individuals [3–7] and endoscopy organizations [8–14]. The problem is that no one has paid attention, as is brutally obvious from a recent survey of 69 graduates from US fellowship programs [15]. Most had had some experience of ERCP (range 12–320 cases, median 140).

One-third stated that their training was inadequate, yet 91% of them proposed to practice ERCP. This is bad medicine, and embarrassing for our profession [16]. We must ensure that those offering ERCP services are competent to do so.

What is 'competence' in ERCP?

There is a wide spectrum of expertise in the performance of ERCP. Competence traditionally describes the point at which a trainee can practice independently. What are the criteria for independent practice? Sadly, our understanding of the complexity of that issue has been slow to develop, and opinions vary widely [17]. Only now are attempts being made to develop meaningful objective methods of assessment.

Issues of training, competence, and assessment for all aspects of endoscopy have been well reviewed recently by Cohen [18] and Freeman [19].

The first ASGE guidelines for ERCP relied almost solely on the numbers of cases experienced during training, and suggested that 100 (including 25 therapeutic) would be adequate [8]. That guideline attempted to put the onus on the training program directors, suggesting that they should not be asked to advise or to arbitrate competency until those 'threshold' numbers had been reached. But this sensible concept was ignored, and formal assessments were rare events. Even when logbooks became routine, it was difficult to assess what contribution the trainee had made (or indeed could have made independently).

A study of the learning curve for ERCP at Duke University was a turning point in the debate. Even after 180–200 cases, trainees were scarcely performing at an 80% level [20].

The latest guideline from the ASGE in 2002 [21] mentions that 200 procedures are not adequate for most trainees to achieve competence, and emphasizes objective end points (such as an 80% biliary cannulation rate) as better minimal standards. The Australians have set the highest hurdle so far, i.e. completion of 200 procedures, unassisted [22]. The British authorities suggested a 90% hurdle in 1999 [13], but the 2004 version [23] replaced numbers completely in favor of a list of needed skills (without precise goals), stating rather quaintly that 'although trainees must aspire to internationally accepted standards for cannulation success—a 90% success rate for uncomplicated cases has been proposed —it is unreasonable to demand this level of performance from trainees by the end of their training . . .'.

Whilst these concepts and guidelines are logical and well-meaning, there have been few attempts so far to document what skill levels are really being achieved. Nor do we know how performance in the training environment translates into independent practice. It is one thing to complete a procedure in the training environment with faculty advice and encouragement, and familiar assistants and equipment, but quite another to do so unaided in a new unfamiliar environment, with pressure to succeed. We need to collect meaningful objective data during training, but also in the early phases of practice.

Cognitive competence

The safe and effective practice of ERCP clearly requires far more than technical skills, as has been well stated repeatedly. Documenting technical competence is difficult, but proving the acquisition of the necessary cognitive skills may be even more so [24]. It has been assumed that formal training in Gastroenterology and Hepatology (e.g. Board certification in the USA) is likely to cover the necessary territory [25], but the specifics of pancreaticobiliary medicine have not been assessed formally. Furthermore, the field is in constant flux and requires ongoing study.

Degree of difficulty and expertise

Not all ERCP examinations are equal. Any case can prove challenging on the day (e.g. due to a duodenal diverticulum), but some are *predictably* more difficult (e.g. known prior Billroth II resection, hilar tumors, or suspected sphincter dysfunction). A five-level scoring system for predicted degree of difficulty was developed [26], and later simplified to three grades (Table 2.1) [26,27]. Grade 1 procedures are those (mainly biliary) interventions which anyone offering ERCP should be able to achieve to a reasonable level of expertise. Grade 2 cases include more complex cases, such as minor papilla cannulations and larger

Table 2.1 Degrees of difficulty in ERCP.

	Diagnostic	Therapeutic
Standard, grade 1	Selective deep cannulation Diagnostic sampling	Biliary sphincterotomy Stones < 10 mm Stents for leaks Low tumors
Advanced, grade 2	Billroth II diagnostics Minor papilla cannulation	Stones > 10 mm Hilar tumors Benign biliary strictures
Tertiary, grade 3	Manometry Whipple Roux-en-Y Intraductal endoscopy	Billroth II therapeutics Intrahepatic stones Pancreatic therapies

Endoscopist	Grade of difficulty		
	1	2	3
Competent	80–90	–	–
Proficient	90+	80+	–
Expert	98+	95+	90+

Table 2.2 Likely success rates (%) of ERCP, correlating the endoscopist's level of skill with the grade of difficulty.

stones. Grade 3 procedures are the most difficult, such as treatments for pancreatitis and intrahepatic stones, and are performed mainly in tertiary referral centers.

The above discussion about competence refers primarily to grade 1 procedures, which are the 'garden-variety' cases that will be encountered in everyday practice. Endoscopists with more training (e.g. a dedicated fourth year in the USA), and those who have honed their skills in practice with the aid of community and academic colleagues, will attempt more complex cases. So-called experts, working in referral centers, will tackle all comers, but will also have very high success rates in the easier cases. These concepts of case difficulty and individual expertise can usefully be combined (Table 2.2).

ERCP training at MUSC

Our trainees select from three levels of training in pancreatico-biliary medicine and ERCP. The simplest is exposure to the service for 2 months, which shows them approximately 80 cases, and the thinking that goes with them. They learn to use side-viewing endoscopes, but are not expected to perform ERCP. The second level is offered to selected fellows in the GI training program (which lasts 3 years). They experience over 300 cases and appear reasonably competent in standard (mainly biliary) procedures when they leave. The third option requires a dedicated fourth year, with another 300+ cases. These endoscopists have mastered standard grade 1 cases, and know enough to attempt some of the more complex procedures.

Towards more structured training

Together, all of these issues in training and assessment point to the need for a much more structured approach, including formalized curricula and enhanced educational resources. The need to be personally involved in so many live cases could be reduced substantially in the future as computer simulators mature and become more widely available [18].

Ongoing competence and re-credentialing

It is logical that endoscopists need a certain ongoing volume of cases to maintain their skills, if not to improve them. There have been no studies to provide guideline figures, but my guess is that it is difficult to remain sharp with less than 50–100 cases per year, even if prior experience has been substantial. Few endoscopists achieve that annual volume in Britain [7], and a survey of US gastroenterologists in 1987 revealed a median number of only 30 ERCPs per year [28].

There is also the issue of the number of ERCP cases in an individual endoscopy unit or hospital. Continuing experience is needed to maintain the necessary nursing skills and equipment; my guess would be a minimum of 100–200 cases per year. Few hospitals achieve those numbers. A British survey reported that only 25% of units performed > 200 cases per year in 1997 [7]. A search of the National Inpatient sample in the USA revealed that ERCPs were done in 2629 hospitals. The average number was 49 per year; only 25% of hospitals performed more than 100, and only 5% more than 200 [29].

Hopefully, ongoing privileging (credentialing) in the future will be based on more than numbers alone [21,23]. Outcomes data should be available, and computer simulators are also likely to play an increasing role. The ASGE suggested in 1995 that intermittent 'proctoring' should be considered [21], a sensible idea that has been ignored completely.

One promising tool is the endoscopy 'report card'.

Report cards

The ASGE has recommended the use of report cards, i.e. summaries of the ongoing practice of individual endoscopists [30], a concept that I support strongly [31]. Endoscopists should keep track of their case volumes and case mix, and their outcomes, and be prepared to share the data when requested (whether by payers, privileging authorities, or patients) [21]. We are becoming accustomed to seeing hospital 'league tables' of the outcomes of major procedures such as cardiovascular surgery and pancreatico-duodenectomy. However, it is clear for endoscopy [32], as for surgery [33], that outcomes are more dependent on the case volume of individual practitioners than on the institutions in which they work. An example of a report card for one long-time ERCPist is shown in Table 2.3. The increasing use of electronic reporting systems will make this process easier, even automatic. Sharing the data between endoscopists eventually will provide benchmarks, and will be a powerful stimulus to improvement.

Report cards are likely to be voluntary at least initially. What is the incentive for less experienced endoscopists to collect data and advertise the fact that they are not super-experts? The answer lies with our patients, who are advised

Table 2.3 Lifetime experience of ERCP > 15 000 cases since 1971. Certifications: Gastroenterology boards (UK); ACLS.

	2002	2003	2004
Annual procedures	422	386	342
Therapy performed	80%	85%	88%
Disease spectrum			
Pancreatitis	115 (27%)	106 (21%)	98 (29%)
Sphincter dysfunction	84 (20%)	118 (27%)	84 (25%)
Tumors	64 (15%)	42 (11%)	43 (13%)
Stones	57 (13%)	52 (13%)	52 (15%)
Benign biliary	54 (13%)	40 (10%)	38 (11%)
Normal	20 (5%)	6 (2%)	10 (7%)
Difficulty scores			
Grade 1	38%	30%	33%
Grade 2	18%	12%	12%
Grade 3	44%	58%	55%
Time taken (minutes)	37 (±19)	39 (±21)	39 (±19)
Biliary cannulation rate	98%	98%	97%
Minor papilla cannulation rate	75%	86%	87%
Stone extraction success	100%	100%	100%
Complications			
Total	*5 (1.2%)*	*15 (4%)*	*17 (5%)*
Mild	4	13	13
Moderate	1	1	2
Severe	0	1	2
Fatal	0	0	0
Pancreatitis	3	11	12
Infection	2	3	2
Bleeding	0	1	1
Other	0	0	2

increasingly to ask their potential interventionists about their experience. Some patients will certainly hesitate if their practitioners are not able or willing to provide data when requested. Well-trained and skillful practitioners should wear their data as badges of quality.

An ERCP diploma?

A strong case can be made for a diploma which attests to ERCP competence. Eventually this will be accepted and embraced by the standard national examination authorities, but we should show the way. I envisage three main elements.

1 A written examination covering
- a knowledge base of pancreatic and biliary medicine;
- safety issues in ERCP practice;
- endoscopic and radiological interpretation.

2 Logbook documentation of all cases and achievement of defined threshold standards (e.g. cannulation rates, risks, etc.).

3 Proctoring of three cases by an outside expert, covering all aspects of the cases, including preparation, consent, performance, and documentation.

This examination would focus on standard grade 1 procedures, and be used to certify completion of training. It could be applied either at the training unit, or, by default, at the institution at which privileges are sought. A shorter version could be used also (along with the report card data and maybe computer simulation testing) for re-credentialing. One could envisage also an analogous diploma in 'Advanced ERCP' for those aspiring to recognition as expert referral resources. These examinations would be voluntary, like the report cards, but the acquisition of a diploma would provide the individual endoscopist with a significant practice advantage.

Conclusion

ERCP has tremendous potential for benefit, but can cause devastating complications. We must provide the training and credentialing framework to ensure that it is offered optimally. Structured training and continuing objective assessment of competence (through collection of real data) will be key elements for future success.

A diploma of competence in ERCP could become a powerful force for improving the quality of ERCP services.

References

1 NIH State-of-the-Science Conference Statement. ERCP for diagnosis and therapy, 14–16 January 2002. *Gastrointest Endosc* 2002; 56: 803–9.
2 Cotton PB, Williams CB. (1996). *Practical Gastrointestinal Endoscopy*, 4th edn. Blackwell Science, Oxford.
3 Sivak MV, Vennes JA, Cotton PB, Geenen JE, Benjamin SB, Lehman GA. Advanced training programs in gastrointestinal endoscopy. *Gastrointest Endosc* 1993; 39: 462–4.
4 Wicks ACB, Robertson GSM, Veitch PS. Structured training and assessment in ERCP has become essential for the Calman era. *Gut* 1999; 45: 154–6.
5 Baillie J. ERCP training for the few, not for all. *Gut* 1999; 45: 9–10.
6 Hellier MD, Morris AI. ERCP training—time for change. *Gut* 2000; 47: 459–60.
7 Allison MC, Ramanaden DN, Fouweather MG, Davis DKK, Colin-Jones DG. Provision of ERCP services and training in the United Kingdom. *Endoscopy* 2002; 32: 693–9.
8 American Society for Gastrointestinal Endoscopy. (1986). *Guidelines for Advanced Endoscopic Training*. ASGE, Publication no. 1026. ASGE, Manchester, MA.
9 American Society for Gastrointestinal Endoscopy. (1991). *Principles of Training in Gastrointestinal Endoscopy*. ASGE, Manchester, MA.

10 American Society for Gastrointestinal Endoscopy. Maintaining competency in endoscopic skills. *Gastrointest Endosc* 1995; 42: 620–1.

11 American Society for Gastrointestinal Endoscopy. Guidelines for credentialing and granting privileges for gastrointestinal endoscopy. *Gastrointest Endosc* 1998; 48: 679–82.

12 American Society for Gastrointestinal Endoscopy. Quality improvement of gastrointestinal endoscopy. *Gastrointest Endosc* 1999; 49: 842–4.

13 Joint Advisory Group on Gastrointestinal Endoscopy. (1999). *Recommendations for Training in Gastrointestinal Endoscopy*. British Society of Gastroenterology, London (www.bsg.org.uk/training/jag_99.html).

14 American Society for Gastrointestinal Endoscopy. Guidelines for advanced endoscopic training. *Gastrointest Endosc* 2001; 53: 846–8.

15 Kowalski T, Kanchana T, Pungpapong S. Perceptions of gastroenterology fellows regarding ERCP competency and training. *Gastrointest Endosc* 2003; 58: 345–9.

16 Sivak MV Jr. Trained in ERCP. *Gastrointest Endosc* 2003; 58: 412–14.

17 Waye JD, Bornman PC, Chopita N, Costamagna G, Ganc AJ, Speer T. ERCP training and experience. *Gastrointest Endosc* 2002; 56: 607–8.

18 Cohen J. (2004). Endoscopic training and credentialing. In: *Advanced Endoscopy*, e-book/annual (ed. Cotton, PB) (www.gastrohep.com).

19 Freeman ML. Training and competence in gastrointestinal endoscopy. *Rev Gastroenterol Disord* 2001; 1: 73–86.

20 Jowell PS, Baillie J, Branch S, Affronti J, Browning CL, Bute BP. Quantitative assessment of procedural competence: a prospective study of training in endoscopic retrograde cholangiopancreatography. *Ann Intern Med* 1996; 125: 983–9.

21 American Society for Gastrointestinal Endoscopy. Methods of granting hospital privileges to perform gastrointestinal endoscopy. *Gastrointest Endosc* 2002; 55: 780–3.

22 Conjoint Committee for Recognition of Training in Gastrointestinal Endoscopy. (1997). *Information for Supervisors: Changes to Endoscopic Training*. The Conjoint Committee for Recognition of Training in Gastrointestinal Endoscopy, Sydney.

23 Joint Advisory Group on Gastrointestinal Endoscopy. (2004). *Guidelines for the Training, Appraisal and Assessment of Trainees in Gastrointestinal Endoscopy, 2004* (www.Thejag.Org.Uk/JAG_2004pdf).

24 Wigton RS. Measuring procedural skills. *Ann Intern Med* 1996; 125: 1003–4.

25 The Gastroenterology Leadership Council. Training the gastroenterologist of the future: the gastroenterology core curriculum. *Gastroenterology* 1996; 110: 1266–300.

26 Schutz SM, Abbott RM. Grading ERCPs by degree of difficulty: a new concept to produce more meaningful outcome data. *Gastrointest Endosc* 2000; 51: 535–9.

27 Cotton PB. Income and outcome metrics for objective evaluation of ERCP and alternative methods. *Gastrointest Endosc* 2002; 56 (Suppl. 2): S283–90.

28 Wigton RS, Blank LL, Monsour H, Nicolas JA. Procedural skills of practicing gastroenterologists: a national survey of 700 members of the American College of Physicians. *Ann Intern Med* 1990; 113: 540–6.

29 Varadarajulu S, Kilgore M, Wilcox CM, Eloubeidi M. Relationship between hospital ERCP volume, length of stay and technical outcomes. *Gastrointest Endosc* [in press].

30 American Society for Gastrointestinal Endoscopy. Quality assessment of ERCP. *Gastrointest Endosc* 2002; 56: 165–9.

31 Cotton PB. How many times have you done this procedure, Doctor? *Am J Gastroenterol* 2002; 97: 522–3.

32 Petersen BT. ERCP outcomes: defining the operators, experience, and environments. *Gastrointest Endosc* 2002; 55: 953–8.

33 Birkmeyer JD, Stukel TA, Siewers AE, Goodney PP, Wennberg DE, Lucas FL. Surgeon volume and operative mortality in the United States. *N Engl J Med* 2003; 349: 2117–27.

CHAPTER 3

Fundamentals of ERCP

JOSEPH LEUNG

Synopsis

Endoscopic retrograde cholangiopancreatography (ERCP) was first described in 1968 and we have recently celebrated the 30th anniversary of endoscopic sphincterotomy. This diagnostic and therapeutic modality has impacted significantly in the management of patients with many different benign and malignant pancreatico-biliary problems. A successful ERCP requires the co-ordination and cooperation of a dedicated and committed team of endoscopists, nurses, and assistants, as well as an organized and functioning unit. It takes many years to learn, and repeated practice, in order to master the skill of ERCP and to do it safely. It is important to understand the indications, contraindications, limitations, and complications of individual procedures when offering ERCP to our patients. Although successful ERCP has replaced surgery as a treatment option for some difficult pancreatico-biliary diseases, we have also seen problems and complications arising as a result of endoscopic treatment. Prospective collection of data and selected randomized controlled studies with long-term follow-up are necessary to evaluate the true value of this technology in the overall care of our patients.

Introduction

Imaging of the pancreatico-biliary system

Methods for imaging the pancreatic and biliary ductal systems continue to evolve. Correct application of ERCP (and other procedures) requires an up-to-date knowledge of all of these modalities.

ERCP

ERCP is a direct contrast study of the pancreatico-biliary system. It is useful in the diagnosis and treatment of diseases involving the pancreas and bile ducts, such as stones, benign and malignant strictures, and developmental anomalies.

It is superior to indirect cholangiography (oral or IV), especially in cases with obstructive jaundice, which leads to raised intrabiliary pressure and impaired biliary excretion of contrast.

Moreover, intrahepatic bile duct pathologies can be demonstrated by ERCP using occlusion cholangiography. Pathology in the gallbladder and cystic duct abnormalities can also be visualized, although ERCP is not the best imaging study for gallbladder disease.

ERCP vs. PTC

Comparative investigation of direct cholangiography studies, i.e. ERCP and percutaneous transhepatic cholangiography (PTC), should take into consideration the individual patients and the expertise of the operator; however, ERCP is considered less invasive than PTC.

ERCP has the added advantages of allowing duodenoscopy and pancreatography, which are helpful in the diagnosis of ampullary pathology and pancreatic abnormalities. ERCP can be performed in the presence of ascites and/or malignancies involving the liver, contraindicating PTC. In addition, bile and pancreatic juice can be collected for cytological and microbiological examination during ERCP procedures.

MRCP

The development and refinement of magnetic resonance cholangiopancreatography (MRCP) have produced excellent quality pictures of the anatomy of the pancreatico-biliary system. It is non-invasive and can give images comparable to ERCP when performed well. Limitations are few and the diagnostic value is high, and it may replace diagnostic ERCP, especially in the investigation of jaundice. MRCP, however, lacks therapeutic potential.

EUS

Endoscopic ultrasonography (EUS) allows good visualization of the distal common bile duct (CBD), with an excellent diagnostic accuracy for ductal stones. It provides superb views of the pancreas, and is useful in defining underlying pancreatic pathology. Fine-needle aspiration cytology further complements the diagnostic capability of EUS in pancreatico-biliary diseases.

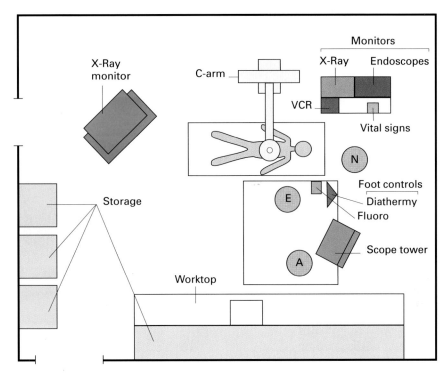

Fig. 3.1 Room set-up and floor plan. A, assistant; E, endoscopist; N, nurse.

Section I: Preparation for ERCP

Room set-up and floor plan (Figs 3.1 and 3.2)

Correct layout of the ERCP room is easier if it is located in a purpose-built endoscopy suite with in-house fluoroscopy facilities, rather than a shared facility in the radiology department. A purpose-built room with fluoroscopy offers the advantage of a better floor plan, organization, and ready access to stored accessories required for the procedures. Daily activities can be better organized and there is less hassle in moving equipment and endoscopists.

Space

The ERCP room should be large enough to house the endoscopy equipment, monitors, and the fluoroscopy unit. There should be ample room for the endoscopists and nurse/assistant(s) to manipulate accessories. Additional space is required for trainees and interested observers. Space should be available for anesthetic support and resuscitation equipment when needed. Ideally, there should be no cables or tubing on the floor that may hinder movement of carts or

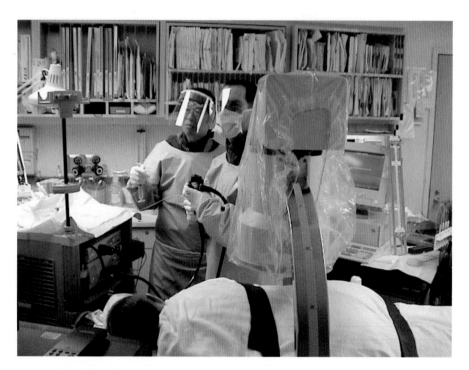

Fig. 3.2 Space for endoscopist and trainee or assistant. Accessories organized and within easy reach of endoscopist.

trolleys. Accessories should be organized and stored to facilitate easy retrieval during procedures.

Position of monitors and endoscopy cart (Fig. 3.2)

Some units have the endoscopy monitor mounted on the endoscopy cart at the head of the patient, which means the endoscopist has to turn to the right, away from the patient, in order to observe the endoscopy image. This bodily rotation tends to change the position and orientation of the scope and is best avoided. It is better to have the fluoroscopy and endoscopy monitors placed side by side facing the endoscopist, on the opposite side of the X-ray table (Fig. 3.3).

Because of the position of the fluoroscopy machine, the monitors may need to be placed at a 15–20° angle off to the right of the endoscopist for easy observation. The monitors are best ceiling mounted or supported on a stand placed at eye level. The endoscopist should adopt a comfortable position to avoid twisting and turning of the body, which may predispose to scope displacement or straining of the back and neck. The endoscopy tower is usually placed on the right behind the endoscopist, with sufficient room left in between for the manipulation of accessories.

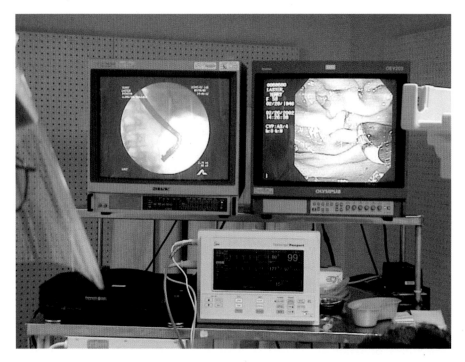

Fig. 3.3 Monitors for endoscopy, fluoroscopy, and vital signs are placed together at eye level.

Essential equipment for ERCP

Side-viewing duodenoscopes

Standard 3.2 mm and large 4.2 mm channel video endoscopes are now used routinely for diagnostic and therapeutic procedures. Smaller pediatric duodeno-scopes (with a 2.0 mm channel) are available for examination in neonates. The standard adult duodenoscope can be used in children above the age of two. Older non-immersible scopes cannot be properly reprocessed and are therefore not recommended for ERCP because of the risk of cross-contamination. A jumbo-size duodenoscope (5.5 mm channel) can be used as part of the mother and baby scope system, but it is more difficult to manipulate.

Forward-viewing scopes

Upper GI endoscopes may be used occasionally in patients with altered anatomy such as previous choledochoduodenostomy, Billroth II gastrectomy, or in patients with hepaticojejunostomy to facilitate intubation of the afferent loop.

Medication

A combination of sedatives and analgesics is used to provide conscious sedation during the ERCP procedure. Medications drawn up in syringes should be clearly labeled to avoid making mistakes during drug administration.

Sedatives and analgesics

Standard medications used for IV conscious sedation include demerol (meperidine) or fentanyl, and valium (Diazemuls) or midazolam (Versed). The dose requirement is titrated according to the patient's response. For an average sized adult, we usually start with 25–50 mg of meperidine *or* 25–50 µg of fentanyl, and 2.5–5 mg of valium *or* 1–2 mg of midazolam. Additional injections are given during the procedure as needed. IV benadryl 25–50 mg or IV phenergan may be given to enhance the sedative effects.

Anesthesia

General anesthesia with IV propofol is used increasingly for complex ERCP procedures, especially in anxious patients, those with cardio-pulmonary compromise, those who use chronic narcotics or excessive alcohol, and others with a history of poor response to standard sedation.

Smooth muscle relaxants

Glucagon (0.25–0.5 mg) or Buscopan (20–40 mg) is given intravenously in increments to relax the duodenum and to facilitate cannulation.

Reversal agents

Reversal agents including naloxone (Narcan 0.4 mg) and flumazenil (1 mg) should be readily available to reverse the effects of sedation.

Monitoring during conscious sedation

A qualified nurse (or anesthetist) should be assigned to administer medications, and to monitor the patient during the ERCP procedure. This person should have no other responsibilities. Medications are given in incremental doses based on the patient's response and condition in order to avoid oversedation. Vital signs including blood pressure, pulse, EKG, and oxygen saturation should be monitored continuously.

Supplemental oxygen can be given via a nasal cannula at a flow rate of

2 liters/min; this has been shown to prevent hypoxia. Care must be taken to avoid giving excess oxygen which may lead to respiratory depression in patients with COPD. Measuring the end-expiration CO_2 level using capnography is carried out in some centers.

Contrast agents

The most commonly used contrast media such as conray 280, urografin, hypaque, and renografin contain iodine. Contrast media used for ERCP include both hyperosmolar ionic medium and isosmolar, non-ionic medium. Isosmolar non-ionic contrast agents are more expensive but should be used in patients allergic to iodine. In addition, it is advisable to give these patients steroid prophylaxis and benadryl prior to the procedure to prevent contrast reaction.

Contrast should be drawn up in clearly labeled syringes prior to the procedure and be ready for use. It is preferable to have at least two 20 ml syringes filled with contrast of normal and half normal strength. A 20 ml syringe is used for contrast injection because it is easy to handle, contains sufficient volume of contrast, and permits injection by the endoscopist. Normal strength contrast should be used for initial cannulation for better visualization of the pancreatic duct. Half normal strength contrast is used to identify ductal stones in patients with dilated bile ducts.

Syringes for aspiration and irrigation

An empty 20 ml syringe is used to aspirate bile for culture and cytology. Sterile water is used to flush the catheters prior to insertion of hydrophilic wires or exchanges.

Organization and storage of accessories (Fig. 3.4)

There is a wide range of ERCP accessories. These include cannulas, sphincterotomes, guidewires, baskets, balloons, dilators, nasobiliary catheters, stents, biopsy forceps, injection needles, and more complex devices such as mechanical lithotriptors.

The accessories should be categorized and organized, and stored to allow easy retrieval as well as stock-keeping. A limited supply of commonly used items should be clearly labeled and displayed on shelves like books in a library.

Similar items are best grouped together and more specialized items kept separately. A detailed catalogue list and location of all accessories should be kept for quick reference. It is helpful to establish a preprocedure 'game plan' so that the necessary accessories can be retrieved and readied for use.

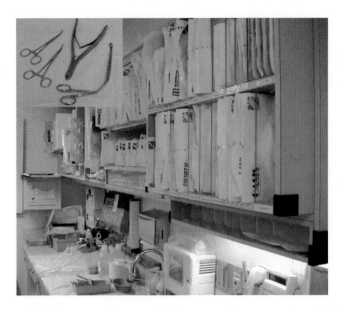

Fig. 3.4 Organize accessories within easy reach for retrieval. Do not stack up, 'file' like books in a library with large clear/'correct' labels. Categorize in groups. Special accessories and tools.

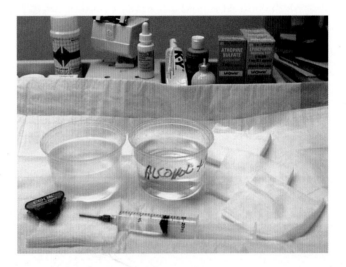

Fig. 3.5 Organization of worktop: water with simethicone for irrigation; 30% alcohol; 4 × 4 gauze; 20 ml syringe with blunt needle adaptor; 1 : 10 000 epinephrine; clips.

Organization of the worktop (Fig. 3.5)

To minimize cross-contamination of unopened accessories it is preferable to separate the clean and soiled items onto different worktops. Long accessories tend to uncoil and they are best organized with a clip.

A small pot of 30% alcohol is useful for cleaning the gloves (finger tips) to remove any sticky contrast or bile. Alcohol also reduces friction at the biopsy valve and facilitates insertion of accessories. Gauze pads are used for cleaning and wiping. Sterile water with simethicone can be flushed down the channel to suppress bubbling in the duodenum to improve visualization.

Fluoroscopy for ERCP

ERCP is ideally performed with the help of a radiologist, but more commonly with the help of a trained radiology technician. Endoscopists who personally operate the fluoroscopy unit during the procedure should receive basic fluoroscopy training and appropriate local licensing.

Fluoroscopy units (Fig. 3.6)

Conventional X-ray machines, as used for barium studies, are adequate for ERCP examinations. High-resolution digital fluoroscopy units produce better pictures but they are also much more expensive. A portable digital C-arm unit can be used but the resolution may be inferior to the full digital unit. It is preferable to use a machine with an under-couch X-ray tube. The X-ray machine should be capable of taking spot films. Digital units can store the images onto a computer for subsequent retrieval and review. Hard copies of selected images can be printed for reporting and filing. It is essential to know the magnification

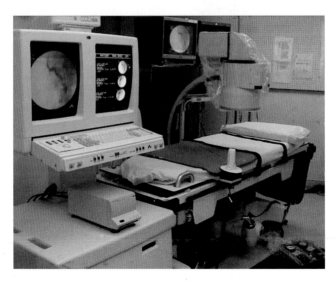

Fig. 3.6 Fluoroscopy machine with under-couch tube. Digital C-arm for designated ERCP room. Full fluoroscopy unit if shared facilities in Radiology. Remote control and foot pedal. Image capture.

factor of the machine for correct interpretation of X-ray findings, and for meas-uring the size of stones and the length of strictures.

A high-resolution monitor is necessary as diagnostic interpretation and therapeutic procedures are often performed in real time under fluoroscopic guidance. The X-ray table should have an electrical remote control for fine adjustment in positioning and preferably be able to tilt in two directions. Apart from built-in shielding, additional pieces of lead can be placed over the side and head end of the table to protect staff from scattered radiation.

KV and mA

These are the settings on the X-ray machine that determine the penetration of the X-ray beam and quality of the image generated. Most digital machines can automatically adjust the setting according to individual patients.

Split screen

The area of interest seen on fluoroscopy can be reduced to allow fine focus on a smaller area. This gives greater detail and reduces the radiation exposure.

Magnified view

A magnified view gives an enhanced image of the area of interest, but it also dou-bles the radiation exposure. It is sometimes necessary for proper localization of the tip of a guidewire or accessories during manipulation in the pancreas or for selective ductal cannulation.

Orientation of fluoroscopic images

The orientation of the fluoroscopic image on the monitor varies depending on the individual endoscopist's personal preference. Some prefer to orientate the image in the conventional way of viewing X-ray films. Some, however, prefer to orientate the fluoroscopic image according to the anatomical position, i.e. right side of the screen corresponds to right side of the patient lying in a prone position (Fig. 3.7).

Personnel protection (Fig. 3.8)

Individuals working with or around the fluoroscopy machine should be pro-tected from scattered radiation by using standard lead aprons (lead thickness 0.2–0.5 mm). If a one-sided lead apron is used, it is important to keep the apron

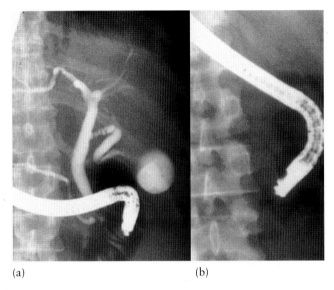

(a)   (b)

Fig. 3.7 Control film and ERCP. (a) Control film to look for calcification or air in biliary system. (b) ERCP showing the pancreatico-biliary system and gallbladder.

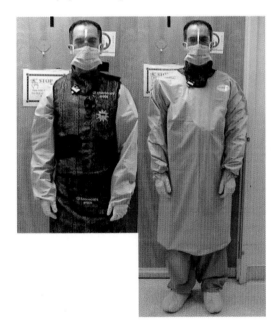

Fig. 3.8 Personnel protection—OSHA regulation. Gowns, gloves (double), shoe cover, face shields or mask, lead apron and collar, X-ray badge, and lead lining for room and warning signs.

facing the fluoroscopy unit during screening. Individuals who need to turn around during fluoroscopy should have both front and back protection. To reduce the weight of the lead apron on the shoulder, a skirt and a vest can be used. A lead collar should be worn to protect the thyroid gland, and lead glasses are recommended, especially if a fluoroscopy unit with an over-couch tube is used. Individuals should also wear their X-ray badge on the outside for monitoring purposes. It is necessary to use external lead shielding of the reproductive organs for young or female patients.

Other protective gear

Apart from radiation protection, standard staff should wear a face shield or mask, impervious gowns, gloves, and shoe covers as appropriate.

Positioning of the patient

ERCP is usually performed with the patient lying prone. It is important, however, to note that gravity will favor filling of specific parts of the pancreaticobiliary system with the patient in different positions. Turning the patient during ERCP examination may sometimes be necessary to eliminate overlapping shadows from superimposed bowel gas, bony structures, or the duodenoscope. This can also be achieved to some extent by rotation of a C-arm. Head up or down tilting of the X-ray table helps gravity drainage to fill the intrahepatic system or the distal common duct.

At the end of the procedure, additional radiographs may be taken with the patient in a supine position. A change of position allows gravity to fill the more dependent portion of the right intrahepatic system and also the tail of the pancreas.

Positioning the patient in the right oblique position moves CBD off the spine and may reveal the cystic duct which sometimes overlaps with the CBD. This position may also allow a better examination of the gallbladder.

In rare circumstances, ERCP may be performed with the patient in a supine position. The endoscopist will have to adjust the position by rotating more to the right, or even work facing away from the X-ray table.

Radiological interpretation

Scout film (Fig. 3.7)

A control film of the right upper abdomen should be taken with the scope in place prior to injection of contrast. With the patient lying prone and the scope in a short scope position, radiopacities or calcifications that lie above and to the right of the scope represent calcifications either in the gallbladder, liver parenchyma, or proximal bile ducts. Calcifications to the bottom left of the scope generally represent pancreatic calcification or, rarely, stones in the distal CBD. The presence of air within the bile ducts may be seen as an air cholangiogram and suggests a patent communication between the bile duct and the gut, such as a patent stent, a fistula, or a bilioenteric anastomosis.

Contrast studies

Most diagnostic and therapeutic interventions are performed under fluoroscopic control; however, radiographs or stored images should be taken for documentation. Hard copy radiographs give better resolution compared to the fluoroscopic images and may reveal more detailed information.

If common duct stones are suspected, early filling films should be taken during injection of contrast. This may demonstrate a 'meniscus' sign where the stone is outlined by contrast within the duct. Excess contrast should be avoided as this tends to mask the small stones in a dilated duct.

With the patient lying prone, the left hepatic system is more dependent and usually fills more quickly than the right side. If the cystic duct is patent, contrast may preferentially fill the gallbladder. The posterior segments of the right hepatic system are non-dependent in the prone position but may be filled more readily by turning the patient to a supine position.

Drainage films

Delayed films after removing the duodenoscope are sometimes indicated if there is a clinical suspicion of a drainage problem, e.g. papillary dysfunction or stenosis. Drainage films may be taken with the patient in the right lateral position or in the Trendelenburg position.

The normal rate of drainage is affected by many factors and precise normal limits have not been established. Delayed drainage is, however, suspected if significant opacification of the bile duct persists after 45 min, and after 10 min for the pancreatic duct.

It is necessary to take hard copy spot films to document any therapeutic interventions. Alternatively, serial digital images are stored and retrieved at the end of the procedure for reporting and filing.

The pancreatogram

Normal anatomy The pancreas is a retroperitoneal organ lying across the abdomen at the level of L1 and L2. Pancreatic calcifications on the control film suggest chronic pancreatitis and rarely pancreatic neoplasm. A good quality pancreatogram should demonstrate the main pancreatic duct up to the tail with adequate filling of the second generation branch ducts. Excess contrast injection will result in acinarization or a parenchymogram.

The pancreatic duct normally has a smooth, slightly wavy course from the papilla tapering towards the tail. In the head a branch duct is seen draining the uncinate process. In addition, the accessory duct (Santorini's duct) drains through the minor papilla.

In 5% of cases a prominent branch duct runs parallel to the main pancreatic duct giving the appearance of a bifid pancreas. Several branch ducts join the main pancreatic duct at irregular intervals, usually at right angles to the main duct. The branch ducts taper and themselves branch off into smaller ducts.

The diameter of the pancreatic duct varies according to the age and size of the patient. Elderly patients may have a slightly larger duct. The maximum diameter of a normal pancreatic duct is 6 mm in the head, 5 mm in the body, and 3 mm in the tail. Care must be taken to correct for magnification, which is usually 30%.

Pathological changes The pancreatic duct may appear normal in mild pancreatitis. In acute pancreatitis the pancreatic duct may appear slightly irregular with changes and irregularities of the side branches. Presence of a cyst or pseudocyst may cause complete obstruction of the pancreatic duct with or without communication with the duct.

The Cambridge Classification is used to document the severity of chronic pancreatitis (Fig. 3.9) as seen on a pancreatogram:

• Mild pancreatitis: a normal main pancreatic duct with three or more abnormal side branches.

• Moderate pancreatitis: an abnormal main duct with irregularities in three or more abnormal side branches.

• Severe pancreatitis: irregularity with strictures and dilation of the main duct, with filling defects suggestive of stones or filling of cavities or cysts.

There is no direct correlation between the radiological abnormalities and the functional loss in chronic pancreatitis because the pancreas has a good functional reserve. Leakage of contrast from a transected pancreatic duct with non-filling of the upstream duct is diagnostic of traumatic pancreatitis.

Cancer in the head of the pancreas may cause stricturing of the main pancreatic duct with uniform dilation of the side branches and the main duct upstream of the obstruction. In addition, the retropancreatic portion of the CBD may be involved, giving rise to the characteristic 'double duct stricture' sign. Displacement or stretching of the side branches may suggest an underlying tumor in the pancreas.

Congenital anomalies In patients with pancreas divisum, there is non-fusion of the dorsal and ventral ducts. The small isolated ventral pancreas drains through the main papilla. The dorsal (Santorini's) duct drains the bulk of the pancreas through the minor papilla.

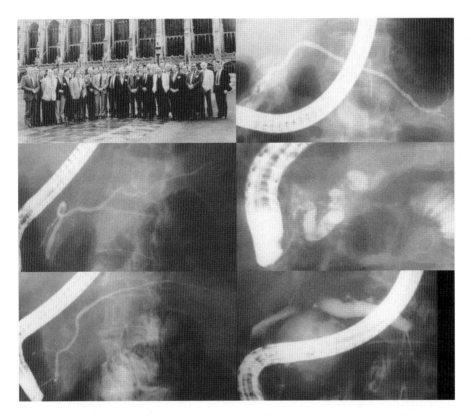

Fig. 3.9 Cambridge Classification of pancreatitis. Mild, three or more abnormal side branches. Moderate, abnormal main duct and side branches. Severe, stricture and dilation, stones, and cyst.

The cholangiogram

A good cholangiogram should visualize the entire intra- and extrahepatic bile ducts, the cystic duct, and the gallbladder (when present).

Normal anatomy The upper limit of normal for the diameter of the CBD varies somewhat with age but is approximately 7 mm (corrected for magnification). Contrary to common belief the bile duct does not dilate progressively as a result of cholecystectomy. Variations in ductal caliber can occur particularly in the retropancreatic portion and at the bifurcation.

Examples of normal anatomical variations include a long common channel seen in patients with congenital cystic dilation of the bile ducts, a low insertion of the cystic duct into the CBD, and anomalous origins of the intrahepatic ducts.

In cases with biliary obstruction, the level of obstruction may be defined by ERCP, with contrast filling the distal CBD. Filling of the proximal ducts depends on the tightness of the stricture but usually can be achieved by performing an

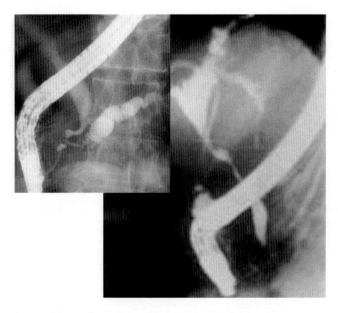

Fig. 3.10 Malignant biliary obstruction. 'Classical appearance' on cholangiopancreatography: double duct stricture, rat tail and shoulder deformity, and hilar strictures.

occlusion cholangiogram. Contrast is injected under pressure by inflating a balloon below the obstruction to fill the more proximal obstructed system.

Pathological strictures Malignant CBD strictures appear as smooth or irregular narrowings with upstream dilatation (Fig. 3.10). These may be caused by cancers of the head of the pancreas (double duct stricture sign), gallbladder, or bile duct, or by lymphadenopathy at the liver hilum. Malignant bile duct strictures at the liver hilum are classified according to the Bismuth Classification:
• Type I stricture is confined to the common hepatic duct with > 2 cm from the bifurcation.
• Type II stricture involves the common hepatic duct with < 2 cm from the bifurcation.
• Type III strictures involve the right and left hepatic ducts.
• Type IIIa is involvement of the right side and IIIb is involvement of the left side.
• Type IV is multiple intrahepatic segmental involvement.
  Malignant bile duct strictures can sometimes be difficult to distinguish from primary sclerosing cholangitis, which classically shows multiple strictures and diffuse irregularity of the extra- and intrahepatic biliary system.
  In contrast, benign postsurgical strictures usually appear as smooth short-segment stenoses. An air-filled periampullary diverticulum may compress the

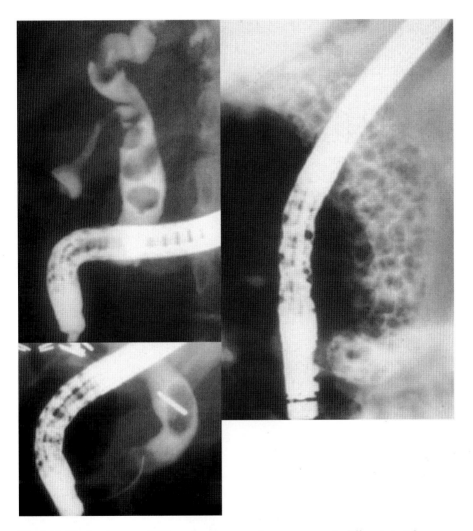

Fig. 3.11 Cholangiogram—CBD stones. Common duct stones seen in different size, shape, and number. Stones can form around a migrated surgical clip.

distal common duct giving rise to a pseudostricture formation. In these cases, the distal bile duct is seen to 'open up' when air is removed from the diverticulum.

Bile duct stones (Fig. 3.11) Stones within the bile duct may be demonstrated initially as a meniscus sign upon contrast injection and subsequently as filling defects. They are round or faceted depending upon their origin. It may be necessary to change the scope position into a long scope position to expose the mid-/distal CBD, an area otherwise overlapped by the scope. Rarely, parasites such as *Clonorchis sinensis* or *Ascaris lumbricoides* may be seen as unique filling defects in the extra- or intrahepatic bile ducts.

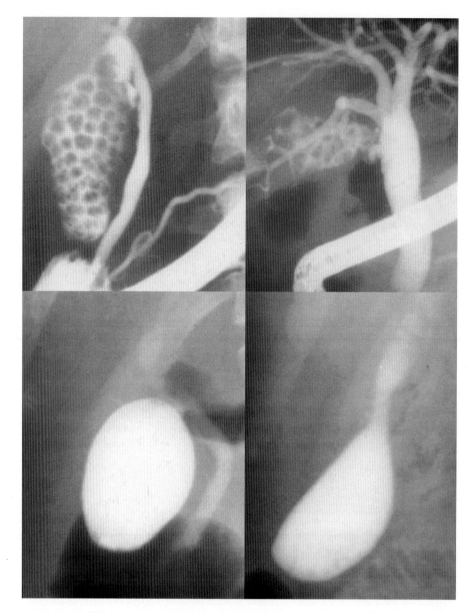

Fig. 3.12 ERCP for gallbladder stones. Gallstones may be obvious on cholangiogram. Note aberrant duct which resembles cystic duct. Always check delayed film of gallbladder for small stones.

Gallbladder ERCP is not an ideal examination of the gallbladder. If the gallbladder is filled, a delayed film of the gallbladder should be taken after 30–45 min. This allows time for the contrast to mix with bile for better definition of gallstones (Fig. 3.12). Failure to fill the gallbladder despite adequate filling of the intrahepatic ducts suggests cystic duct obstruction. Stone impaction in the cystic duct may cause edema and compression of the common hepatic duct giving rise to Mirizzi's syndrome.

Underfilling and delayed drainage With an adequate intrahepatic cholangiogram, underlying parenchymal liver diseases may be inferred from abnormal appearance of the intrahepatic ducts. Crowding of tortuous intrahepatic ducts may suggest liver cirrhosis. Stretching of a particular intrahepatic duct may be seen around space-occupying lesions such as abscesses, tumors, or cysts in the liver.

Underfilling of the bile ducts or 'streaming effect of contrast' may suggest an apparent narrowing in the distal bile duct. Inadequate filling due to stricture or obstruction may fail to detect intrahepatic pathologies such as stones in patients with hepatolithiasis. Functional obstruction at the papilla is difficult to diagnose, but is suspected if there is delayed drainage of contrast (> 45 min).

The clinical diagnosis of papillary stenosis or sphincter of Oddi dysfunction depends on the presence of abnormal liver function tests with or without a dilated bile duct associated with right upper quadrant abdominal pain. Manometric studies are necessary to confirm the diagnosis in patients without obvious duct dilation or liver test abnormalities. Bile leaks and fistulas complicating biliary tract surgery can be readily identified on cholangiography.

Section II: Diagnostic and therapeutic ERCP

Diagnostic ERCP

Scopes

ERCP is performed using side-viewing duodenoscopes with a 2.8, 3.2, or 4.2 mm channel. All of these scopes readily accept a 5 Fr or 6 Fr catheter and accessories. The larger channel duodenoscopes accept accessories up to 10–11.5 Fr diameter and are used for both diagnostic and therapeutic purposes. The larger instrument channel allows aspiration of duodenal contents even with an accessory in place, and also permits the manipulation of two guidewires or accessories simultaneously.

Accessories (Fig. 3.13)

The cannula or diagnostic catheter is a 6 or 7 Fr Teflon tube which tapers to a 3–5 Fr tip. It is used for injection of contrast into the ductal systems. A variety of cannulas are available with different tip designs. A commonly used example is the bullet tip or fluorotip catheter, which has a small metal or radiopaque tip at

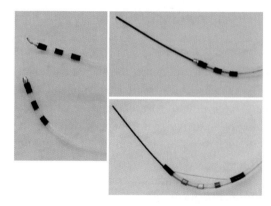

Fig. 3.13 Accessories: cannula, guidewire, and papillotome.

the end to facilitate orientation and cannulation on fluoroscopy. Other catheters may have a tapered tip which facilitates cannulation. Some catheters have two lumens, which allow both injection of contrast and manipulation of a guidewire. Most allow the passage of standard (0.035 inch) guidewires.

Preparation of patient

Most ERCP examinations are performed on an outpatient basis provided that the patient is physically fit and recovery facilities are available. Rarely, ERCP is performed as an inpatient procedure for patients with significant comorbidities or those in whom therapeutic procedures or surgery may be necessary.

Informed consent

ERCP is a complex procedure with significant potential hazards. It is important that the patient understands the potential benefits, risks, limitations, and alternatives. Written, informed consent should be obtained in the presence of a witness.

Fasting

The patient is instructed to fast overnight, or for at least 4 h prior to the procedure. Outpatient procedures are preferably performed in the morning to allow more time for recovery.

Antibiotics

Antibiotics are given for endocarditis prophylaxis according to local and national guidelines. ERCP can cause clinical infection if the procedure does not relieve the obstruction and if cleaning and disinfection regimens are not ideal. Antibiotics are given prophylactically when difficulty in drainage is anticipated, e.g. in patients with multiple strictures (hilar tumors or sclerosing cholangitis) or pseudocysts. Antibiotics should also be given immediately if obstruction is not relieved.

ERCP procedure

Intubation and examination of the stomach

When the patient is adequately sedated, a self-retaining mouth guard is placed and the patient is supported in a left lateral/semiprone position. This position facilitates intubation and examination of the upper GI tract with the side-viewing duodenoscope.

With the patient in the prone position, slight left rotation of the scope is required to correct for the change in axis. Gentle downward tip angulation allows examination of the distal esophagus. Once in the stomach, the gastric juice is removed by suction to minimize the risk of aspiration. The stomach is inflated slightly to allow an adequate view of the lumen.

The endoscope is slowly advanced with the tip angled downwards looking at the greater curve and distal stomach. With further advancement, the scope will pass the angular incisura. The cardia can be examined by up angulation and withdrawal of the scope.

Once past the angular incisura the tip of the scope is further angled downwards and the pylorus is visualized. The scope is positioned so that the pylorus lies in the center of the field. The tip of the endoscope is then returned to the neutral position as the pylorus disappears from the endoscopic view, the so-called 'sun-setting sign'.

Gentle pushing will advance the scope into the first part of the duodenum. The scope is angled downwards again and air is insufflated to distend the duodenum. Care must be taken to avoid overinflating the duodenum as this causes patient discomfort and makes the procedure more difficult. Careful examination is performed to rule out any pathologies such as ulcers or duodenitis. The scope is pushed further to the junction of the first and second part of the duodenum.

At this point, the scope is angled to the right and upwards, and by rotating the scope to the right and withdrawing slowly, the tip of the scope is advanced into the second part of the duodenum. This paradoxical movement shortens the scope using the pylorus as a pivot, bringing it into the classical 'short scope position'. The markings on the duodenoscope should indicate 60–65 cm at the incisors.

With the patient prone, and the scope returned to a neutral position, the papilla can be easily visualized, in the middle of the second portion of the duodenum. The landmark for identification of the papilla is the junction where the horizontal folds meet the vertical fold. Duodenal diverticula may cause difficulties with cannulation as the papilla may be located on the edge or rarely inside a diverticulum.

Approaching the main papilla

A control film of the right upper abdomen is taken to look for calcification and for air in the biliary system, prior to injection of contrast.

Cannulation is performed in the short scope position allowing better control over angulations and tip deflection. In some difficult cases or in attempted minor papilla cannulation, the long scope approach may be adopted. Excess bubbles in the duodenum can be removed by injecting a diluted simethicone solution down the channel. Duodenal contractions may be reduced with the use of antispasmodic medication.

The presence of a periampullary diverticulum does not normally increase the technical difficulty of cannulation, unless the papilla is displaced or located inside the diverticulum (Fig. 3.14).

The normal papilla appears as a pinkish protruding structure and the size may vary. Abnormalities result from previous stone passage, stone impaction, or tumor.

Cannulation of the papilla

Cannulation is best performed in an 'en face' position. The cannula should be flushed and primed with contrast to remove any air bubbles prior to insertion into the duodenoscope. Air injected into the biliary system could mimic stones. Flushing excess contrast in the duodenum should be avoided since hypertonic contrast stimulates duodenal peristalsis.

A combination of 12 different maneuvers can be used for positioning the tip of the cannula for cannulation. These include up/down and sideways angulation, rotation of the endoscope, use of the elevator, and pushing in and pulling back of the scope. Suction collapses the duodenum and pulls the papilla closer to the endoscope. Air insufflation pushes it away. Most beginners find pancreatography easier to obtain than cholangiography. The pancreatic duct is normally entered by inserting the cannula in a direction perpendicular to the duodenal wall, in the 1–2 o'clock orientation (Fig. 3.15).

Fine adjustments of the position and axis of the cannula are helpful. Excessive pressure in the papilla is best avoided because pushing may distort the

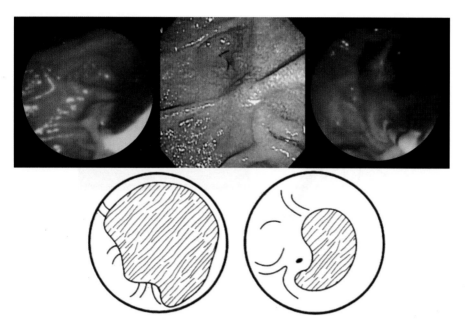

Fig. 3.14 The obscure papilla. Look for bile! Lift the overhanging fold. With prior papillotomy, biliary orifice is often more cephalad. Note relationship of papilla to duodenal diverticula. Probing or suction to change shape of diverticulum and axis to reveal the papilla.

papilla and increase the difficulty with cannulation. Cannulation of the CBD is usually achieved by approaching the papilla from below, in line with the axis of the CBD. It may be helpful to lift the roof of the papilla, and to direct the cannula towards 11 o'clock (Fig. 3.16).

Full strength contrast should be used initially, and is injected under fluoroscopic control. The pancreatic duct should be filled until the tail and some side branches are visualized. Avoid overfilling and acinarization as this increases the risk of post-ERCP pancreatitis. When filling the CBD, start with full strength contrast and consider switching over to dilute contrast when stones are visualized. If deep cannulation is successful, aspirate bile before injecting contrast to avoid excess contrast masking small stones in a dilated biliary system.

The left hepatic ducts usually fill before the right because they are dependent with the patient lying prone. The gallbladder is usually filled except in cases with cystic duct obstruction. Multiple spot films are taken during contrast injection. It may be necessary to change the scope position to expose the portion of the common duct hidden behind the scope.

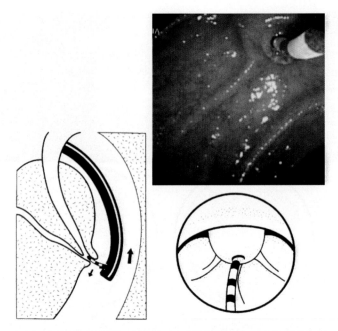

Fig. 3.15 Selective pancreatic duct cannulation. Cannula perpendicular to duodenal wall. Aim at 1–2 o'clock position. 'Drop' the cannula by withdrawing tip of scope, relax up angulation or lower elevator. Use hydrophilic guidewire.

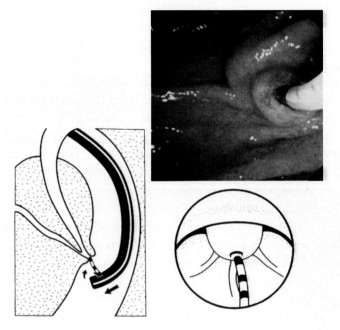

Fig. 3.16 Selective CBD cannulation. Stay close to papilla, approach from below, lift roof of papilla. Cannula directed at 11–12 o'clock position, use papillotome if needed.

At the end of the procedure the endoscope is withdrawn and air is suctioned from the stomach to minimize discomfort. The patient is then turned to a supine position and more radiographs are taken in different projections (as previously described).

In patients with a partially filled gallbladder, immediate diagnosis of gallstones may be difficult due to inadequate mixing of contrast with bile. Delayed films of the gallbladder (after about 45 min) may reveal small stones after allowing time for the contrast to mix with bile.

Ease and success in cannulation

Success of diagnostic ERCP depends on the experience of the endoscopist and the presence or absence of pathology. Successful cannulation of both ductal systems is commonly achieved in 85–90% of cases with experts achieving rates of over 95%. The success rate is lower in patients with previous gastric surgery, e.g. Billroth II gastrectomy.

Minor papilla cannulation

The minor papilla is located proximally and to the right of the main papilla. It can be identified as a small protruding structure. It may not be obvious or may appear as a slightly pinkish nipple between the duodenal folds. When prominent, it can sometimes be mistaken for the main papilla; however, it does not have a distinct longitudinal fold and the small opening usually resists cannulation.

Cannulation of the minor papilla is indicated in patients with suspected or proven pancreas divisum and when cannulation of the pancreatic duct fails at the main papilla. Cannulation of the minor papilla is usually best performed in a long scope position using a 3 mm fine metal tip cannula. Bending the tip of the cannula to form an angle facilitates cannulation.

It is important to identify the correct location of the orifice before any attempt is made to inject contrast, as trauma from the cannula may result in edema and bleeding and obscure the opening.

If the papilla or orifice is not obvious, it is useful to give secretin by slow IV infusion and wait 2 min to observe the flow of pancreatic juice. During injection, it is important to monitor the contrast filling by fluoroscopy as the tip of the cannula is often hidden by the endoscope in the long scope position.

Complications of diagnostic ERCP

The complication rate for diagnostic ERCP is very low in experienced hands. In addition to the specific risks related to ERCP, the procedure also carries the risks of any endoscopic procedure including those related to sedation and scope perforation.

Respiratory depression and other complications

Adverse drug reactions and respiratory depression due to excess medication may occur. This complication is best prevented by giving sedation slowly in small increments, and by assessing the overall response of the patient. Proper monitoring of blood pressure, pulse, and oxygenation helps to avoid this complication. The use of oxygen at 2 liters/min given via a nasal catheter helps to prevent hypoxia. Glucagon may increase the blood sugar level in diabetic patients and the anticholinergic effect of Buscopan may cause tachyarrhythmia. These unwanted side-effects should be monitored.

Pancreatitis

Pancreatitis is the commonest serious complication of ERCP. The serum amylase often increases transiently following pancreatography and may be of little clinical significance. The incidence of clinical pancreatitis is 0.7–7%. The risk is higher when the pancreas is overfilled, in patients with sphincter of Oddi dysfunction with manometry, and in those with pancreatic manipulation.

Cholangitis

The risk of cholangitis after ERCP is small, but may occur in patients with bile duct obstruction due to stones or stricture, especially when biliary drainage cannot be established. The risk of sepsis is high in patients with acute cholangitis when the intraductal pressure is raised by excess injection of contrast. The risk can be reduced by aspirating bile before injecting contrast.

The most common bacteria causing biliary sepsis include Gram-negative bacteria, i.e. *Escherichia coli*, *Klebsiella*, and *Enterobacter*, and Gram-positive enterococci. An improperly reprocessed duodenoscope may carry a risk of cross-infection with other bacteria such as *Pseudomonas* spp.

Failed cannulation and special situations

What to do with a difficult intubation

Failure to insert the duodenoscope Side-viewing scopes are usually easier to pass into the esophagus than standard forward-viewing scopes because of the rounded tip. Difficulty may be encountered if the patient is anxious or struggling due to inadequate sedation. Careful explanation and reassurance prior to the procedure help to alleviate the patient's anxiety.

It is sometimes difficult for patients to swallow in the prone position. Supporting the patient in the left lateral position during scope insertion may help to overcome this problem. Check that the scope angulations are appropriate and advance the tip of the scope over the tongue and against the posterior pharyngeal wall; scope insertion is facilitated by asking the patient to swallow.

Do not push if resistance is encountered. It is important to synchronize your push with the patient's swallow. If in doubt, rule out any obstructing factors with a forward-viewing endoscope. In rare cases, it may be necessary to guide the scope with the left index finger in the oropharynx.

Lost in the stomach Negotiating the stomach with a side-viewing duodenoscope is sometimes confusing. A side-viewing endoscope can function like a forward-viewing endoscope if the tip is deflected downwards. Orientation is easier if the patient is in the left lateral (rather than the prone) position.

Rotation of the patient into the prone position changes the axis of the stomach, and the tip of the scope often ends up in the fundus. Air is insufflated to distend the stomach until an adequate view of the lumen is obtained and to locate the greater and lesser curves.

Downward angulation facilitates examination of the lumen and further passage of the endoscope. If the tip of the scope catches against the mucosa, upward angulations will lift the tip away. It may be necessary to rotate the scope gently to the right to align it with the axis of the stomach.

Passage of the scope is made by a series of up and down tip deflections and pushing movement. Advance the tip until the distal antrum and pyloric opening are seen.

Position the pyloric opening in the center of the endoscopic view and then return the tip of the scope to the neutral position and gently push the scope through into the duodenum. It is important to note any changes in the orientation of the pyloric opening while changing the tip position since sideways angulations/ rotation may be necessary to compensate for a change in axis.

In a J-shaped stomach secondary to deformity, it may be necessary to deflate the stomach and even to apply abdominal pressure to assist scope passage. If the pyloric opening is tight or deformed, backing the tip of the scope by downward tip deflection or, rarely, sideways angulations may help to 'drive' the scope into the duodenum. Again, intubation of the pylorus is much easier in the left lateral position.

Insufflate a small amount of air to distend the duodenum to identify the junction of the first and second part before advancing the endoscope. Passage through a tortuous or deformed duodenum may again require downward tip deflection and checking the axis or orientation before upward tip deflection while pushing to advance the scope.

Once the tip of the scope has passed the D1/D2 junction, return the scope to a 'short scope' position by up and right angulations of the tip and rotation to the right, while pulling back the scope gently. The patient should now be placed to lie in a prone position. The papilla is normally seen when the scope is returned to the neutral position after this shortening maneuver, with the markings of 65–70 cm at the incisor level in the majority of patients. If examination of the stomach is performed with the patient in a prone position, initial rotation of the scope to the left will compensate for a change in the axis and make the examination easier.

Failure to identify the papilla

Tip of endoscope is too proximal The tip of the scope falls short of the second part of the duodenum. This failure to shorten into a 'short scope' position is usually due to duodenal deformity caused by existing ulceration or scarring, previous ulcer surgery, or nearby tumor. The malpositioning of the scope is obvious on fluoroscopy. Advance the scope further by pushing gently with downwards and sideways angulations to negotiate the bends into the third portion of the duodenum before withdrawing the endoscope.

Rotation to the right may be necessary to maintain the scope position and prevent it from slipping back into the stomach. Sometimes cannulation has to be performed in a distorted and long scope position because of duodenal deformity. Care should be taken while pushing the scope through a stenosed duodenum (especially in cases with tumor infiltration) to avoid a perforation.

Tip of scope is too distal The tip of the scope is inserted into the third part of the duodenum. This is sometimes encountered in a very short patient or as a result of over-energetic pushing of the endoscope. Fluoroscopy is useful for checking the position of the scope. In this situation, relax the angulations and withdraw the scope slowly back into the second part of the duodenum, looking for the landmarks of the papilla. In a short patient (or child), the marking on the scope may read 50 or 55 cm and the scope may appear very straight on fluoroscopy. It may be necessary to push in and angle the tip of the scope upwards to gain a better position for cannulation.

Obscured papilla The papilla usually appears as a prominent structure normally located at the junction where the longitudinal mucosal fold meets the horizontal folds in the second part of the duodenum. In rare cases the papilla may appear as a flat and inconspicuous pinkish area. Excess fluid or bubbles in the duodenum sometimes obscure the papilla. Examination can be improved by squirting anti-foam agents, such as simethicone solution, and aspiration. The papilla may be obscured by an overhanging duodenal fold. Using the cannula to lift up or push away the covering mucosal fold will expose the papilla.

If the papilla cannot be identified, it is useful to look for the presence of a duodenal diverticulum in the second part of the duodenum. The papilla may lie on the edge, or sometimes within it. Pushing on the edge of the diverticulum may move the papilla into a more favorable position for cannulation. Excess air in the duodenum may distend the diverticulum, thus pulling the papilla away. Deflating the duodenum by suction helps to bring the papilla back into the duodenal lumen or into a better axis for cannulation.

In patients with previous sphincter surgery or sphincterotomy, the biliary orifice is usually separate from the pancreatic orifice, and is found in a more cephalad position. A suprapapillary fistula may drain the bile duct and cannulation may fail at the main orifice. It is important to check for a fistulous orifice which may be hidden by duodenal folds.

What to do if cannulation is difficult

Abnormal papilla Cannulation may be difficult in pathological situations such as an ampullary tumor or when severe acute pancreatitis results in local edema. Cannulation is still possible if the orifice is seen. For an ampullary tumor, the orifice may not be obvious if the tumor replaces the whole papilla. It is important to avoid trauma to the tumor with the cannula since this often precipitates bleeding which makes cannulation more difficult if not impossible. It is worth spending a moment to observe the papilla and to identify the likely opening before attempting cannulation. The orifice may be located in the distal or inferior aspect of the papilla. Sometimes bile seen draining from the papillary orifice helps with localization. Blindly probing the papilla may create a false passage or result in intratumor injection of contrast or even a perforation.

Failed common duct cannulation This may result from failure to identify the papilla or a failure to inject contrast due to poor positioning (access) or orientation (axis). Cannulation is best performed in a short scope position, which allows better control over the tip of the duodenoscope. Avoid excess body or left wrist movement since these may affect the scope position. It is useful to insert the cannula and be ready for cannulation before performing fine adjustment of the scope position. Locking the wheel that controls sideways angulations helps to minimize movement.

Cannulation is best performed with the papilla positioned in the center of the endoscopy field. Proper alignment is achieved by a combination of up/down and left/right angulations, rotation of the tip of the scope, and pulling back or pushing the tip of the scope further into the duodenum. Suction to collapse the duodenum may pull the papilla closer to the scope. These movements, together with lifting the cannula using the elevator, will help to align the papilla for cannulation.

If the cannula is seen to approach the papilla from the side, adjust the right or left angulation to put the papilla back into a central position. If the pancreatic duct is repeatedly cannulated, the tip of the cannula should be directed upwards towards the 11–12 o'clock position by advancing the scope further into the second part of the duodenum, so that the tip of the cannula approaches the papilla from below, and using the elevator to direct the cannula upwards in the axis of the CBD. Use the cannula to lift the roof of the papilla before attempting further insertion.

Putting a curl on the tip of the cannula may facilitate cannulation. In addition, looping the cannula gently in the duodenum may help to align its tip with the axis of the CBD. Too much pressure on the cannula may impact the tip amongst the folds in the papilla and impede the flow of contrast. Forceful injection of contrast may result in a submucosal injection.

A metal tip cannula (bullet tip) is sometimes better than a standard Teflon cannula. The smooth radiopaque metal tip facilitates cannulation under fluoroscopy. Injection of a small amount of contrast during attempted cannulation to outline either ductal system will help in correct orientation or alignment. If cannulation from below proves difficult because the cannula keeps sliding over the surface of the papilla, it is useful to first angle the tip of the scope up close to the papilla and impact the tip of the cannula against the roof of the papilla before pushing the scope to change its axis. This so-called 'kissing technique' serves to align the cannula in the orifice of the bile duct before repositioning in order to achieve deep cannulation.

If cannulation is still unsuccessful, a bowed double or triple lumen sphincterotome offers additional upward lift for cannulation of the CBD. Most endoscopists bow the sphincterotome in the duodenum before attempting cannulation. In this way, there is less control over the tip and cannulation is similar to fishing for the papilla with a 'hook'. It may be preferable to use the tip of the sphincterotome initially like a standard cannula for cannulation. When a change in axis is desired, the wire is then tightened (this is difficult if the wire is still within the channel), lifting the tip of the sphincterotome in the axis of the bile duct. In addition, the sphincterotome is gently pushed out while advancing the tip of the scope further down into the second part of the duodenum. Sometimes sideways angulation is necessary to achieve a correct alignment with the axis of the bile duct. Frequent injection of small amounts of contrast during manipulation helps to guide the sphincterotome.

When conventional methods of deep cannulation fail, a guidewire can be used to cannulate the bile duct. It is helpful to have contrast present in the pancreatic duct to guide the direction of the guidewire. We prefer to use a 0.025 or 0.035 inch hydrophilic-coated guidewire (e.g. Metro tracer wire from Wilson Cook). The flexible tip guidewire is inserted through a catheter or a sphincterotome and 5 mm of the tip is pushed gently in the direction of the CBD. It is important that the endoscopist or an experienced assistant performs the initial gentle probing (or exploration) at the papillary orifice with the guidewire as the feel and control of the catheter/guidewire are important.

When the tip of the guidewire is advanced without any resistance, the catheter is passed over the guidewire into the ductal system. Passage of the guidewire into the pancreatic duct can be easily identified on fluoroscopy. When the guidewire and catheter (or sphincterotome) are inserted into the bile duct, the wire is then removed and bile is aspirated back into the catheter to confirm the position before contrast is injected to outline the biliary system. The use of tapered tip cannulas and precut sphincterotomy increases the risk of submucosal injection and perforation, especially when performed by inexperienced endoscopists.

With a displaced papilla, it may sometimes be difficult to get into a correct axis with the papilla close to the endoscope. A cannula or sphincterotome can be positioned in the correct axis for cannulation even when the tip of the scope is further away from the papilla in a 'long' position. With a bulging papilla due to edema or an impacted stone, the orifice of the papilla may be pointing downwards. It is helpful to advance the tip of the scope further into the duodenum and to approach the papilla from below in a long scope position. Using a bowed sphincterotome passed distal to the papilla and hooking the tip into the orifice is another way to achieve cannulation. Suction to decompress the duodenum may also pull the papilla closer to the endoscope.

Failed pancreatic duct cannulation The most common cause is an improper axis. The pancreatic duct is best entered by directing the cannula perpendicular to the duodenal wall in the 1 o'clock position. It is sometimes necessary to withdraw the tip of the scope, relaxing the upward angulation together with adjustment of the sideways angulation and lowering the elevator to drop the cannula. Taking a radiograph in cases with an apparent failed cannulation may sometimes reveal a small ventral pancreas.

Pancreas divisum may account for non-visualization of the body and tail of the pancreas which can only be demonstrated by injecting contrast through the minor papilla. Obstruction due to carcinoma of the head of the pancreas may be misinterpreted as a ventral pancreas. Pancreatic stones may obstruct the pancreatic duct and prevent proper filling. Pancreatic cannulation may be facilitated by using a flexible tip guidewire.

Pancreatic duct cannulation may fail in cases with pancreas divisum since there may be no ventral duct.

Failed accessory (minor) papilla cannulation Identification of the accessory or minor papilla can sometimes be difficult. The minor papilla is located in the second part of the duodenum, to the right and proximal to the main papilla. It may be prominent in cases with obstruction of the main pancreatic orifice or with underlying pancreatitis. Cannulation of the minor papilla is necessary in patients with suspected pancreas divisum to outline the dorsal pancreatic duct. Cannulation is best performed in a long scope position and with the scope tip angled slightly to the right. This maneuver will put the accessory papilla in the center of the endoscopy field. In most cases, the minor papilla is not obvious and cannulation is difficult.

It is useful to give secretin by slow IV infusion and to wait 2 min to observe for flow of pancreatic juice from the minor papilla. Once the papilla is identified, cannulation is attempted with a fine metal (3 mm) or needle tip cannula. Bending the tip facilitates cannulation. It is important to avoid traumatizing the mucosa with the tip of the cannula, as bleeding may obscure the orifice. In the long scope position, the tip of the cannula may be hidden behind the endoscope on fluoroscopy but contrast is seen flowing across the spine when the dorsal duct is filled.

In difficult cases, cannulation can be attempted using a 0.018 inch flexible tip guidewire contained in a fine tip Teflon cannula, using the tip of the guidewire to explore the orifice. Once the guidewire is inserted into the dorsal pancreatic duct, the cannula is advanced over the guidewire and contrast is injected through the cannula after removal of the guidewire.

It is worth remembering that cannulation of the main pancreatic duct via the main papilla may fail even in patients without pancreas divisum. If no obvious flow of pancreatic juice is observed at the minor papilla after injection of secretin, it is wise to re-examine the main papilla. A good flow of pancreatic juice at the main papilla suggests that the patient does not have pancreas divisum and further cannulation attempts should be made at the main papilla.

Failure to obtain deep CBD cannulation This usually results from a failure to align with the correct axis of the bile duct. Pushing the tip of the cannula may distort the papilla. The scope is adjusted so that the papilla is in the central position. If the cannula is seen coming from below pointing towards the right or the anterior wall of the CBD, withdraw the cannula and relax the upward angulation of the scope. The direction or axis of the cannula can be altered by pulling back the scope until the curve of the cannula is in line with the axis of the CBD. Slight left angulation of the tip of the scope may help to slide the tip of the cannula into the CBD.

Manipulation is best performed with intermittent injection of contrast to outline the direction/axis of the CBD on fluoroscopy. Using a cannula with a metal or radiopaque tip will help in correct positioning. Care is taken to avoid repeated injection or overfilling of the pancreatic duct. If the bile duct axis cannot be defined, it may be necessary to use a sphincterotome as previously described.

If the bile duct is defined, a guidewire can be used to facilitate deep cannulation. The guidewire is inserted initially into the bile duct and the cannula or sphincterotome is advanced over the guidewire. The guidewire is then removed and bile is aspirated back into the syringe before contrast is injected to fill the bile duct. Sometimes, stone impaction at the papilla or tumor involvement may prevent deep cannulation of the CBD. A stiffer instrument such as a sphincterotome can be used to dislodge the impacted stone.

Precut sphincterotomy to assist in CBD cannulation

Precut sphincterotomy can facilitate deep cannulation of the bile duct, and is used when standard cannulation fails in the presence of known bile duct pathology (e.g. impacted stone or tumor). Since precutting carries significant hazards, and other safer techniques are available, it should be used only with great caution. There should be a specific indication and a strong need to gain access into the bile duct, such as palliation of malignant jaundice. Precut sphincterotomy should not be performed for a diagnostic ERCP or as an alternative to a good biliary cannulation technique.

Needle-knife precut technique

Precutting with the needle-knife is performed in two ways, either by inserting the knife into the papilla and gently moving upwards, or by incising downwards from above the papilla. Prior insertion of a stent into the pancreatic duct protects the pancreatic orifice and may minimize the risk of pancreatitis. Precut needle-knife sphincterotomy over a stent is also used to perform accessory sphincterotomy for pancreas divisum.

Selective cannulation of the intrahepatic system (IHBD)

In a standard short scope position, the angulation of the scope, curvature of the cannula, and shape of the CBD all favor cannulation of the right hepatic system. Selective cannulation of the right hepatic system is facilitated by the use of a J-tipped guidewire or a straight guidewire contained in a curved catheter, although a curved cannula may sometimes lodge in the cystic duct.

Cannulation of the left hepatic system is more difficult, especially if there is stricture of the left hepatic duct. A straight tip catheter or a right angle tip nasobiliary tube can be used to aim the guidewire. Inflating an occlusion balloon in the mid common duct and using it as a fulcrum may help to direct the tip of a guidewire into the respective left and right hepatic ducts.

If the axis of the CBD is straight, the tip of the catheter or nasobiliary tube is positioned in the distal CBD pointing towards the left side, and a straight guidewire is inserted and directed towards the origin of the left hepatic duct. Rotation of the tip of the endoscope to the left may help to deflect the guidewire into the left hepatic system.

If the axis of the CBD is curved, the guidewire usually ends up in the right hepatic duct. It may be useful to try and direct the tip of the catheter or nasobiliary tube against the wall of the common hepatic duct on the right side, using the common hepatic duct to deflect the tip of the guidewire into the left system. Also, unwinding a looped guidewire gently at the bifurcation may deflect the tip, thus flipping the guidewire into the left hepatic duct.

If withdrawal of the loop and tip deflection fail, it may be helpful to continue pushing the looped guidewire which may back itself into the left hepatic duct. Once the tip of the guidewire is inside the left system, the guidewire is advanced to gain a more secure position before the catheter or nasobiliary tube is advanced over the guidewire into the left hepatic duct. It is important to remember that the distal 3 cm of a guidewire is floppy and advancing a catheter over this portion of the guidewire may be difficult.

Pushing a stiff catheter may deflect the guidewire and thus the catheter into the right hepatic system. It is therefore necessary to pass the guidewire further into the desired portion of the intrahepatic system before advancing the catheter over the stiffer portion of the guidewire. Pushing the tip of the scope further into the duodenum may straighten the axis of the bile duct and increase the chance of directing the guidewire into the left hepatic duct. Selective cannulation can be performed using wires with a J or curved tip and a torque control to deflect the wire into the respective ductal system.

Cannulation of the papilla in a Billroth II situation (Fig. 3.17)

Previous gastrectomy or gastroenterostomy changes the anatomy of the stomach. The approach to the papilla is not through the usual route via the pylorus. Instead the papilla is approached from below via the afferent loop of the gastroenterostomy.

It is worth remembering that the orifice of the afferent loop is usually located to the right of the anastomosis. Rotating the scope for a proper orientation, and turning the patient to the supine position, may help facilitate passage of the endoscope.

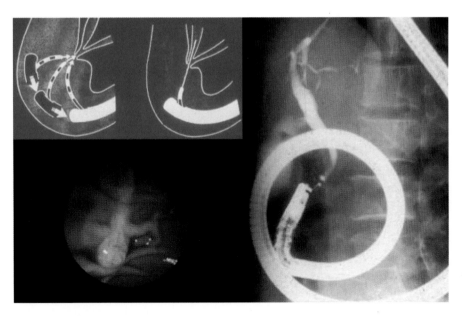

Fig. 3.17 Billroth II cannulation. Approach via afferent loop. Straight catheter from a distance to obtain correct axis.

In difficult cases, intubation of the gastroenterostomy is performed by backing the scope into the correct loop. Sometimes biopsy forceps may help the passage or advancement of the scope into the afferent loop. Passage of the scope down the small intestine is similar to doing a colonoscopy with a side-viewing endoscope.

The presence of bile in the lumen does not always predict the afferent loop. It is helpful to monitor the passage of the endoscope on fluoroscopy to determine the direction and position of the scope. It is unlikely that the scope is in the afferent loop if the tip is down in the pelvis on fluoroscopy. The length of the afferent loop may vary and affect the success of reaching the papilla.

In situations where difficulty is encountered or the relevant segment is not clearly defined, it is worth taking a biopsy close to the gastroenterostomy where the bleeding can serve to identify the jejunal segment that has been explored. If intubation with a side-viewing scope fails, it may be necessary to use a forward-viewing colonoscope to examine and intubate the afferent loop. If the papilla is successfully identified, it may be useful to place a Savary guidewire through the colonoscope and leave it in place to guide subsequent intubation with the side-viewing duodenoscope.

The papilla is inverted in the afferent limb and the closed off duodenum appears as a blind stump. Cannulation of the papilla in the inverted position can be difficult. The pancreatic duct is cannulated more readily than the bile duct which comes down in a cephalic and steep axis. A straight cannula gives a better axis for cannulation. For CBD cannulation it is helpful to pull back the scope so that the tip is further away from the papilla and cannulation is performed from a distance. This position tends to align the tip of the cannula in the axis of the bile duct.

In most situations the common duct is cannulated with the help of a straight guidewire. Pushing the tip of the cannula against the duodenal wall may deflect the tip of the guidewire in the axis of the CBD. It is useful to have contrast in the pancreatic duct to guide the direction of the guidewire. If no contrast is present in either system, it may be necessary to probe the papilla gently with the tip of a guidewire (with about 1 cm of the guidewire protruding from the tip of the catheter).

If the guidewire can be inserted deeply into the papilla without any resistance, the catheter is advanced over the guidewire. The guidewire is then removed and a syringe is used to suck back from the catheter to confirm its position before the injection of contrast. Bile aspirated in the syringe indicates that the bile duct has been cannulated. Aspirate air from the catheter before injecting contrast. When filling the system, begin with normal contrast and inject very slowly. Part of the residual air within the catheter may be pushed into the ductal system, which may pose a problem if injected into the pancreas. Air bubbles injected into the bile duct may mimic stones.

Therapeutic ERCP

Standard endoscopic sphincterotomy or papillotomy (Fig. 3.18)

Endoscopic sphincterotomy is a therapeutic application of ERCP, designed to cut the sphincter muscle and open the terminal part of the CBD using diathermy. It was first described in 1973, and is now widely accepted as a therapeutic alternative to surgical management of CBD stones. Endoscopic sphincterotomy is simple, cheap, and more acceptable to patients than surgery. The procedure involves cutting the papilla and sphincter muscle of the distal CBD; therefore papillotomy is an incomplete term and the term sphincterotomy is more appropriate.

Preparation of patients The preparation of patients for sphincterotomy is the same as for diagnostic ERCP. It can be performed as an outpatient procedure except for patients who have coexisting cholangitis, pancreatitis, or significant coagulopathy. Selected patients may need overnight observation in the hospital after sphincterotomy and stone extraction.

Laboratory tests Preliminary laboratory tests including blood counts, liver biochemistry, and coagulation profile should be taken prior to the procedure. Coagulopathy is corrected when necessary by IV vitamin K injection or transfusion of

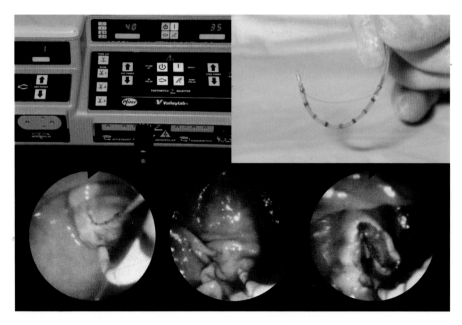

Fig. 3.18 Standard biliary papillotomy. Single lumen papillotome. Double lumen papillotome over a guidewire. Use blended current, stepwise cut in 11–12 o'clock direction. Avoid excess tension on wire.

fresh frozen plasma. Patients are advised to stop taking aspirin and NSAIDs and anticoagulants are withheld for 5 days prior to elective sphincterotomy to avoid bleeding complications. For patients who require continued anticoagulation, for example those with prosthetic heart valves, admission for conversion to intravenous heparin may be required. The procedure is performed after withholding heparin for 4 h. Anticoagulation therapy is restarted after the procedure.

Antibiotics may be given to patients with coexisting cholangitis and those with significant biliary stasis.

We prefer to use the larger 4.2 mm channel endoscope for therapeutic procedures because it can accept larger accessories.

The sphincterotome (or papillotome) Sphincterotomes are available in different designs with some specially designed for altered anatomy following gastric surgery (e.g. Billroth II). In general, the sphincterotome is a single, double or triple lumen Teflon catheter containing a continuous wire loop with 2–3 cm of exposed wire close to the tip. The other end of the wire is insulated and connected via an adaptor to the diathermy or electrosurgical unit. The diathermy unit provides both cutting and coagulation currents, either separately or in combination (blended mode). The power setting on the diathermy machine can be adjusted. The early single lumen sphincterotome allowed injection of contrast through a single lumen, but leakage occurred around the side ports for the wire. Double lumen sphincterotomes allow injection of contrast or passage of a guidewire through a separate lumen and can be used for both diagnostic cannulation and sphincterotomy (Fig. 3.18).

More recent sphincterotomes (e.g. DASH system, Wilson Cook) have a side-arm adaptor that allows contrast injection and insertion of a (0.025 or 0.035 inch) guidewire at the same time. The adaptor can be tightened to close an O-ring around the guidewire to prevent spillage of contrast. The O-ring can be loosened to allow free passage of a guidewire through the sphincterotome. Triple lumen sphincterotomes allow both injection of contrast and passage of a guidewire independently.

Most sphincterotome wires tend to deviate to the right when bowed or tightened, potentially resulting in a deviated cut with an increased risk of complications (i.e. bleeding, perforation, and pancreatitis). It is often necessary to shape the wire to ensure that it remains in the 12 o'clock position when bowed to minimize the risk of complications. When a double or triple lumen sphincterotome is used, it is helpful to insert a guidewire to stabilize the sphincterotome and maintain access into the ductal system during sphincterotomy.

A diagnostic ERCP is performed to define the anatomy of the biliary system and to confirm the presence of stones. Using standard techniques the sphincterotome is inserted deeply into the CBD and its position confirmed either by injecting contrast or wiggling the sphincterotome under fluoroscopy. This is to prevent inadvertent cannulation and cutting of the pancreatic duct. The sphincterotome is withdrawn until only one-third of the wire lies within the papilla. The wire is then tightened so that it is in contact with the roof of the papilla. Excess tension on the wire should be avoided to prevent an uncontrolled or 'zipper' cut. The position of the wire is adjusted and maintained by the elevator bridge and up/down control of the endoscope.

Electrosurgical unit A blended (cutting and coagulation) current is passed in short bursts to cut the roof of the papilla in a stepwise manner in the 11–1 o'clock direction. The power setting on different diathermy units varies depending on the energy output of individual units, and has to be adjusted accordingly. For the Olympus diathermy (UES series), the power is set at 3–3.5 with a blended current; the setting on a Valley-lab diathermy machine is 3 of cutting and 6 of coagulation, or a power setting of 30–40 W with a blended I current. The ERBE unit has a unique design that initially coagulates followed by cutting the papilla; the sphincterotomy can be performed in a more controlled fashion.

Whitening of the tissue upon passage of current is indicative of the beginning of the cut. If the tissue does not blanch within a few seconds, it is necessary to reduce the length of wire in contact with the papilla. It is important to avoid increasing the power setting of the diathermy unit without adjusting or repositioning the wire.

Adequacy of sphincterotomy A gush of bile is usually seen flowing from the bile duct when the sphincter is cut. The sphincterotomy is then completed to its full length which is usually 1–1.5 cm. The safe length of a sphincterotomy depends on the configuration of the distal CBD and shape of the papilla.

However, it should not go beyond the impression of the common duct on the duodenal wall in order to avoid a perforation. The size of a sphincterotomy can be gauged by pulling a fully tightened (bowed) knife from within the distal bile duct to assess resistance to passage. An alternative method is to size the sphincterotomy by pulling an inflated occlusion balloon through the opening. Any deformity of the balloon would suggest resistance to its passage.

Wire-guided sphincterotomes An advantage of the double or triple lumen sphincterotome is that it can be inserted over a guidewire especially in cases with difficult cannulation. The guidewire also serves to anchor and stabilize the sphincterotome during sphincterotomy. A properly insulated guidewire should be used to prevent the current from jumping between the diathermy wire and the guidewire, leading to an ineffective cut or injury to the liver. Most of the currently available guidewires with hydrophilic coating, such as the JAG wire (Microvasive) or Metro Tracer wire (Wilson Cook), can be used for this purpose.

Periampullary diverticula and sphincterotomy Diverticula do not increase the risk of sphincterotomy unless the papilla is located on the edge or inside a large diverticulum. Cannulation may be technically more difficult and the risk of perforation is increased as a result of a deviated cut.

Distorted anatomy A previous Billroth II gastrectomy increases the technical difficulty of ERCP and sphincterotomy. Although a forward-viewing scope may facilitate entry into the afferent loop, most experts prefer to use a side-viewing duodenoscope because of the additional elevator control. The success of sphincterotomy in patients with Billroth II gastrectomy is lower than that for patients with normal anatomy. Since the approach to the papilla is through the afferent loop, the orientation of the papilla on endoscopy is reversed. Special sphincterotomes can be employed or a needle-knife may be used to cut the papilla over a biliary stent.

Precut sphincterotomy for impacted stone

In general, deep cannulation of the CBD may fail in 5% of patients, but could be higher because of stone impaction at the ampulla. The biliary orifice is often displaced more distally because of the bulging papilla. In such cases, a precut sphincterotomy can be performed using a needle-knife which is basically a bare wire that protrudes for 4–5 mm at the end of a Teflon catheter. A lower power setting on the diathermy unit is often sufficient for precut sphincterotomy.

It is relatively safe to cut directly onto the bulging intraduodenal portion of the papilla. The needle-knife is either placed right at the orifice and the cut is made upwards by lifting the knife, or the knife is used to cut down onto the papilla by dropping the elevator. The risk of pancreatitis is minimal because the impacted stone pushes the wall of the bile duct away from the pancreatic duct. Once access to the bile duct is achieved, the sphincterotomy can be extended with the needle-knife or using a standard sphincterotome. The impacted stone sometimes may pass spontaneously into the duodenum after an adequate sphincterotomy. Fine control of the needle-knife is difficult and carries an increased risk of bleeding and perforation. It should not be undertaken lightly by an inexperienced endoscopist or used as an alternative to good ERCP cannulation techniques.

Indications for sphincterotomy and results

Endoscopic sphincterotomy is useful for the removal of residual or recurrent common duct stones in patients with a prior cholecystectomy. The success rate of removing stones ≤ 1 cm in diameter exceeds 95% in expert hands. Patients with large stones may require special treatment such as mechanical lithotripsy (as discussed in a later section).

In elderly or high-risk patients with the gallbladder *in situ*, sphincterotomy for CBD stone obstruction is indicated, especially in those presenting with acute cholangitis. Interval cholecystectomy may be performed but long-term follow-up suggests that cholecystectomy may not be necessary if gallbladder stones are absent. Even for those with gallbladder stones the majority of patients remain asymptomatic on long-term follow-up. Only about 10% of patients develop subsequent biliary symptoms and require further intervention.

Urgent endoscopic drainage with sphincterotomy and/or insertion of a nasobiliary catheter is effective in reducing the overall mortality of suppurative cholangitis. A prospective randomized controlled study confirmed the benefits of urgent endoscopic drainage over emergency surgery.

Sphincterotomy and removal of an impacted ampullary stone are beneficial in patients with severe acute gallstone pancreatitis. A randomized controlled study demonstrated that urgent ERCP and sphincterotomy resulted in a significant reduction in mortality and complications compared to a control group.

Precut sphincterotomy may be indicated in patients with difficult cannulation to gain access to the bile duct for endoscopic biliary stenting. Sphincterotomy also facilitates easier exchange of accessories and double stent placement. It is less commonly applied to treat patients with documented papillary stenosis or sphincter of Oddi dysfunction.

Complications of sphincterotomy

The results of sphincterotomy are operator dependent. An endoscopist must have sufficient skill and experience with ERCP before attempting sphincterotomy in order to minimize the risk of complications. Bleeding, pancreatitis, and perforation can have serious consequences.

Postsphincterotomy bleeding Some bleeding may be observed at the time of sphincterotomy in 2–5% of cases. Clinically significant bleeding is more likely in cases with a deviated cut, a large sphincterotomy, and in patients with coexisting coagulopathy. Active bleeding can be controlled by compressing the sphincterotomy with a balloon inflated inside the distal bile duct against the tip of the duodenoscope. Pure coagulation current may be applied to control the bleeding. Injection therapy with 1:10 000 dilution of epinephrine delivered into the apex and side of the sphincterotomy and adjacent tissue using a sclerotherapy needle is also very effective in controlling the bleeding. Injection therapy may give rise to tissue edema and potential biliary stasis. It is therefore necessary sometimes to insert a nasobiliary catheter or a stent to drain the bile duct. There may be a risk of pancreatitis if epinephrine is injected close to the pancreatic orifice.

In rare situations major hemorrhage may result from cutting an aberrant branch of the retroduodenal artery. The resultant massive bleeding is difficult to control with endoscopy and may require emergency surgery or radiological embolization of the bleeding vessel. Surgical treatment for postsphincterotomy bleeding is not straightforward since it may be difficult to identify the exact bleeding site and the coagulated tissue does not hold sutures well. The risk of rebleeding is high in patients with clotting disorders and these should be corrected and monitored for up to 7–10 days after the sphincterotomy. Patients should continue to withhold aspirin or NSAIDs for another 5 days to prevent recurrent bleeding.

Pancreatitis Pancreatitis may result from inadvertent cutting of or edema around the pancreatic orifice. It can also occur from repeated injection of contrast into the pancreas or excess coagulation during biliary sphincterotomy.

Post-ERCP pancreatitis can be reduced by ensuring drainage of the pancreatic duct using a temporary 3 Fr stent or a 5 Fr nasopancreatic catheter.

Cholangitis Acute cholangitis is a rare but important early complication following sphincterotomy. This may occur when contrast is injected into an obstructed biliary system but drainage cannot be established. Antibiotics should be given promptly, but the risk is best minimized by ensuring drainage of the biliary system with an indwelling stent or nasobiliary catheter.

Perforation Perforation is a rare complication of sphincterotomy and may occur as a result of a deviated cut or excessive cutting of the papilla. Patients complain of pain and retroperitoneal free air may be demonstrated on fluoroscopy. If recognized during ERCP, it may be useful to decompress the bile duct with a nasobiliary catheter or an indwelling stent to reduce leakage and the risk of retroduodenal abscess formation. If perforation is suspected after the procedure, CT scan of the abdomen is the most sensitive test in detecting the presence of retroduodenal air.

The patient should be kept nil by mouth with nasogastric tube decompression. Intravenous fluids and broad spectrum antibiotics are given to prevent infection. Patients often respond to conservative management and bowel rest, and surgical treatment is usually not necessary. However, early consultation is wise and percutaneous drainage of retroduodenal fluid collection may be necessary to prevent abscess formation.

What to do if the sphincterotomy fails to cut

Before the sphincterotomy, it is important to check that the electrosurgical or diathermy unit is working properly, the patient's grounding plate is connected, and the correct adaptor is used for the sphincterotome. Poor contact of the grounding plate can be improved using electroconducting gel or gauze soaked with normal saline (not sterile water) placed between the patient and the grounding plate.

If the electrical connections are correct and functional, an apparent failure to cut may be the result of having too much wire in contact with the tissue. Withdraw the sphincterotome until only about one-third of the wire is left inside the bile duct. Too little wire in contact with the tissue also produces an ineffective cut. Too much coagulation current leads to formation of a coagulum adherent to the wire and increases the resistance and difficulty in cutting the papilla. It may be necessary to remove the sphincterotome and clean the wire before further cutting or to insert the unbowed sphincterotome into the duct to clear the coagulum. Poor contact between the wire and the tissue may also result in ineffective cutting.

As the sphincterotomy is being performed, it may be necessary to gently tighten the wire and lift the sphincterotome with the elevator to maintain contact with the papilla. Whitening of the tissue indicates the beginning of a cut. A lot of smoke without cutting means that insufficient wire is in contact with the tissue or there is too much coagulation. Gently moving the wire to separate the cut edge of the papilla will facilitate further cutting and ensure proper contact with the tissue. In patients with a thick papilla due to stone impaction or a tumor, it may take some time for the wire to cut through. An impacted stone at the papilla may prevent adequate tissue contact.

Too much tension on the wire may result in a sudden jump when the sphincter muscle is completely severed. This uncontrolled or 'zipper' cut is due to excess tension on the wire cutting the relatively thin-walled distal bile duct and is associated with an increased risk of bleeding and perforation.

The risk of a half cut

When excess coagulum forms, it may be necessary to remove the sphincterotome and to clean the wire. Tissue edema and charring around the sphincterotomy site may make subsequent cannulation of the CBD more difficult. There is a potential risk of dissection through a false tissue plane or submucosal injection of contrast. Using a wire-guided sphincterotome and exchanging over a guidewire prevent this potential complication. Indeed, inserting a guidewire within the bile duct serves also to stabilize the sphincterotome and facilitates exchanges and positioning of the sphincterotome.

What to do with a deviated cut

The risk of bleeding or perforation is increased if the biliary sphincterotomy is performed outside of the 'safety zone', i.e. in the 11–1 o'clock direction. There is a tendency for most sphincterotomy wires to deviate to the right when being tightened, thus increasing the risk of complications.

It is important to check the wire prior to the sphincterotomy. Some sphincterotomes have a stabilizing metal plate or differential catheter thickness that allows the wire to exit in the 12 o'clock position (at least in theory). If the wire comes out in a poor direction or orientation, it is necessary to train or shape the wire.

The purpose of training the wire is to ensure that it remains in the central position when being tightened. It is performed by turning the tip of the sphincterotome by 90° so that the wire is on the left side of the catheter tip, curling the tip of the sphincterotome with the fingers while at the same time tightening the wire. This helps to put a memory on the tip of the sphincterotome which keeps the wire in the central position when tightened.

Sphincterotomes come in different designs and shapes, and have different wire lengths. The longer 3.5 cm wire sphincterotomes are more flexible and can be shaped readily and tend to remain in a more neutral position when being tightened. The drawback is that cutting has to be performed with the papilla positioned further away from the tip of the endoscope to avoid the risk of short-circuiting the wire at the elevator. Sphincterotomes with a shorter wire tend to be stiffer and deflect to the right side more readily. One way to compensate for wire displacement is to use sideways angulation to the left, lean the body to the left, or rotate the left wrist to the left, thus displacing the scope to compensate for the malpositioning of the wire. This maneuver makes use of the side of the wire to cut. An alternative is to angle the tip of the scope downwards away from the papilla and angle left to align the wire in a better axis.

It is necessary to check the direction of the wire frequently during the sphincterotomy to ensure that it stays within the accepted axis. There is a tendency for the wire to fall back into an existing cut despite manipulation, and continuing a misdirected cut will increase the risk of complications. In a displaced papilla, sometimes it may be necessary to over-relax the wire or to push instead of tightening to form a loop on the left side. In this position the wire is more likely to make an acceptable contact with the papilla in the correct axis for the sphincterotomy, although the control over the wire is less. A sphincterotome with a rotatable wire (Autotome, Microvasive) may help in correcting the axis of the cut, especially with a distorted papilla.

In order to maintain a proper position for the sphincterotome during sphincterotomy, some endoscopists prefer to use a long-nose sphincterotome so that the wire can be steadied and maintained within the bile duct to minimize the risk of losing the position during cutting. A long-nose sphincterotome is, however, difficult to use for cannulation since the wire is still within the endoscope and cannot be used to provide tension and tip deflection. The use of a double or triple lumen sphincterotome placed over a special coated guidewire may serve the same purpose. Whilst it is best to perform the sphincterotomy in the short scope position, correct orientation may require pushing the scope into a long position.

Sphincterotomy in Billroth II cases

The approach to the papilla is different in patients with a prior Billroth II gastrectomy. The papilla is seen upside-down when approached from below through the afferent loop. Most of the conventional accessories, including standard sphincterotomes, tend to point away from the bile duct orifice and axis when tightened. This increases the risk of failure as well as complications. The use of a 'reverse' sphincterotome, in which the tip of the sphincterotome and

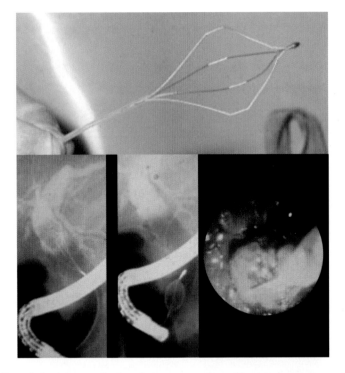

Fig. 3.19 Dormia basket, open basket above stone and trawl back to engage stone. Stone removed with traction and angulation of scope tip. For medium or small sized stones. Avoid pulling scope to remove the stone. Potential risk of basket/stone impaction.

wire is shaped such that it points in the correct direction of the bile duct axis, may be helpful.

Control of the orientation of the sphincterotome is sometimes difficult. The best technique is to place an indwelling stent into the distal bile duct and to use a needle-knife to cut onto the stent in the axis and direction of the bile duct. This provides a correct orientation for the cut and protects the pancreatic duct from injury.

Stone extraction (Figs 3.19 and 3.20)

With an adequate sphincterotomy, most stones < 1 cm will pass spontaneously. However, the expectant policy carries a risk of cholangitis due to stone impaction and current practice is to remove the bile duct stones to achieve duct clearance at the time of sphincterotomy.

Equipment Accessories useful for stone extraction include double lumen balloon catheters, wire baskets, and mechanical lithotriptors. The large

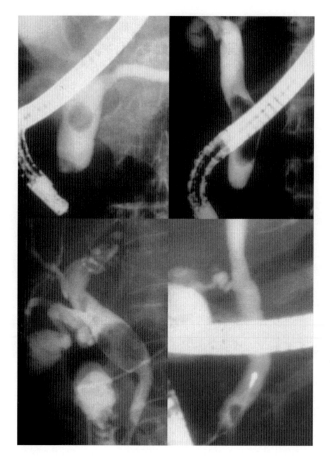

Fig. 3.20 Ease of stone extraction depends on the size of the exit passage, i.e. distal CBD and papillotomy, and the size of the stone.

through-the-scope mechanical lithotriptor will require the large (4.2 mm) channel duodenoscope.

Procedure The stone extraction balloon catheter is an 8 Fr double lumen catheter with a balloon (8, 12, or 15 mm diameter) at the tip. It is useful to ensure that the balloon inflates correctly prior to insertion. The tip of the balloon catheter is stiff and cannulation may be difficult. It may be helpful to gently curl the tip of the catheter to facilitate cannulation or insert it over a guidewire. The catheter is inserted deeply into the bile duct and the balloon is inflated above the stones. It is useful to try and remove individual stones separately starting at the distal end of the common duct.

With an adequate sphincterotomy, the stone can be pulled down and expelled from the CBD using downward tip deflection of the scope. Care is taken to avoid pulling the balloon too hard against the stone as this may rupture the balloon. As the balloon can be deformed, the balloon may slip past the stones resulting in stone impaction. Stone extraction is best confirmed by observing stone passage from the sphincterotomy. Alternatively, an occlusion cholangiogram can be performed to document complete clearance of the bile ducts.

Stones can also be removed using a wire basket. The basket is made of four wires and shaped such that the wires open like a trap to engage the stones. The basket is inserted and opened beyond the stones and withdrawn in a fully opened position. The basket is moved gently up and down or jiggled around the stone to trap it. When the stone is engaged the basket is closed gently and pulled back to the papilla. The tip of the endoscope is angled up against the papillary orifice and tension is applied. The stone is extracted by downward tip deflection and right rotation of the endoscope. If necessary, the maneuver is repeated to remove the stone. A newer design has eight wires on the top (Flower basket, Olympus) which result in a small mesh size between the wires, and is useful for trapping smaller stones or fragments.

Mechanical lithotripsy

Large > 15 mm, common duct stones are difficult to remove, especially if considerable discrepancy exists between the size of the stone and the diameter of the exit passage, i.e. a narrowed distal bile duct, a small sphincterotomy, and in those who had only balloon sphincteroplasty for stone extraction (Fig. 3.21). Extension of the sphincterotomy is not always possible and may carry an increased risk of bleeding and perforation. Lithotripsy facilitates stone extraction and common duct clearance by crushing the stones using strong wire baskets before extraction.

There are different designs for lithotripsy baskets—one type requires cutting the handle of the basket and removing the endoscope prior to stone fragmentation, e.g. Soehendra lithotriptor (Wilson Cook Medical, Winston Salem, NC). This consists of a 14 Fr metal sheath and a self-locking crank handle. The lithotriptor can be used with large lithotripsy baskets or standard stone extraction baskets. These are typically four wire hexagonal baskets measuring 2 cm by 3 cm or 3 cm by 5 cm in diameter (Fig. 3.22).

Another type is a pre-assembled through-the-scope lithotripsy basket which can be inserted through a therapeutic duodenoscope, e.g. BML lithotripsy baskets (Olympus Co, Tokyo, Japan). The BML lithotriptor has three layers—a strong four wire basket, a Teflon catheter, and an overlying metal sheath. The reusable version requires assembly by inserting the Teflon catheter initially through the metal sheath and then loading the basket retrogradely on to the Teflon catheter. The wires are soldered together on to a shaft which is connected to the crank handle. Contrast is injected via the Teflon catheter. The opening

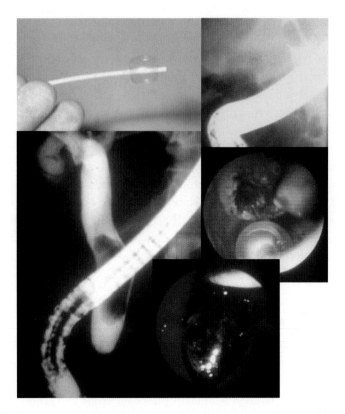

Fig. 3.21 Balloon stone extraction. Extraction of small stones in small ducts after papillotomy; stone expelled by retracting balloon. Large stones can be removed if axis is correct. Risk of stone impaction with inadequate papillotomy.

and closing of the basket are controlled with the handle. Stone engagement is performed with the Teflon catheter and basket. The metal sheath is usually advanced over the Teflon catheter up to the level of the stone when lithotripsy is required. Traction is applied to the wires by turning the control wheel in order to crush the stone. As the control does not have a built-in locking mechanism, traction should be applied slowly and continuously to allow time for the wires to cut through the stone.

The reusable system can be taken apart after lithotripsy for cleaning and sterilization. The disposable version comes with the lithotripsy basket, Teflon catheter, and metal sheath all built into one. The set-up is designed to break at the connection between the basket and the crank handle. The basket wires are also designed to break at the tip to prevent having a broken basket around an impacted stone in the bile duct. The larger lithotripsy baskets, or BML-3Q or 201 equivalent, have a slightly thicker metal sheath that goes through a 4.2 mm channel scope; contrast injection is possible. The smaller basket, or BML-4Q or

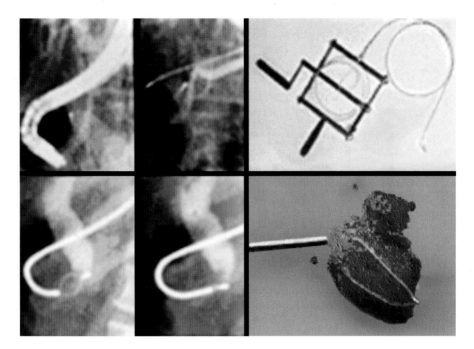

Fig. 3.22 Mechanical lithotripsy (Soehendra lithotriptor). 'Life-saver', metal sheath inserted over basket wires. Stone crushed with a crank handle. For unexpected stone and basket impaction.

203 equivalent, goes through a 3.2 mm channel scope but contrast injection is difficult because of the small size (Fig. 3.23).

The Monolith (Microvasive, Boston Scientific, Natick, MA) is a single-piece disposable mechanical lithotriptor with the basket, metal sheath, and crank handle all built into one. The basket is inserted to engage the stones in the bile duct. Traction to the wires is applied by a self-locking pistol grip mechanism. Three sizes of baskets are available and the commonly used basket size is 2 cm by 4 cm.

Procedure The Soehendra lithotriptor is used when unexpected stone and basket impaction occurs during routine stone extraction and that is why it is often called the 'life-saver'. The handle of the basket is cut and the duodenoscope is removed. The metal sheath is then railroaded over the basket wires. It is helpful to retain the Teflon sheath to facilitate insertion of the metal sheath and to prevent the bare wires from being caught at the tip of the sheath. A tape can be used to round off the tip of the sheath to prevent injury to the posterior pharynx. The metal sheath is advanced all the way to the level of the stone under fluoroscopic control. The basket wires are then tied around the shaft of the handle and traction is applied slowly. This allows time for the wires to cut through and break up

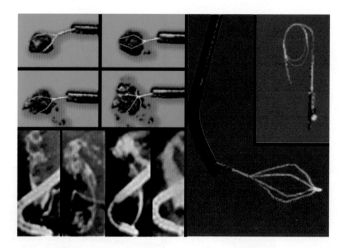

Fig. 3.23 Mechanical lithotripsy (BML through-the-scope lithotriptor). Three layer system with strong wire basket. Teflon sheath and metal sheath connected to crank handle. Large stone is engaged in basket and crushed by traction on wire. Multiple lithotripsy may be necessary to break up a large stone to aid in duct clearance.

the stone. This device is the best method to salvage a complication of stone and basket impaction. It is important to remember that stone may be trapped in a standard basket which is not designed for lithotripsy. Therefore, traction applied too quickly to the wires may break the basket and not the stone.

The BML lithotripsy basket can be used in anticipation of lithotripsy for large common duct or intrahepatic stones above a strictured bile duct. Initial cannulation of the common duct is performed with the basket after an adequate sphincterotomy or balloon sphincteroplasty. The metal sheath is retracted within the scope channel and only the Teflon catheter and basket are used to engage the stone. The basket is opened beyond the stone and pulled back to engage the stone. Trapping of large stones may be difficult because of a lack of space within the bile duct for basket manipulation. Shaking the basket may not work. If necessary, the metal sheath is advanced up the Teflon catheter to provide more stiffness for manipulation of the basket. Gentle twisting or rotation of the scope may facilitate movement of the basket wires around the stone. Advancing the scope further into the duodenum straightens the axis of the basket and the bile duct and facilitates stone engagement. When the stone is properly trapped in the basket, the metal sheath is advanced up to the stone by adjusting the control on the shaft of the lithotripsy basket. Traction is applied to the wires by turning the control wheel to crush the stone. In the case of a very hard stone, the basket wires may be deformed after stone fragmentation. It should be removed and the wires shaped to reform the basket before further stone engagement. As the stone fragments may still be relatively large, repeated stone crushing is necessary to facilitate stone extraction and duct clearance. As discussed above, the disposable systems BML-201, 202, 203, and 204 are used in a similar fashion.

The Monolith lithotriptor is inserted through the duodenoscope, the metal sheath is advanced into the bile duct, and the basket is opened and pulled back to engage the stone. Contrast can be injected to define the position of the stone. Once the stone is engaged, traction is applied to the wires to crush the stone. As the basket wires can become deformed, reshaping the wires is necessary before lithotripsy is repeated. Mechanical problems including failure of proper opening of the basket and damage to the scope elevator have been reported.

Results The new lithotripsy baskets are strong and successful mechanical lithotripsy depends mostly on effective trapping of the stone. Lithotripsy may fail in the presence of stone impaction or if there is insufficient room in the CBD for manipulation of the basket. Partial fragmentation of a very large stone may be possible, although the wires may tend to slip around the stone. Repeated stone crushing is necessary to break up the large fragments. The reported success rate of mechanical lithotripsy for large stones ranges from 85% to 90%, improving the overall common bile duct clearance rate to over 95%.

Complications of lithotripsy

The Soehendra lithotriptor provides effective crushing of the stone in unexpected cases with stone and basket impaction. However, when a standard basket is used for stone extraction, the basket wires may break in the duodenum resulting in stone and a broken basket impacted in the bile duct. Such cases may require surgical common duct exploration to deliver the impacted stone and basket. Special precautions including slow application of traction to the wires may prevent this complication.

With the BML system, the baskets are made to break at the connection of the shaft with the handle. When this happens, Olympus has made a special metal oversheath and a crank handle similar to the design of the Soehendra lithotriptor. The standard metal sheath of the lithotriptor basket is replaced by this special metal sheath before stone fragmentation is continued. We do not recommend adapting the Soehendra lithotriptor handle to the BML basket for lithotripsy.

Perforation is an uncommon event and rarely occurs as a result of the stiff basket perforating the bile duct. Excessive force in removing the impacted basket and stone may result in bruising of the pancreatic orifice and a potential risk of pancreatitis. Incomplete CBD clearance without adequate drainage may result in cholangitis due to retained stone fragments. Forceful extraction of large stone fragments should be avoided to minimize the risk of scope trauma to the

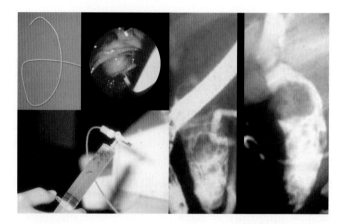

Fig. 3.24 Nasobiliary catheter drainage. Preshaped 6.5 Fr catheter with side-holes. Inserted with/without prior papillotomy. Bile duct decompressed by aspiration via nasobiliary drain. Useful for unstable patients, multiple large stones, and coagulopathy.

duodenum, which may result in duodenal perforation especially in patients with a deformed duodenum.

Endoscopic nasobiliary catheter drainage for bile duct obstruction (Fig. 3.24)

There are several ways to decompress an obstructed biliary system. In patients with acute suppurative cholangitis secondary to stone obstruction, endoscopic sphincterotomy and insertion of a nasobiliary catheter provide effective decompression with dramatic improvement of the clinical condition. The nasobiliary catheter is relatively easy to insert and is well tolerated for a few days. It allows sequential cholangiography, bile culture, and irrigation. Nasogallbladder drains have been inserted with the help of special guidewires for the drainage of acute cholecystitis.

Procedure Following a diagnostic ERCP, deep cannulation of the bile duct is obtained using a 0.035 inch guidewire. A nasobiliary catheter is a 6.5–7 Fr polyethylene tube (260 cm in length) with a preformed tip and multiple side-holes in the distal 10 cm. It can be inserted into the biliary system over the guidewire with or without a prior sphincterotomy. Direct cannulation is sometimes possible using a nasobiliary catheter with a right angle tip. The guidewire helps to bypass the obstructing stones and to position the tip of the nasobiliary catheter deep in the bile duct.

Once the nasobiliary catheter is in place, the endoscope is withdrawn slowly leaving the catheter and guidewire in the bile duct. This exchange is performed under fluoroscopic control to avoid excess looping of the catheter in the

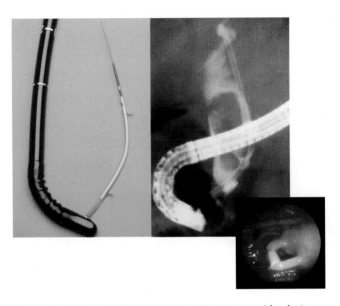

Fig. 3.25 Stenting for cholangitis and CBD stones. 10 Fr stent provides drainage and prevents stone impaction. Drainage through and alongside stent. Short-term drainage. Definitive drainage for high-risk patients.

duodenum. A nasopharyngeal or nasogastric suction tube (rerouting tube) is inserted through a nostril and brought out through the mouth.

The end of the nasobiliary catheter is inserted through this tube until the proximal end of the catheter appears in the nasopharyngeal tube. The nasobiliary catheter together with the nasopharyngeal tube is pulled back through the nose. Care is taken to avoid looping and kinking of the nasobiliary catheter in the posterior pharynx. The nasobiliary catheter is then connected to a three-way adaptor and the bile ducts are decompressed by aspirating bile. A bile specimen is sent for culture. The final position of the nasobiliary catheter is checked under fluoroscopy and anchored by taping to the face. The catheter is then connected to a drainage bag.

Temporary stenting may be helpful when large stones cannot be extracted (Fig. 3.25).

Endoscopic plastic stent insertion for malignant biliary obstruction (Fig. 3.26)

The technique of endoscopic insertion of biliary stents was first described in 1979. It is now an established method for the palliation of malignant obstructive jaundice. This is especially useful in patients with carcinoma of the pancreas as fewer than 20% of patients are appropriate for surgical resection, and less than 1% survive for more than 5 years.

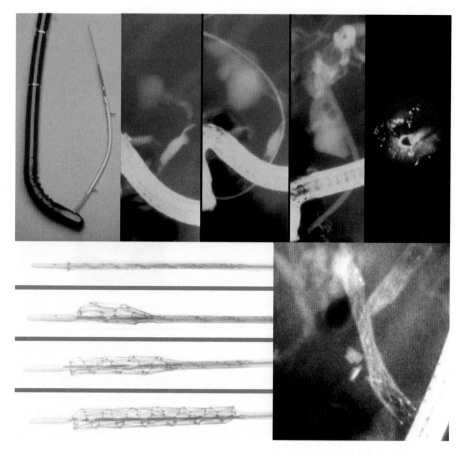

Fig. 3.26 Endoscopic stenting for malignant jaundice. Plastic stents: guidewire, inner catheter to negotiate stricture. Stent deployed with help of pusher. Metal stents: stent collapsed on introducer. Stent deployed through stricture by pulling back on covering sheath.

Equipment Side-viewing duodenoscopes with a 3.2 mm channel are necessary for insertion of 7–8 Fr stents. Larger 4.2 mm channel endoscopes are available for insertion of 10 and 11.5 Fr stents. The most commonly used plastic stents are straight with flap anchorage systems.

The standard applicator system consists of a 0.035 inch guidewire (480 cm) with a 3 cm flexible tip, and a 6 Fr radiopaque Teflon (260 cm in length) guiding catheter with a tapered tip to facilitate cannulation. Some guiding catheters have two metal rings (placed 7 cm apart) at the distal end for ease of identification and for measuring the length of the stricture.

The outer pusher tube is made of Teflon (8, 10, and 11.5 Fr) and used for positioning the stent during deployment. Stents are made of 7, 10, or 11.5 Fr radiopaque polyethylene tubes. They vary in length between the two anchoring flaps (5, 7, 9, 10, 12, 15 cm). There is no inner catheter for the 7 Fr stenting system.

Other stents have double pigtails that serve to anchor the stent to prevent upward or downward migration. However, the straight stent with side flaps is preferred because it maintains its position with infrequent dislocation. It provides maximal flow and minimizes the risk of blockage compared with the double pigtail stents, which have a smaller lumen and side-holes.

Preparation of patient The resectability of the underlying cancer or lesion and the clinical condition of the patient should be carefully assessed prior to stenting. Initial investigations include liver function tests, abdominal ultrasound, and CT scanning to define the nature and level of obstruction. Endoscopic ultrasound and fine-needle aspiration biopsy are also useful for staging and diagnosis of the underlying cancer. MRCP may be necessary in cases of hilar obstruction to outline the obstructed ductal system.

Coagulation defects are corrected by IV vitamin K_1 and/or fresh frozen plasma. Prophylactic antibiotic may be given before the procedure.

Procedure Preparation and sedation of the patient are the same as for standard ERCP procedures. A diagnostic ERCP is performed and the level of obstruction is defined. Sphincterotomy is not necessary for placement of a single stent but is useful to facilitate insertion of multiple stents, and may prevent the complication of pancreatitis following stenting for hilar strictures caused by pressure of the stents against the pancreatic orifice.

Initial cannulation and insertion of the guidewire past the stricture can be performed using standard accessories. It is preferable to use a guidewire with a hydrophilic tip for easy passage through the stricture. Brush cytology can be taken by exchanging the cytology brush over the guidewire. The guiding catheter is then exchanged over the guidewire to bypass the obstruction. The guidewire is then removed and additional bile samples can be aspirated for culture and cytology. The length of the stricture is determined on cholangiography with the help of radiopaque ring markers.

A suitable length stent is chosen so that the proximal flap of the stent lies about 1 cm above the obstruction. The optimal length of the stent can be determined by measuring the separation between the proximal obstruction and the level of the papilla on the radiographs. It can be estimated with reference to the scope diameter or by using the radiopaque markers on the inner catheter. The correct length of the stent is determined by correcting for the magnification factor of the fluoroscopy unit. The stent length can also be determined by retracting the guidewire between the two points and measuring the distance traveled on the outside of the catheter.

The stricture may be dilated (when particularly tight) prior to stent insertion with graded dilators or pneumatic balloon dilators (4, 6, 8 mm) inserted over the guidewire. The stent is loaded onto the catheter or guidewire and then positioned through the obstruction with the help of the pusher tube. The stent is deployed by removing the inner catheter and guidewire. Bile is seen draining through the stent into the duodenum. The pusher is then removed.

One-step introducer system A modified introducer system combines the inner catheter and pusher into a single system using a Luer lock mechanism. A suitable length stent is preloaded on to the introducer system, inserted over the guidewire, and positioned through the obstruction. Once the inner catheter is in position, the pusher and inner catheter are unlocked and the stent is pushed and deployed across the obstruction by withdrawing the inner catheter and guidewire.

Bilateral stenting for hilar obstruction

Hilar tumors pose difficult technical problems. Whether it is necessary or desirable to drain all obstructed ducts remains controversial. When one duct is dominant, draining it alone may be sufficient. To drain both the right and left hepatic systems, it is necessary to insert two guidewires separately. Correct anchorage of the guidewires is necessary because of the potential for dislodgement during exchange of accessories. This can be achieved using either a hemostat to clip the wire to the biopsy valve or a special anchoring unit that comes with a particular stenting system.

We recommend performing routine balloon dilation of hilar strictures prior to stent insertion as they are often very tight. It is better to start with the left hepatic system due to the more difficult access and axis with stent insertion.

Once the left stent is in place, another straight stent is introduced into the right side to drain part or all of the right hepatic ducts. Care is taken not to push the first stent into the bile duct during insertion of the second stent. In general, successful drainage of the left hepatic system alone may result in improvement of the liver function. The left hepatic duct branches off after 2 cm in contrast to the right hepatic duct which branches off after 1 cm.

Multiple segment obstruction is more likely to occur on the right side. Successful drainage and recovery of liver function are therefore more difficult due to the limited volume of liver tissue drained by the individual segmental hepatic ducts. Some endoscopists recommend multiple stents in all cases to achieve complete drainage.

Every attempt should be made to avoid overfilling the intrahepatic system to minimize the risk of sepsis. If endoscopic drainage fails, percutaneous trans-

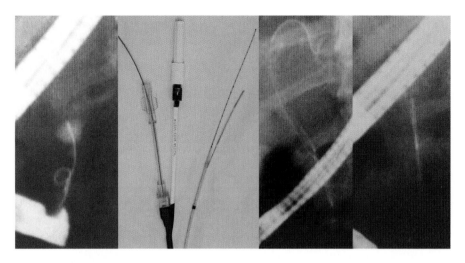

Fig. 3.27 Brush cytology for distal CBD stricture. Double lumen cytology brush. Guidewire to negotiate stricture. Brush pushed out above obstruction and withdrawn back through stricture for cytology. X-ray documentation.

hepatic drainage of the obstructed system may be considered and the combined percutaneous and endoscopic approach (or rendezvous approach) may be helpful on rare occasions.

Brush cytology for bile duct strictures (Fig. 3.27)

Single lumen system Brush cytology can be taken after passing a guidewire through the obstruction. The sheath of the cytology brush can be inserted over the guidewire through the stricture. The guidewire is then removed and the cytology brush inserted through the sheath. The sheath is then pulled back to allow the brush to emerge into the dilated proximal system. The brush and catheter are then pulled back through the stricture. An X-ray is taken to document the position of the brush through the stricture. Care is taken to ensure that the guidewire tip remains above the obstruction.

After the brush has been pushed and pulled through the stricture several times, the catheter sheath is advanced back into the proximal dilated system, the brush is removed, and the tip is prepared for cytology. The guidewire is then replaced and the cytology sheath is exchanged for the inner catheter. The rest of the stenting procedure is completed in the usual manner.

Using the single lumen cytology system, cell loss is inevitable because the brush is pulled back through the whole length of the catheter. It is useful to aspirate bile from the catheter to collect any dislodged cells within the catheter to improve the diagnostic yield.

Double lumen system Double lumen cytology brush systems allow the guidewire to pass through the central lumen of a tapered tip catheter and the cytology brush exits from the side lumen near the tip. With the brush in the retracted position, the catheter is inserted over the guidewire through the obstruction. With the help of radiopaque markers, the cytology brush is advanced from the catheter into the dilated proximal system. The entire apparatus is then moved back and forth through the area of the stricture to obtain samples. An X-ray is taken for documentation.

The brush is then withdrawn into the catheter and the whole set-up is exchanged over the guidewire without having to pull back the brush completely. This set-up ensures access is maintained across the stricture by the guidewire for the ease of subsequent stenting or drainage and also avoids cell loss. When the brush is withdrawn, the tip of the brush is cut off and saved in the cytology solution. It is useful to remove the stylet and to flush air or water through the channel of the brush to remove any fluid inside for cytological examination.

Assessment of response to biliary stenting

The clinical course of the patient is a good guide to the function of the stent. With successful drainage, pruritus usually disappears in 1–2 days as jaundice begins to resolve. Serum bilirubin declines by a mean of 2–3 mg/dl per day. With distal bile duct obstruction, bilirubin levels may return to normal after 1–2 weeks. Incomplete or slow recovery of liver function may be related to prolonged obstruction which affects hepatocyte function or may be due to inadequate or incomplete drainage because of multiple segment involvement, as in hilar obstruction. The presence of an air cholangiogram suggests stent patency which can also be assessed by an EHIDA scan. Delayed appearance of radioisotope in the biliary system and intestine, with appearance of radioisotope in urine, suggests stent blockage.

Results of biliary stenting The success rates for biliary stenting vary depending on the level of obstruction. They are high for mid- or distal CBD obstruction and lower for hilar obstruction. The success rates for draining both the right and left hepatic systems are low in patients with bifurcation lesions. Failure of endoscopic stenting may be due to tumor compression and/or distortion of the duodenum, marked displacement of the papilla, or failure of insertion of the guidewire through a very tight stricture.

Complications of stenting

Early complications Early complications of stenting include pancreatitis, bleeding if a sphincterotomy is performed, cholangitis in patients with bifurcation tumors, and early stent blockage by blood clots. Guidewire perforation through a soft and necrotic tumor has been reported.

Late complications Late complications are largely due to stent blockage by bacterial biofilm and biliary sludge, resulting in recurrent jaundice and cholangitis. Stent dislocation and traumatic ulceration of the duodenum by the distal tip of the stent may occur. Acute cholecystitis secondary to stenting is a rare complication.

Recurrent jaundice is a major late complication of endoscopic stenting. Tumor extension may account for a small proportion of cases. The most important cause is clogging of the lumen of the stent by biliary sludge. Sludge consists largely of calcium bilirubinate and small amounts of calcium palmitate, cholesterol, mucoprotein, and bacteria. Bacterial infection is important in initiating sludge formation through adherence and formation of a bacterial biofilm. The likely source of bacteria is ascending infection from the duodenum via the stent or descending infection through the portal system. The bacteria are mostly large bowel flora.

Different methods have been tested to prevent stent blockage. Larger lumen stents delay the onset of clogging. Stent exchange at regular intervals also prevents the clinical risk of blockage. Antibacterial plastics and prophylactic antibiotics have not produced any clinically significant benefits. An alternative solution to the blockage of plastic stents is to use self-expandable metal mesh stents.

Self-expandable metal stents

Self-expandable metal stents (SEMS) were introduced as a means of prolonging stent patency. SEMS expand to 1 cm diameter and do not become obstructed by bacterial biofilm. However, metal stent occlusion does occur, but mostly as a result of tumor/tissue ingrowth or overgrowth.

Stent configurations The commonly used SEMS have an open mesh design. Variations include the Wallstent, the Diamond Stent, the Spiral Z-Stent, the Za-Stent, and the more recently introduced Zilver Stent. SEMS are made of surgical-grade stainless steel or nitinol, a nickel–titanium alloy that provides a high degree of flexibility and is kink resistant. However, nitinol is less radiopaque than stainless steel and additional radiopaque (gold or platinum) markers are put on the stents to improve radiopacity to facilitate proper positioning during deployment. Covered SEMS are now available. One example is the Wallstent (Microvasive) which has a polymer (Permalune) coating on the inside of the stent except for the proximal and distal 1 cm. This membrane is designed to prevent tumor ingrowth and prolong stent patency.

Lengths of stents SEMS usually come in two or three different expanded lengths (e.g. 4.8, 6.8, and 8.0 cm for the Wallstents, 5.7 and 7.5 cm for the Spiral Z-Stents). The Wallstent foreshortens after deployment to about two-thirds of its collapsed length when it is fully expanded. The Spiral Z- and Zilver Stents do not shorten after deployment.

Introducer system for SEMS In general, the wire mesh metal stents are collapsed and restrained on a 6–6.5 Fr introducer catheter by an 8–8.5 Fr overlying plastic sheath. Smaller 7/7.5 Fr introducer systems are now available. Sterile water or saline is initially injected to flush the system to minimize friction between the stent and the restraining sheath and to facilitate stent deployment. The whole system is placed over the guidewire and advanced through the obstruction.

   With the stent correctly positioned across the stricture, the overlying sheath is pulled back while the handle is held steadily to hold the introducer catheter and guidewire in position. The stent is deployed slowly in a stepwise manner. Stent deployment can be monitored under fluoroscopic control using the radiopaque markers. Adjustment of the stent position may be necessary before complete deployment, especially for stents that foreshorten, e.g. the Wallstent. It is also easier to pull back than to advance a partially deployed stent through the stricture or obstruction.

   Metal stents are usually placed with the distal tip in the duodenum for distal bile duct obstruction. Due to the limited lengths available, the stent can be placed completely inside the CBD for proximal or mid-duct strictures. It is important to avoid leaving the distal tip of the stent just at the level of the papilla as this can cause discomfort and dysfunction.

Balloon dilation of biliary strictures (Fig. 3.28)

Both malignant and benign bile duct strictures may present with obstructive symptoms. Patients with dominant extrahepatic strictures complicating primary sclerosing cholangitis (and some with chronic pancreatitis) may respond to balloon dilation of the strictures with or without use of biliary stents. A stenosed choledochoduodenostomy may be safely and effectively dilated using a pneumatic balloon dilator. Similarly, balloon sphincteroplasty using a pneumatic

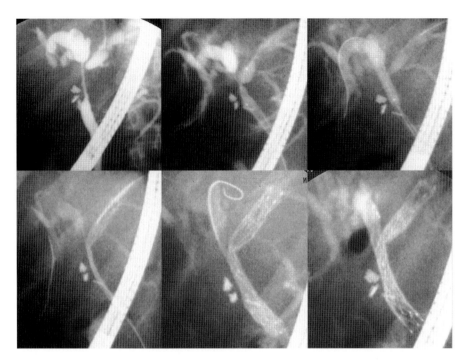

Fig. 3.28 Balloon dilation and bilateral Z-Stent for hilar obstruction. Dual guidewires. Balloon dilation of right and left hepatic duct stricture. Z-Stent inserted into left hepatic duct and then right hepatic duct.

balloon has been employed to facilitate removal of small CBD stones without a sphincterotomy.

Equipment Balloon dilation is best performed with a large channel endoscope. Additional accessories include the pneumatic balloons. These are made of non-compliant polyethylene with two types available. One type goes over a guidewire while the other type, the TTS (through-the-scope) balloon, does not require a guidewire. Balloons come in different sizes and lengths: 4, 6, or 8 mm in diameter and 2–6 cm long.

Procedure A prior sphincterotomy is not necessary but may facilitate the intro-duction of large balloon catheters and exchange of accessories. A flexible tip guidewire is inserted with the help of a catheter and negotiated through the stric-ture. The catheter is removed and the dilation balloon is railroaded over the guidewire across the stricture. The balloon is positioned so that the stricture lies at the midpoint of the balloon. The presence of radiopaque markers helps in positioning the balloon.

The balloon is then inflated with dilute (10%) contrast and the pressure adjusted according to the type of balloon and the manufacturer's recommendation. The dilation is performed under fluoroscopy and a waist is seen at the midpoint of the balloon upon inflating the balloon. Effective dilation is achieved when the waist disappears.

The patient may experience pain during insufflation of the balloon. The balloon is usually kept inflated for 30–60 s and then deflated. It is helpful to reinflate the balloon and note the opening pressure when the waist disappears on the balloon. With successful dilation, the opening pressure should be lower with repeat dilation. The balloon is then completely deflated, the guidewire removed and contrast injected while the balloon catheter is pulled back to assess the effect of dilation.

Balloon dilation facilitates stent insertion in patients with malignant biliary strictures. The short-term effects of balloon dilation for benign biliary strictures are good but long-term follow-up shows some restenosis. Repeat dilation at regular intervals may be necessary to keep the stricture open. Some endoscopists advocate the use of temporary stenting (with multiple stents) to keep the stricture open and repeat dilation and stent exchange every 3 months for up to a year. Intrahepatic bile duct stones have been successfully removed following balloon dilation of intrahepatic strictures.

Endoscopic management of bile leaks

Bile leaks may arise from the cystic duct stump after a cholecystectomy or from injury to the CBD during surgery. Patients usually present with persistent bile drainage or formation of a biloma. As bile tends to flow in the path of least resistance, an intact papilla maintains a positive intrabiliary pressure and may perpetuate the leak. Eliminating or bypassing the sphincter mechanism may reduce the intrabiliary pressure.

Alternatively, an indwelling nasobiliary catheter or stent which bypasses the sphincter may serve to decompress the biliary system and promote healing of the leak. A small leak can be closed off easily by nasobiliary catheter drainage for a few days. Bile leak associated with CBD damage may require placement of an indwelling stent across the leak for up to 4–6 weeks. It is important to check for residual damage or stricture of the CBD after removal of the stent.

Outstanding issues and future trends

ERCP now plays a very important role in the imaging and therapy of different pancreatico-biliary problems. Many different technologies are being developed to shorten the time of the procedure by improving access and success with selective deep cannulation, thus minimizing manipulation within the ductal systems.

ERCP is, however, not without risk and serious complications have been reported. Acute pancreatitis remains an important complication of this procedure and can occur even after a simple diagnostic cannulation. Although we are able to identify individuals who are at increased risk, currently available methods are not very effective in preventing this complication. Prophylactic pancreatic stenting to improve drainage is promising but this procedure itself requires considerable skill and experience.

MRCP with improved resolution may well replace diagnostic ERCP. However, ERCP will continue to play a role in the management of pancreaticobiliary diseases because of its therapeutic applications. There is a potential concern that, with the limited number of cases and the high skill level required of a biliary endoscopist, we may see a significant reduction in the number of trained endoscopists in the future. We are already seeing a reduction in the number of training positions and the expectation of additional (third-tier) training before an endoscopist becomes qualified to perform these procedures. The question of whether training with simulators may improve the skill of the biliary endoscopist remains to be addressed.

References

1 Cotton PB, Williams CB. (1996). *Practical Gastrointestinal Endoscopy*, 4th edn. Blackwell Publishing, Oxford.
2 Leung JWC, Ling TK, Chan RC *et al*. Antibiotics, biliary sepsis, and bile duct stones. *Gastrointest Endosc* 1994; 40: 716–21.
3 Sung JJ, Lyon DJ, Suen R *et al*. Intravenous ciprofloxacin as treatment for patients with acute suppurative cholangitis: a randomized, controlled clinical trial. *J Antimicrob Chemother* 1995; 35 (6): 855–64.
4 Lee JG, Leung JW. Endoscopic management of common bile duct stones. *Gastrointest Endosc Clin N Am* 1996; 6: 43–55.
5 Leung JWC, Chung SCS, Mok SD, Li AKC. Endoscopic removal of large common bile duct stones in recurrent pyogenic cholangitis. *Gastrointest Endosc* 1988; 34: 238–41.
6 Chung SC, Leung JW, Leong HT, Li AK. Mechanical lithotripsy of large common bile duct stones using a basket. *Br J Surg* 1991; 78: 1448–50.
7 Sorbi D, Van Os E, Aberger FJ, Derfus GA, Erickson R, Meier P *et al*. Clinical application of a new disposable lithotripter: a prospective multicenter study. *Gastrointest Endosc* 1999; 49: 210–3.
8 Chan ACW, Ng EKW, Chung SCS *et al*. Common bile duct stones become smaller after endoscopic biliary stenting. *Endoscopy* 1998; 30: 356–9.
9 Lau JYW, Ip SM, Chung SCS *et al*. Endoscopic drainage aborts endotoxaemia in acute cholangitis. *Br J Surg* 1996; 83: 181–4.
10 Lai ECS, Mok FPT, Tan ESY *et al*. Endoscopic biliary drainage for severe acute cholangitis. *N Engl J Med* 1992; 326: 1582–6.
11 Leung JWC, Chung SCS, Sung JJ *et al*. Urgent endoscopic drainage for severe acute suppurative cholangitis. *Lancet* 1989; 1: 1307–9.
12 Sugiyama M, Atomi Y. The benefits of endoscopic nasobiliary drainage without sphincterotomy for acute cholangitis. *Am J Gastroenterol* 1998; 93: 2065–8.

13 Lee DW, Chan AC, Lam YH *et al*. Biliary decompression by nasobiliary catheter or biliary stent in acute suppurative cholangitis: a prospective randomized trial. *Gastrointest Endosc* 2002; 56: 361–5.
14 Leung JW, Del Favero G, Cotton P. Endoscopic biliary prostheses: a comparison of materials. *Gastrointest Endosc* 1985; 31: 93–5.
15 Libby E, Leung J. Prevention of biliary stent clogging: a clinical review. *Am J Gastroenterol* 1996; 91: 1301–8.
16 Sung J, Chung SCS. Endoscopic stenting for palliation of malignant biliary obstruction. *Dig Dis Sci* 1995; 40: 1167–73.

CHAPTER 4

ERCP Communications, Recording, and Reporting

PETER B. COTTON

ERCP in context

There is much more to ERCP than knowing how to perform the procedures. At a macro level, it is necessary to be able to place the procedure appropriately within the broad spectrum of biliary and pancreatic diseases, and to appreciate the many ways of approaching them. Achieving this wisdom is the goal of specialist training, but remains an imperative throughout our careers as the world of medicine changes and as we ourselves help to change it. This evolution requires, and is greatly facilitated by, the development of active collaboration between all of the interested disciplines, especially gastroenterology, surgery, and radiology, which is the vision behind the Center concept [1].

Teamwork

At the micro, everyday, level, it is essential to realize that ERCP is a team event, requiring careful coordination between the endoscopist and the assistants (nurses and radiology technicians), and any trainees. Teams work better together if the goals are clear, and when the efforts of all members are respected. There is potential for confusion when the room is crowded with extra people, such as medical and nursing students, anesthesia staff, interested visitors, and even equipment vendors. It is wise and polite to make sure that you know everyone's name (and role) before getting started. Some hospitals have initiated a 'time out' at the beginning of all operative procedures, like the cockpit drill for pilots that is mandatory before any take-off or landing. This is intended to double-check that we have the correct patient, that key facts (e.g. allergies) have been noted, and that we have a clear plan of action.

It is also important for everyone in the room to maintain focus on the job in hand, keeping irrelevant conversation to a minimum, especially if the patient is under conscious sedation. The need for appropriate behavior in the endoscopy room has been well emphasized by one of the leaders of our profession [2].

Our experience in watching and performing ERCP around the world has shown that the teamwork and interpersonal communications essential for this collaboration are often threatened by lack of a common lexicon, or consistent 'ERCP speak'. Devices, sites, and actions can be described in many different ways. For example 'needle out' can be interpreted as advancing the needle out of the catheter, or, just the opposite, i.e. out of the patient. Is the 'distal pancreas' the head or the tail? Does 'fluoro further right' mean to the patient's right, or to our right? Such confusions can have serious results, and would not be permitted in the cockpit of an aircraft.

ERCP speak

To reduce the potential for confusion, we suggest trying to develop and use a structured lexicon of communication, such as:

1 Endoscopist to assistant/nurse
   - push/pull wire
   - push/pull guide catheter
   - basket open/close
   - snare open/close
   - bow/relax sphincterotome
   - exchanging, push/accept wire
   - pull everything out
   - show needle/hide needle
   - balloon up/balloon down
   - inject contrast
   - aspirate
   - start to deploy (metal stent)
2 Endoscopist to trainee

Controlling the endoscope
   - angle up/down
   - angle right/left
   - rotate right/left
   - bridge up/down
   - push/pull scope
   - brake on/off

Controlling devices
   - push/pull catheter/device
3 Endoscopist to radiology technician
   - fluoro on/off
   - take (hard-copy radiograph)
   - magnify image/mag off

- shutters in/out top and bottom/right/left
- flip image right/left
- rotate C-arm towards me/away from me
- tilt table head up/head down

4 Endoscopist to sedationist/anesthesiologist

All instructions should be equally clear, including dosing.

Confirming commands and feedback

Endoscopists need to know that their requests have been heard and acted upon, at least when this is not obvious visually. For example, we like to be told when medicines have been given (e.g. glucagon, Buscopan, or secretin).

Teams need positive educational feedback. Thank everyone when the procedure has been completed, and, if things have not gone completely smoothly, take the opportunity immediately (and politely) to suggest how improvements can be made.

Recording and reporting

The procedure is not complete until it has been documented appropriately, so that everyone knows what has been done and why. Inadequate documentation can result in much uncertainty, and future diagnostic and therapeutic actions may be compromised.

Endoscopy reports

There are some published guidelines regarding the content of endoscopy reports [3,4]. Reports should include key details of the patient, referring source(s), indications (including relevant clinical history, labs, and imaging), preparation (including fitness assessment, need for antibiotics, allergy issues, and the process for patient education and consent), the site and timing of the procedures, the doctors and staff involved, the sedation/analgesia used and tolerance, instruments, extent of the endoscopic survey, cannulation attempts, opacifications, findings on fluoroscopy, adjuvant diagnostic procedures (e.g. biopsy, manometry), diagnoses made and excluded, treatments attempted and their immediate outcomes, unplanned events (complications), accessories consumed, total duration and fluoroscopy time, recovery, disposal, patient education, and follow-up plans.

A great deal of work has gone into trying to develop consensus on a common lexicon for endoscopy. The minimum standard terminology (MST) is the best known and studied [5], and is used increasingly in electronic reporting systems.

These systems drive compliance in reporting by prompting appropriate entries, and may even disallow saving or printing a report until certain mandatory fields are completed.

By contrast, there has been no consistency, and no formal recommendations, concerning the number and variety of images that should be recorded during ERCP, either endoscopic or radiological.

Endoscopic image documentation

It would seem logical to document pertinent landmarks (e.g. the papillary area), any lesions or unusual mucosal findings, and the appearances before and after therapeutic procedures, e.g. sphincterotomy. These images are now easy to capture, and to annotate, with electronic reporting systems. DICOM technical standards are being widely adapted [6–8]. Video-recording onto tape, or digitally, provides a much more complete document, but can generate storage and retrieval problems. Most units have many boxes of videotapes that have been recorded with enthusiasm, but are either ignored ever after or become a source for frustration when trying to find key sequences for teaching purposes. This problem will be solved eventually with high-capacity digital video storage units, which can be searched by keywords as well as by patient name.

Radiological image documentation

The permanent X-ray images of ERCP found in radiology files (or, increasingly, on CD-ROMs) are often woefully inadequate. Radiologists are rarely involved during the actual procedures; image capture is at the whim of the endoscopist and a radiology technician who is often not familiar with ERCP. The usual result is an inadequate number and variety of images, with only haphazard documentation of the important findings and events. This may lead to errors of interpretation at the time, and at subsequent consultations when no other information is available.

Radiological aspects of ERCP are mentioned in other chapters of this book in specific contexts. Other books have included some discussion of radiological equipment and techniques [3,9,10], but we have been unable to find any general recommendations for the number and types of images to be captured. Here we suggest some minimum standards for radiographic documentation.

Checklist for radiological filming

1   Check that the system has the correct name, date, and timings.
2   Take an abdominal scout film with the endoscope in the second part of the

duodenum. This ensures that the field is clear (e.g. of monitoring wires), the patient position is adequate, and that any unusual densities (e.g. pancreatic or vascular calcification, foreign bodies) are recognized before any contrast confuses the view.

3   Take films during the filling phase of both biliary and pancreatic systems (when clinically relevant) to detect any small lesions and stones.

4   Document complete filling (without overfilling) of all of the relevant ductal systems. This may require turning the patient (or a C-arm), or moving the endoscope (particularly to see the mid-part of the bile duct and the region of the pancreatic neck).

5   Document any lesion or suspicious area.

6   Record all the phases of intraductal procedures to show correct positioning of guidewires, cytology brushes, stents, sphincterotomes, etc.

7   Record any possible or definite deviations, such as extraluminal air, intravascular contrast, guidewire perforation, acinarization, and submucosal or extravasated contrast.

8   Record images prone and supine after removing the endoscope to see how much contrast has drained, and to provide a reference for future studies (e.g. of stent position). The gallbladder is usually best seen with the patient supine with the head elevated.

Radiographic interpretation

Rarely is there a radiologist in the ERCP room or available quickly nearby, and so most endoscopists have to interpret the fluoroscopy and hard-image findings in real time to make immediate decisions about the need for further manipulations, and for endoscopic therapy.

In most institutions, the captured images are reported later by one of many general radiologists, without reference to the endoscopist, and often even without access to the procedure report. This situation is fraught with potential error, with clinical and medico-legal risk. Several studies have now documented these discrepancies [11–13].

Reporting errors by endoscopists and radiologists can be reduced by:

1   Teaching ERCP trainees about radiological techniques and interpretation.

2   Complying with guidelines for capturing images, as suggested above.

3   Making sure that the reporting radiologist receives a copy of the complete ERCP report.

4   Minimizing the number of radiologists involved, and having joint meetings to discuss interesting cases and discrepancies. Those involved in each institution should meet to consider the local situation, and to initiate a process to improve collaboration and quality control.

Transmitting the information

The procedure document(s) is of limited value unless it reaches the right people. The primary target is the referring physician, who will put the information in context and make future care plans. In practice, it is not always easy to find that target. Patients often reach specialist centers by a roundabout route, which they may not repeat in reverse when they leave. Thus it is very important to clarify which doctor(s) the patient will see for continuing care, and to ensure that he/she is on the list of people to receive reports (along with the actual referral source and any primary provider, if different). Speed is a key parameter of reporting. Phone calls or emails are often very helpful, and the days of snail-mail reporting must be numbered.

What about the patient? It is good medical practice to explain what has been done to any accompanying person immediately after the procedure, but it is sometimes more difficult to ensure that the patient is fully informed, not least when he/she is discharged while still somewhat sleepy in the warm glow of recovery. Some endoscopists give patients a copy of the procedure report, but it is perhaps better to provide a simplified version. Newer endoscopy reporting systems can be programmed to print this out, with the key features and conclusions, including the main recommendations, and plans for follow-up.

Most patients like to receive photographic prints of their procedures, and some are given videos. For ERCP, it is desirable to give patients a CD-ROM of the radiographs, since many of them will have several subsequent consultations.

ERCP reporting: conclusion

ERCP procedures, even when indicated and well performed, may ultimately fail to help patients if the findings and results are not documented clearly and completely, and do not reach those making subsequent treatment decisions. Endoscopists should consider how to improve their own reporting practices, and how to help their radiologist colleagues to play a more useful role.

References

1 Cotton PB. Interventional gastroenterology (endoscopy) at the crossroads: a plea for restructuring in digestive diseases. *Gastroenterology* 1994; 107: 294–9.
2 Boyce HW. Behavior in the endoscopy room. *Gastrointest Endosc* 2001; 53: 133–6.
3 Cotton PB, Williams CB. (1996). *Practical Gastrointestinal Endoscopy*, 4th edn. Blackwell Scientific, Oxford.
4 American Society of Gastrointestinal Endoscopy. (1992). *Defining the Endoscopy Report*. American Society of Gastrointestinal Endoscopy, Manchester.
5 Korman LY, Delvaux M, Crespi M. The minimal standard terminology in digestive endoscopy: perspective on a standard endoscopic vocabulary. *Gastrointest Endosc* 2001; 53: 392–6.

 6 Aabakken L. (2004). Digital documentation in endoscopy. In: *Endoscopy Practice and Safety* (ed. Cotton, PB) (www.gastrohep.com).

 7 Fujino MA, Ikeda M. (1996). Electronic image management. In: *Gastroenterologic Endoscopy*, Vol. 1, 2nd edn (ed. Sivak, MV), pp. 103–14. W. B. Saunders, Philadelphia.

 8 Heldwein W, Rosch T. (2002). Reporting terminology and image documentation in endoscopy. In: *Gastroenterological Endoscopy* (ed. Classen, M, Tytgat, GNJ, Lightdale, CJ), pp. 754–9. Thieme, Stuttgart.

 9 Taylor AJ, Bohofoush III, AG. (1997). *Interpretation of ERCP with Associated Digital Imaging Correlation*. Lippincott-Raven, Philadelphia.

10 Martin DF, Tweedle D, Haboubi NY. (1998). *Clinical Practice of ERCP*. Churchill Livingstone, London.

11 Thomas M, Geenen JE, Catalano MF. Importance of real time interpretation (INTERP) of ERCP films over conventional static images: medicolegal implications. *Gastrointest Endosc* 2004; 59: AB183.

12 Khanna N, May G, Cole M, Bass S, Romagnuolo J. Post-ERCP radiology interpretation of cholangio-pancreatograms appears to be of limited benefit and may be inaccurate. *Gastrointest Endosc* 2004; 59: AB186.

13 Sweeney JT, Shah RJ, Martin SP, Ulrich CD, Somogyi L. The impact of post-procedure interpretation by radiologists on patient care: should it be routine or selective? *Gastrointest Endosc* 2003; 58: 549–53.

CHAPTER 5

Common Bile Duct Stones and Cholangitis

ENDERS K. W. NG AND SYDNEY CHUNG

Synopsis

Common bile duct (CBD) stones can be classified into primary stones (those that form within the bile ducts) and secondary stones (those that originate from the gallbladder). They can cause pain, jaundice, cholangitis, or biliary pancreatitis. Endoscopic sphincterotomy (ES) is an established method for the removal of CBD stones. Stones < 1 cm in diameter can be extracted easily with baskets or balloon catheters. Large (> 2 cm) or giant stones require some form of lithotripsy (mechanical or intraductal with laser/electrohydraulic lithotripsy) to facilitate duct clearance.

Patients presenting with acute cholangitis secondary to biliary stones carry a significant morbidity and mortality. Broad spectrum antibiotic therapy is necessary to cover against the mixed bacterial infection. The presence of complete biliary obstruction and infection may lead to suppurative cholangitis with an increased risk of fatality. The clinical outcome is improved with urgent endoscopic biliary decompression using a nasobiliary catheter or an indwelling biliary stent. Successful removal of CBD and intrahepatic stones may require stricture dilation and lithotripsy. Combined percutaneous and endoscopic drainage procedures ensure complete duct clearance and prevent stone recurrence.

Background

Incidence of CBD stones

Choledocholithiasis is a common clinical problem worldwide. It has been estimated that 10–15% of patients undergoing cholecystectomy for symptomatic gallstones harbor concomitant stones in their CBD [1]. Primary ductal stones formed *de novo* also add a further small percentage to the overall prevalence.

Traditional management

After the first successful CBD exploration by Courvoisier in 1890, surgical lithotripsy was the treatment of choice for choledocholithiasis for nearly a century [2].

Non-operative approach to CBD stones

The introduction of ES in 1974 [3] and the rapid development of minimal access surgery in the late 1980s have completely revolutionized the approach to CBD stones. As laparoscopic cholecystectomy is the first-line treatment for gallstones nowadays, endoscopic removal of biliary tree calculi has become the most appealing and widely embraced technique for removal of choledocholithiasis.

Pathogenesis

Classification of CBD stones

Bile duct stones can be broadly classified into two types according to the site of origin.

Primary CBD stones

Primary ductal stones are stones that develop *de novo* in the intrahepatic ducts or common duct. They are far more common in the Asian populations than in the West. The reason for such a geographical difference is enigmatic. These stones are often brownish-yellow in color with a soft muddy consistency (Fig. 5.1); biochemically, they consist of calcium bilirubinate mixed with variable amounts of cholesterol and calcium salts. While the etiology remains conjectural, bacterial infections and biliary stasis are considered the two most important causative factors.

Bacteriology of primary CBD stones Gastrointestinal tract microorganisms such as *Escherichia coli*, *Klebsiella*, *Proteus*, *Bacteroides*, and *Clostridium* have been isolated from the bile of patients with primary duct stones [4]. In addition, bacterial cytoskeletons are invariably seen in primary duct stones under electronic microscope [5]. These bacteria may have a contributory role by producing enzymes that catalyze deconjugation of bilirubin and lysis of phospholipids, which in turn promote the precipitation of calcium bilirubinate and initiate

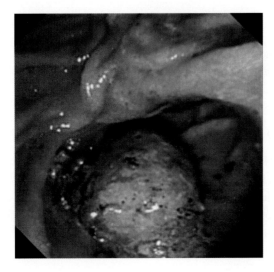

Fig. 5.1 Typical brown pigment stone retrieved by ERCP.

stone formation. Among all the bacteria isolated, *Clostridium perfringens* has been found to produce the highest beta-glucuronidase enzyme activity, which is 34-fold higher than that for *E. coli*, *Corynebacterium* spp., *Enterococcus* spp., and *Klebsiella* spp. [6]. On the other hand, the biliary stasis theory is supported by the fact that intrahepatic ductal strictures and proximal dilation are commonly seen among patients with primary duct calculi [7]. Nevertheless, whether these strictures are the cause or consequence of the intrahepatic ductal calculi remains unresolved.

Secondary CBD stones

Secondary common duct stones are supposed to have originated from the gallbladder. Conceivably their composition is identical to that of gallstones, which are mainly yellowish cholesterol or black pigment calculi with a hard and crispy consistency. It is unclear why gallstones migrate into the common duct in some patients. In one study the size of the cystic duct has been reported as the single most important determinant [8].

Clinical presentations

Asymptomatic biliary stones

A considerable proportion of patients with common or intrahepatic ductal calculi are asymptomatic. The stones may be found incidentally during investigation for unrelated abdominal conditions. The presence of coexisting ductal stones is sometimes noted by abdominal ultrasound scan when patients are being worked up for cholelithiasis.

Symptomatic biliary stones

Obstructive jaundice

Intermittent jaundice is said to be a typical feature of choledocholithiasis, when the stone impacts and disimpacts at the papilla or the distal CBD leading to fluctuating jaundice and serum bilirubin levels. Continuous obstruction from stone impaction in the distal common duct may manifest as progressive jaundice.

Pain

Dull right upper abdominal pain due to increased biliary tree pressure may also be experienced as a result of stone impaction.

Clinical cholangitis

When bacterial infection superimposes in the obstructed biliary system, the patient presents with the typical Charcot's triad (fever, pain, and jaundice) of cholangitis. Nevertheless, cholangitis may not necessarily present with all three features, and the diagnosis should not be dismissed lightly just because the patient is afebrile or not jaundiced.

Biliary pancreatitis

Small stones may pass spontaneously through the ampulla of Vater. The passage of stones across the papilla may induce a transient rise in the pancreatic duct pressure and trigger intrapancreatic activation of enzymes resulting in acute pancreatitis. Patients with acute pancreatitis typically present with epigastric pain radiating to the back, associated with nausea and vomiting. A serum amylase level exceeding 1000 IU/liter is considered to be diagnostic of pancreatitis.

Oriental cholangitis or recurrent pyogenic cholangitis

Patients with primary intrahepatic duct stones may present with recurrent attacks of cholangitis. Characteristically, there are multiple strictures, with stone formation proximal to the stricture in the dilated portion of one or more segments of the intrahepatic ducts. Jaundice may not be obvious if only segmental

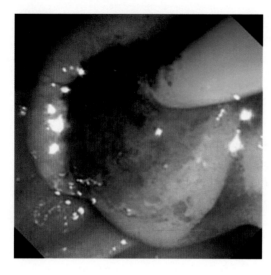

Fig. 5.2 Characteristic muddy bile and sludge discharging through the papilla of a patient with oriental cholangiohepatitis.

branch ducts of one liver lobe are involved. This condition is more commonly seen in South-East Asia and thus is called oriental cholangitis or cholangiohepatitis (Fig. 5.2).

Diagnosis

Clinical diagnosis

For patients presenting with jaundice, acute cholangitis, or pancreatitis, the diagnosis of CBD or intrahepatic duct stones is not difficult because the pathology often declares itself with typical clinical or biochemical features.

However, it may be difficult to diagnose asymptomatic biliary stones, and these may be suspected or identified because of a subtle derangement of liver function tests. Some patients may only have a mild elevation of serum alkaline phosphatase, without any changes in the bilirubin level.

Imaging

The presence of CBD stones can be determined by non-contrast or contrast studies.

Abdominal ultrasound scan

Abdominal ultrasound is the first-line imaging investigation if biliary tree calculi are suspected. In addition to seeing echogenic materials within the biliary tree,

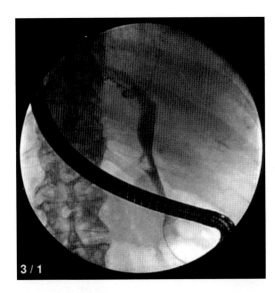

Fig. 5.3 A triangular shaped stone in the CBD revealed by ERCP.

the status of the CBD, intrahepatic bile ducts, and gallbladder can be determined.

Endoscopic retrograde cholangiopancreatography (ERCP)

The diagnosis is confirmed by contrast studies of the biliary system with ERCP or other forms of imaging. Although ERCP has been the gold standard for demonstrating biliary tract calculi, the procedure itself is invasive and carries a considerable risk of complications (Fig. 5.3).

Magnetic resonance cholangiogram (MRC) for CBD stones

MRC has evolved over the last decade and may potentially replace or supplement ERCP in the diagnosis of choledocholithiasis. In a recent prospective study by Calvo *et al.*, 61 patients with suspected biliary tree calculi according to Cotton's criteria (high probability in 49 patients, intermediate probability in nine patients) were subjected to MRC within 72 h prior to diagnostic ERCP. MRC correctly identified CBD stones in all three patients with choledocholithiasis in the intermediate probability group, as well as 29 out of the 32 patients in the high probability group [9]. Overall sensitivity and specificity of MRC were 91 and 84%, respectively. The global efficacy was estimated at 90%. It appears to be a promising technique, especially in cases with equivocal serum biochemistry or sonographic findings (Fig. 5.4). However, MRC is purely diagnostic and a separate therapeutic session needs to be arranged if choledocholithiasis is found, rendering it a less favored option for patients with a high suspicion for CBD stones.

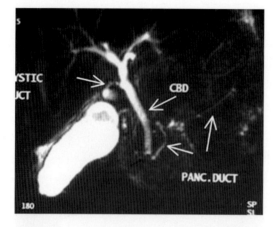

Fig. 5.4 Magnetic resonance cholangiogram showing a small stone impacted at the lower end of CBD.

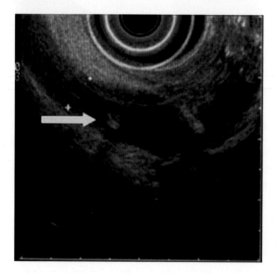

Fig. 5.5 A small common duct stone detected by EUS.

Endoscopic ultrasonography (EUS) for CBD stones

There is now supporting evidence that the accuracy of EUS is as good as, or comparable to, ERCP in diagnosing bile duct stones (Fig. 5.5), with a sensitivity of 84–100% and specificity of 76–100% [10,11]. These data were largely generated by the use of a radial scanning transducer [12]. Whether a linear scanner can achieve similar accuracy in the diagnosis of choledocholithiasis is still under investigation [13]. One major disadvantage of EUS is that it is highly operator-dependent, which may account for the wide variations in sensitivity and specificity being reported in the literature, and which makes the interpretation of data difficult.

Management for CBD stones

While some may advocate the use of medical treatment such as chemical dissolution for the removal of biliary tree calculi, endoscopic or surgical approaches remain the preferred treatments because they are more effective and reliable.

ERCP, sphincterotomy, and stone extraction

CBD stones < 5 mm in diameter may pass spontaneously or can be removed without a sphincterotomy. For stones > 5 mm, ES is the most commonly performed procedure for their retrieval.

Endoscopic sphincterotomy

Choice of endoscopes The preparation, positioning, and sedation of the patient are the same as those for diagnostic ERCP. The choice of duodenoscopes is determined by the anticipated size of the CBD stones. For small stones, where a complex lithotripsy instrument is unnecessary, a regular duodenoscope with a 2.8 mm channel is adequate. However, when the stone is > 1 cm or there is a strong likelihood that lithotripsy will be needed, a bigger duodenoscope, with a 3.2 or 4.2 mm channel, should be used.

Cannulation with sphincterotome Cannulation of the common duct is the same as for diagnostic ERCP. Some patients may have stones impacted at the lower end of the common duct (Fig. 5.6), and the resultant bulging papilla could render cannulation more difficult. A cannulating sphincterotome with an

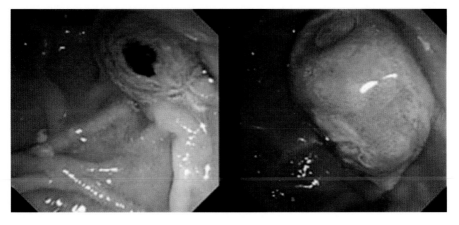

Fig. 5.6 Two cases with impacted stone at the papilla.

adjustable tip may facilitate cannulation of the bile duct in this situation by lifting the roof of the papilla. The use of a hydrophilic guidewire under such circumstances may also help in selective cannulation. Deep cannulation of the bile duct should be confirmed by injecting a small amount of contrast through the sphincterotome or by gently wiggling the sphincterotome under fluoroscopy.

Sphincterotomy A guidewire is inserted through the lumen of the cannulotome once deep cannulation is confirmed, so that access to the bile duct can be assured in subsequent exchange maneuvers. The cutting wire is then bowed so that it is in contact with the roof of the papilla. The incision is made in a stepwise manner in the 11–1 o'clock direction along the longitudinal fold. To avoid an uncontrolled 'zipper' cut, minimal tension is applied to the wire. The electrocautery unit should be set with a high cutting current blended with a low coagulation current. The size of the sphincterotomy can vary but it should be limited to the junction between the duodenal wall and the intraduodenal portion of the ampulla of Vater, which often appears as a semicircular mucosal fold above the papilla.

Stone extraction

After endoscopic sphincterotomy, stones in the biliary tree can be removed with either a basket or a balloon catheter. The authors prefer a dormia basket because it is in general more durable than the fragile retrieval balloons.

Basket stone extraction In brief, the closed basket covered by its plastic sheath is inserted into the common duct through the therapeutic channel of the duodenoscope. Inside the bile duct, the basket is gently opened and contrast is injected to confirm its position and relation to the biliary calculi. Care must be taken when opening the basket because stones in the main duct may be displaced upward and become trapped in one of the intrahepatic ducts. It is also advisable to remove stones lying in the distal CBD before making any attempts to retrieve stones located in the proximal duct. Vigorous shaking of the fully open basket inside the bile duct may help to bring the stones into the basket. Once the stones are captured, the basket is withdrawn slowly without closure. Closure of the basket at this juncture may disengage the stones. When the basket and stones are withdrawn to the level of papillotomy, the duodenoscope is gently pushed in with a right rotational movement. This maneuver helps straighten the tip of the duodenoscope, and exerts a traction force along the axis of the CBD which facilitates the removal of the stones, and avoids damage to the papilla or duodenum. By repeating the above maneuver, multiple ductal stones < 1 cm in diameter can be removed in the same ERCP session (Fig. 5.7).

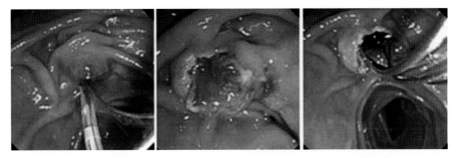

Fig. 5.7 *Left*: a wire-guide papillotome locating inside the low CBD; *Middle*: completion of endoscopic sphincterotomy (ES); *Right*: use of dormia basket for retrieval of CBD stone after ES.

Balloon stone extraction Biliary stones in the CBD of < 1 cm in diameter can be removed with a balloon catheter. The balloon is deflated and inserted into the CBD through the sphincterotomy, and advanced above the stones. The balloon is gently inflated to the size of the bile duct and pulled back gently, displacing the CBD stone distally. With an adequate sphincterotomy, the stone can be pulled against the cut orifice and then expelled by traction on the balloon catheter followed by downward angulation of the tip of the endoscope. The maneuver is repeated and complete clearance of the CBD is confirmed by an occlusion cholangiogram.

Complications

Bleeding, perforation, pancreatitis, and cholangitis are potential complications of ES and stone extraction. The reported incidence varies markedly in the literature, but bleeding is generally the most common complication encountered. Previous studies failed to identify predicting factors for these complications. Most of these studies were univariate or bivariate analyses, which generated inconsistent and often contradictory results [14,15]. Two multicenter studies based on multivariate regression models, however, have shed new light on this complex issue.

Acute pancreatitis

In a prospective survey conducted in the United States between 1992 and 1994, acute pancreatitis was found to be significantly more common if the ES was performed for suspected dysfunction of the sphincter of Oddi, in young patients, using a precut technique, after difficult cannulation, or with repeated and excessive pancreatic contrast injections (Fig. 5.8) [16]. Similar findings were reported in

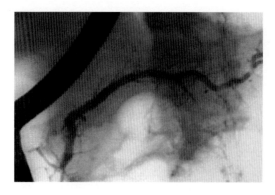

Fig. 5.8 Excessive contrast injection into the pancreatic duct may precipitate acute pancreatitis.

an Italian multicenter study, in which acute pancreatitis was independently predicted by young patient age, pancreatic duct opacification, and a non-dilated CBD [17].

Bleeding

Significant postsphincterotomy bleeding happened more readily if the patient had associated coagulopathy, had cholangitis, or the procedure was performed by an inexperienced endoscopist. Interestingly, bleeding and cholangitis were again associated with small centers with low case volume. These two large-scale and multivariate studies have two points in common: sphincterotomy complications are closely related to indications for the procedure and to the experience or case volume of individual endoscopists or institutions.

Controversies

Sphincterotomy vs. balloon sphincteroplasty

The reported complication rates of ES ranged from 6 to 10%, with a mortality resulting from these complications of 0.4–1.2% [18,19]. Although the percentages appear to be small, the actual number of patients suffering from these complications, as well as the associated prolonged hospitalization, is considerable. Since complications are mostly related to the sphincterotomy, some have advocated the use of endoscopic balloon dilatation (EBD) as an alternative procedure prior to stone extraction.

Balloon sphincteroplasty

EBD was first described by Staritz *et al.* in 1983 [20]. In addition to the lower risk of bleeding and perforation, another apparent advantage of EBD is that the sphincter of Oddi function can be preserved. This has been demonstrated in a number of studies involving sphincter of Oddi manometry [21,22]. However, when EBD was first proposed in the early 1980s, it was not widely embraced due to skepticism concerning its efficacy and the fear of precipitating acute pancreatitis. The incidence of acute pancreatitis reported then was as high as 25% according to some earlier series in which EBD was performed mainly for sphincter of Oddi dysfunction [23,24].

Balloon sphincteroplasty for CBD stones

More recent studies have revealed that EBD is a safe and effective procedure for patients with biliary stones [25,26]. In a randomized trial by Bergman *et al.*, 202 patients were assigned to either EBD or ES prior to removal of the CBD stones [27]. There was no significant difference in overall duct clearance rate, procedure time, early complications, and death associated with the two procedures. The drawback for EBD was that mechanical lithotripsy was more frequently required in these patients. Besides, a considerable number of patients in the EBD group eventually required an ES for ductal clearance.

Sphincterotomy for CBD stones

Although there is concern regarding the safety of ES, a multicenter prospective database study in the United States based on standard criteria for defining complications revealed that morbidities only occurred in 5.8% of the 1921 patients studied [28]. Two-thirds of the events were graded as mild, which required less than 3 days of hospitalization. In addition, this study disproved the dogma that complications are more likely to occur in young patients with normal sized ducts. Out of the 238 patients aged younger than 60 years, only one developed severe complications and there were no fatalities.

Long-term complications of sphincterotomy As the short-term outcome of ES is no longer in question, there is an increasing concern about the long-term effects of sphincterotomy on the biliary system. In a retrospective study by Costamagna *et al.*, 529 patients with successful sphincterotomy and bile duct clearance were evaluated after a follow-up of at least 5 years [29]. Recurrent biliary symptoms or duct stones occurred in only 11.1% of the patients, while the remainder were either asymptomatic or died of unrelated causes. A dilated bile duct > 22 mm was found to be the only independent predictive factor for recurrence. In another population-based cohort study by Karlson *et al.*, the cancer risk of 992 patients who had undergone sphincterotomy over a median follow-up time of 10–11 years was estimated, and was found to be almost the same as that of the normal population.

In conclusion, there is no evidence that ES is unsafe in either the short or long term provided that it is being performed by, or under stringent supervision of, experienced endoscopists. EBD can be an alternative to ES, but currently it should be limited to patients with no more than three stones, each < 10 mm in diameter [30].

ERCP vs. laparoscopic common duct exploration for retained CBD stones

In the era of open cholecystectomy, intraoperative cholangiogram was part of the operation. If CBD stones were suspected with intraoperative cholangiogram, exploration of the common duct was performed, and a variety of techniques were used to remove the ductal calculi. The choledochotomy was closed around a rubber T-tube, and a check cholangiogram was performed about 10 days after the operation to rule out any residual ductal stones. However, with the rapid acceptance of laparoscopic cholecystectomy in the last decade, when and how these concomitant choledocholithiases should be managed is becoming increasingly controversial.

Preoperative ERCP

To perform ERCP for all patients scheduled for laparoscopic cholecystectomy is impractical and the projected numbers of complications and mortality are also unacceptable.

Operative removal of CBD stones

An operative laparoscopic cholangiogram can be performed to rule out CBD stones. If stones are found intraoperatively, transcystic duct lithotripsy or exploration of the common duct is a feasible option with the laparoscope. Success rates for using such an approach to diagnose and clear the common duct stones have been reported to be close to 90% [31,32]. However, these laparoscopic procedures require a much higher level of skill and expertise, which may not be universally available except in some tertiary referral centers.

Factors that predict CBD stones

One possible approach is to identify patients at higher risk of concomitant choledocholithiasis and send them for preoperative cholangiogram and lithotripsy prior to laparoscopic cholecystectomy. A number of studies have reported that deranged liver function, dilated biliary tree on ultrasound scan, and history of jaundice or pancreatitis predict the presence of CBD stones [33,34].

Unfortunately, these studies were unable to generate concrete data that would allow accurate prediction of the biliary tree status preoperatively.

MRC for detection of CBD stones

The emergence of magnetic resonance technology in the 1990s opened up new possibilities for solving this clinical dilemma. Earlier series comparing MRC with conventional ERCP or operative findings have already shown promising data regarding non-invasive diagnosis of common duct calculi [35,36]. In a recent series by Laokpessi et al. on a group of 147 patients with clinical and biological signs of choledocholithiasis, MRC was shown to have a sensitivity of 93% and a specificity of 100% in detecting the ductal calculi [37]. MRC is likely to play an important role in preoperative diagnosis of concomitant CBD stones in equivocal cases, and may allow better planning regarding the mode of stone removal prior to or during laparoscopic cholecystectomy.

Risk scores for prediction of CBD stones

There is as yet no conclusion as to which approach is superior, and the choice of management method depends mainly on the expertise and support available in individual centers. One of the latest developments is to categorize patients into high-, intermediate-, and low-risk groups for CBD stones, and the management approach is dependent upon the risk score of each individual patient [38].

Alternative approaches to CBD stones

Precut sphincterotomy for failed deep cannulation

A needle-knife sphincterotome can be used to incise the lower end of the common duct when guidewire cannulation of the bile duct fails (Fig. 5.9). In a recent prospective study by Binmoeller et al., precut papillotomy was performed on 123 out of 327 patients who had an unsuccessful CBD cannulation [39]. Selective cannulation was achieved in all cases after the procedure, without a significant increase in the rate of pancreatitis and bleeding when compared to those undergoing the conventional pull-type ES.

Complications of precut sphincterotomy

Today, the overall incidence of complications following precut sphincterotomy has been reported to be 7–11%, which is not much higher than that quoted for conventional sphincterotomy [40,41]. However, it cannot be overemphasized

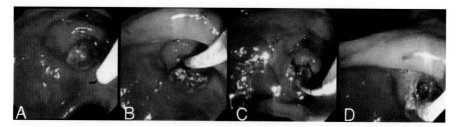

Fig. 5.9 Use of needle-knife for precut sphincterotomy. (A) Needle-knife passed through the duodenoscope. (B) Precut sphincterotomy being performed. (C) Cannulation of the common duct with guidewire after precut sphincterotomy. (D) Completion of the sphincterotomy with pull-type papillotome.

that these figures were mostly produced by experienced endoscopists in world-renowned centers. The mortality and morbidity rates could have been higher if the procedure had been performed by trainees or by the less experienced.

Percutaneous transhepatic cholangiogram and drainage

A percutaneous transhepatic biliary drain (PTBD) can be considered when deep cannulation of the common duct has been unsuccessful. The procedure is usually performed under ultrasound guidance. With the intrahepatic duct punctured, a pigtail catheter of size 7 Fr to 10 Fr can be inserted using the Saldinger technique. This allows immediate decompression and drainage of the system, and the risk of introducing infections to the biliary tree is low. It may not be a procedure of choice if the patient has underlying coagulopathy or if the intrahepatic ducts are not dilated. After a successful PTBD, a cholangiogram can be performed in a later session to delineate the details of the common duct pathology. If stones are found, there are essentially two possible approaches.

Rendezvous procedure (two-hands technique)

A guidewire is passed through the percutaneous catheter down to the common duct and duodenum, which is to be picked up by a snare inserted through a duodenoscope. The guidewire is pulled out from the biopsy valve of the duodenoscope and a wire-guided sphincterotome is threaded over the guidewire into the common duct. Subsequent ES and stone extraction can be performed in the standard manner. In a series reported by Calvo *et al.*, the success rate for clearing the CBD with a rendezvous approach was 93% (13/14) [42]. Only one complication was encountered—a retroperitoneal perforation during sphincterotomy. This approach is an extremely good option for patients with poor surgical risks and refractory choledocholithiasis.

Percutaneous stone extraction

For patients in whom the duodenoscope cannot be advanced into the duodenum, e.g. a history of previous hepatico-jejunostomy, percutaneous stone extraction after serial dilation of the PTBD tract can be considered. The tract needs to be dilated up to at least 18 Fr in order to allow a standard choledochoscope to be inserted into the bile duct. A waiting period of 4–6 weeks is allowed for the dilated tract to become mature and tough enough for subsequent manipulations. Our preference is to insert a choledochoscope into the biliary system and perform a cholangiogram through the endoscope under fluoroscopy. Stones are seen as filling defects, and can be removed by dormia basket. An electrohydraulic lithotripsy device is a useful adjunct for breaking up the stones before they are removed through the percutaneous tract. Another alternative is to dilate the sphincter of Oddi from above, with the stone fragments then being flushed or pushed down into the duodenum using the choledochoscope. In a recent series by the Dutch group, the totally percutaneous approach managed to clear the bile duct in 27 out of 31 patients (87%), and complications only occurred in three patients, with no mortality [43].

The challenge: giant CBD stones

The ordinary endoscopic methods described above are suitable for stones around 1 cm in size. For stones > 1.5 cm in diameter, endoscopic retrieval becomes difficult, if not impossible (Fig. 5.10). Several options are available to tackle the situation.

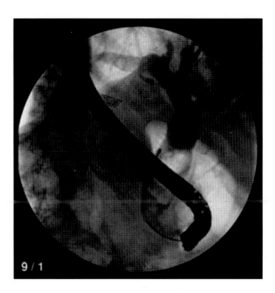

Fig. 5.10 Giant stones inside the CBD.

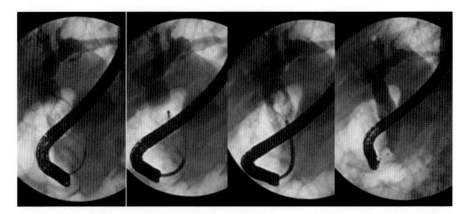

Fig. 5.11 Fragmentation of large CBD stones using basket mechanical lithotriptor.

Basket mechanical lithotripsy (BML)

Mechanical lithotripsy is the most commonly used technique in the authors' center when giant biliary stones are encountered (Fig. 5.11). When unexpected stone and basket impaction occurs, soft stones may be crushed by forceful closure of a standard basket against the Teflon sheath. It is, however, generally not recommended because the basket wire may be distorted or embedded into the stone surface, resulting in a basket trapped inside the common duct. The Wilson Cook Soehendra lithotriptor or Percy McGowan 'fishing reel' system is the device of choice for salvaging such a situation.

Through-the-scope BML using a metal sheath

When performing BML, it is imperative to make sure the stone-engaged basket is placed in the most dilated portion of the common duct. When stone capture is confirmed, the Teflon sheath is gradually withdrawn to facilitate the passage of the metal sheath into the common duct. After the Teflon sheath has been fully withdrawn into the spiral metal sheath, fragmentation of stones is accomplished by closing the basket wire with the captured stone pressed against the metal sheath. This maneuver is monitored mainly under fluoroscopic imaging. Caution is taken to avoid ductal injury when the basket is about to close completely into the metal sheath, as tension on the tip of the BML basket may suddenly change its direction and potentially damage the common duct.

Results of BML

The reported success rate of stone fragmentation by BML ranges from 82 to 100% [44,45]. In a series reported by the authors' center, 55 out of 68 patients

(81%) had complete CBD clearance after lithotripsy of giant stones with BML [46]. Of the remaining 13 patients, one had the stone crushed with the Soehendra lithotriptor, six were successfully managed by electrohydraulic lithotripsy through a 'mother and baby' endoscope, four received an indwelling stent, and two patients underwent surgery. The ductal clearance rate was 92% in another multicenter study of the efficacy of BML in 116 patients, without any significant increase in the incidence of pancreatitis or hemorrhage [47]. Thus far the largest series ever reported was by Schneider *et al.* on a group of 209 patients, in which the overall success rate was 88%, with 79% of the stones > 20 mm in diameter [48]. The reasons for failure in the remaining 12% of patients were either unsuccessful insertion of the basket, or failure to engage the stone because of its size, the common duct diameter, or other technical problems.

Mother and baby choledochoscopy and intraductal lithotripsy

Passing a baby endoscope via the channel of a large-sized duodenoscope is another method for the management of giant CBD stones. Using the baby cholangioscope, an electrohydraulic lithotriptor or laser probe can be applied to shatter the stone under direct visualization. This approach used to require a standard mother and baby system, but the recent release of a per-oral choledochoscope (CHF system, XP20, Olympus) that can go through the 4.2 mm working channel of a regular therapeutic duodenoscope has reduced the cost. Caution should be exercised by the endoscopist controlling the duodenoscope to avoid excessive elevation of the elevator, which may damage the delicate optical fibers inside the choledochoscope and result in premature failure.

Electrohydraulic lithotripsy (EHL)

EHL was first introduced in the 1950s as a method of fragmenting rocks in mines. It was later adapted for medical use, and Koch *et al.* in 1977 were the first to attempt fragmentation of CBD calculi [49]. The mechanism is a cracking force transmitted by hydraulic pressure waves generated under water by the high-voltage sparks discharged across the tip of the EHL probe. Few data are available in the literature regarding the use of EHL for biliary tract stones. The largest series reported thus far had a success rate of 99% in 65 patients [50]. Other smaller series involving less than 10 patients also claimed CBD clearance in all the patients treated [51].

Intraductal laser lithotripsy

The other device that can work through the mother and baby system is laser lithotripsy. Essentially there are three types of laser available. The Nd:YAG laser is no longer in use because of the high risk of ductal injury. The flash lamp pulsed dye lasers, on the other hand, can be delivered with thinner fibers and are superior to the Nd:YAG lasers for intraductal lithotripsy. The reported success rates range from 80 to 94%, and serious complications are uncommon [52,53]. The latest development includes the 'smart dye laser', which is capable of differentiating stone from normal ductal tissue and thus obviates the need for direct visualization during the procedure. This new mode of intraductal lithotripsy can be performed under fluoroscopic guidance without the necessity of a baby cholangioscope. In a series of 38 patients, 37 had successful ductal clearance after being treated by an automatic stone recognition laser system [54]. A slightly lower success rate was reported by Hochberger *et al.* in a group of 50 patients [55]. Major complications were not found in either series.

Stenting and interval endoscopic lithotripsy

For patients whose common duct stones are refractory to endoscopic retrieval, a plastic biliary stent can be inserted as a temporary or permanent measure. It has been shown in several prospective series that elderly patients with difficult stones remained symptom-free after insertion of an endoprosthesis, and thus surgery was avoided. There have also been studies reporting a decrease in the stone size after a period of biliary stenting. In a study by the authors, 46 patients with large CBD stones received plastic stents [56]. Twenty-eight patients had repeat ERCP for stone extraction after a median of 63 days. The size of the stones was significantly reduced, from 11–46 mm (mean 24.9 mm) to 5–46 mm (mean 20.1 mm), and duct clearance was achieved in 25 patients (89%) during the repeat procedure. Similar findings have been reported by Maxton *et al.* and Jain *et al.* [57,58].

Effects of stenting on CBD stones

The exact mechanism causing the change in the size of stones is unclear, but improvement in the solubility of bile after drainage as well as the mechanical friction between stents and calculi are thought to be responsible.

The need for stone extraction after stenting

Temporary drainage and decompression of the biliary system by a plastic stent are a valid option for high surgical risk patients whose stones are too big for endoscopic retrieval at the outset. However, in a prospective randomized trial by Chopra *et al.*, significantly more long-term biliary complications were observed in patients treated with endoprosthesis as compared to those with complete ductal clearance [59]. Thus it is highly advisable to clear all common duct calculi and reserve stenting as a definitive treatment only for those who are extremely unfit for other procedures.

Extracorporeal shock-wave lithotripsy (ESWL)

ESWL can be used for giant stones not amenable to regular ERCP or mechanical lithotripsy. The latest models of ESWL are more patient-friendly and the procedure can be performed under sedation. ERCP and papillotomy are still required in most cases for localization of the stones. A nasobiliary catheter is placed for cholangiography. Alternatively, percutaneous cholangiography can be employed for stone localization. Even if fragmentation by ESWL is successful, the resultant stone fragments are often too big to pass out spontaneously and must be removed by either ERCP or percutaneous cholangioscopy.

Results of ESWL for CBD stones

There are many studies reporting high ductal clearance rates. In a multicenter study conducted in Germany, the success rate was 86%, with a mortality rate of only 1.8% [60]. Other series also reported similar outcomes, with cholangitis being the most frequent complication. The most recent report by Ellis *et al.* studied 83 patients with retained bile duct stones treated by the third-generation lithotriptor. Complete stone clearance was achieved in 69 (83%) patients. Complications included six cases of cholangitis, and one perinephric hematoma which resolved spontaneously [61].

Open surgery

For patients with giant or inaccessible CBD stones who have failed all the treatment modalities described above, surgical exploration and clearance of the common duct should be contemplated if the general condition of the patient allows.

Intrahepatic duct stones

Primary intrahepatic duct calculi, or hepatolithiasis, is a distinct condition that is predominantly found in the Far East. It is characterized by the presence of multiple strictures and brown or black pigment calculi in the intrahepatic ducts. For unknown reasons, it tends to affect the left lobe of the liver more than the right side. Surgical resection of the affected liver segment and creation of drainage are the preferred treatment if the pathology is localized to one side. However, due to the multiple segment involvement and peripheral location of

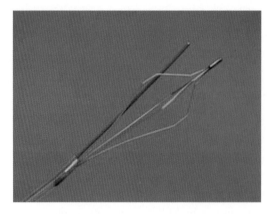

Fig. 5.12 Wire-guided basket.

the strictures and stones, management of this condition remains formidable, and surgical resection is only possible in a small percentage of patients.

ERCP and basket removal

Stones located in the intrahepatic ducts close to the bifurcation of the common hepatic duct can be removed with an ordinary dormia basket. The accessibility of specific segmental ducts is largely dependent on the technique and experience of the endoscopist. More sophisticated endoscopic maneuvers may be required to retrieve intrahepatic calculi lying proximal to a relative stenosis or stricture. Balloon dilators or through-the-scope graded dilators can be applied to dilate these strictures so as to facilitate complete clearance of stones endoscopically.

Wire-guided basket

Endoscopic retrieval of intrahepatic calculi with conventional baskets can be difficult if the stones are located deeply inside the tortuous segmental ducts with multiple or tight strictures. The development of a wire-guided basket has helped to overcome this problem. Earlier prototypes had the guidewire going through the center of the basket, rendering engagement of stones inefficient. The guidewire needed to be removed to permit entrapment of the stones, but repeated cannulation of the same segmental duct sometimes became technically difficult. The wire-guided basket used nowadays has the guidewire passed along the side instead of the center of the basket (Fig. 5.12). Access to the same segmental duct can be guaranteed during capture and retrieval of the intrahepatic stones. Our preliminary experience with this device on four patients with intrahepatic calculi was very good and successful stone retrieval was achieved in all [62].

Percutaneous transhepatic cholangioscopy (PTC)

Although the preferred treatment of primary intrahepatic stones has been removal of the stones via resection of the stenotic bile duct and atrophic segments, surgery may be impossible in patients with multisegmental distribution of the stones. PTC lithotripsy is definitely one possible option whereby the intrahepatic duct stones can be removed from above a stricture using a more straightforward approach [63].

Results of percutaneous treatment of intrahepatic stones

In a study on 165 patients treated with PTC lithotripsy for intrahepatic duct stones, the success rate of complete stone clearance was 80% [64]. Three major causes of incomplete removal of stones were identified: (1) angulation or stricture of the intrahepatic ducts; (2) sludgy bile and stones; and (3) a peripheral location rendering access impossible. After a mean follow-up of 58 months, 43 (32.6%) of the 132 patients with initial clearance developed recurrent stones. Other investigators have reported similar results, and it appears that the risk of stone recurrence tends to increase with time [65]. In a more recent series reported by the Korean group, recurrence of intrahepatic stones after percutaneous cholangioscopic treatment was strongly associated with severe biliary stricture, advanced biliary cirrhosis, and Tsunoda types III and IV hepatolithiasis [66]. As a whole, PTC lithotripsy is an option for patients whose stones are not amenable to endoscopic treatment but who, at the same time, are not suitable candidates for surgical resection due to poor anesthetic risk.

ERCP and sphincterotomy in Billroth II gastrectomy

ERCP is considered to be more difficult in patients with previous Billroth II gastrectomy. The overall complication rates reported in the literature range from 8 to 13% [67,68]. The problems include difficulties in (1) maneuvering the side-view duodenoscope through the afferent loop in a retrograde manner; (2) cannulating the CBD from an inverted position; and (3) carrying out a papillotomy in an upside-down position. Among all the morbidities reported, bowel perforation involving in particular the afferent loop is a considerable and unique complication of ERCP. In one of our recent series, there were 11 perforations in 185 ERCP procedures for patients with a history of previous Billroth II gastrectomy [69]. Nine perforations occurred when the afferent loop was entered, one occurred after sphincterotomy, and another during cannulation. The majority of perforations were found near the duodenojejunal flexure area. The likely mechanism is that the endoscope loops excessively in the jejunum when it is being inserted across the relatively fixed duodenojejunal flexure. Mucosal tear or perforation happens as a result of overstretching of the proximal jejunum during retrograde advancement of the endoscope.

Precautions and alternatives for Billroth II gastrectomy

We believe that the experience of the endoscopist is the key factor for avoiding perforation in this clinical setting. The passage of the endoscope through the afferent loop must be monitored under fluoroscopy. Excessive looping of the duodenoscope should be avoided. If resistance is encountered, the procedure should be stopped and alternative methods for gaining access to the biliary system considered. One option is to drain the bile ducts by PTBD and have the calculi fragmented and removed through the PTBD tract in subsequent sessions. This approach is likely to lengthen the course of treatment because the PTBD tract requires serial dilation, to a size of 16 Fr or 18 Fr, before lithotripsy is possible. Another option is to enter the afferent loop with a forward-viewing endoscope instead of a side-viewing duodenoscope.

Side-viewing vs. forward-viewing scope for ERCP in Billroth II gastrectomy

In a comparative study by Kim *et al.* on the use of these two types of endoscope in patients with previous Billroth II gastrectomies, significantly less bowel perforation was observed in the group having the forward-viewing endoscope, yet the success rate in cannulating the CBD was comparable [70]. However, due to the lack of the bridge elevator, maneuverability of various devices is compromised with the forward-viewing endoscope. Thus we still prefer to use a side-viewing duodenoscope whenever possible because it allows the operator to view the papilla *en face*. Recently, a special wire-guided B-II papillotome with the cutting wire on the reverse side has been introduced [71]. Whether it helps the safety of sphincterotomy in gastrectomized patients remains to be seen.

Cholangitis

Pathophysiology

In the obstructed biliary tree, stagnant bile is a favorable culture medium for bacteria. Ascending infection in the biliary system is one of the mechanisms leading to acute cholangitis.

Effect of biliary obstruction on the reticuloendothelial system

It has been shown in both clinical and animal studies that the phagocytic function of the reticuloendothelial cells surrounding the canaliculi is severely affected in complete bile duct obstruction. Clearance of the bacteria entering with the portal venous blood is therefore compromised, and infection of the stagnant bile inside the obstructed system may take place.

Bacteriology of cholangitis

The infected bile contains a large quantity of bacteria, mostly Gram-negative bacilli, with *E. coli*, *Klebsiella* spp., *Enterobacter* spp., and *Pseudomonas*, sometimes mixed with anaerobes such as *C. perfringens* and *Bacteroides fragilis*, or Gram-positive enterococci.

Effect of raised intrabiliary pressure and cholangiovenous reflux

The intraductal pressure in the biliary tree may rise in the presence of obstruction. As the terminal ends of bile canaliculi are in direct contact with the hepatic sinusoids, a raised intrabiliary pressure will facilitate cholangiovenous reflux of infected materials into the hepatic venous circulation. Under such circumstances the patient may develop bacteremia as well as endotoxemia. The septicemia then triggers a systemic response from the patient's own immune system, including a variety of cytokines, complements, and vasodilators. In severe cases the reaction may be overwhelming, with deleterious effects towards other internal organs, resulting in a phenomenon known as systemic inflammatory response syndrome (SIRS), with multiorgan failure, and considerable mortality.

Clinical presentation

Simple cholangitis: Charcot's triad

Charcot's triad of acute cholangitis includes acute right upper abdominal pain, fever, and jaundice. Nevertheless, not every patient having cholangitis manifests all these features. Jaundice can be subtle if the onset is acute or the obstruction is incomplete, yet the patient could be very ill and septic if there is considerable endotoxemia. Frail or old patients may not experience or complain of any pain even if they are suffering from cholangitis. Overall, fever is the most common and consistent symptom, present in more than 90% of patients. Chills and rigor are not as frequent but their presence is suggestive of bacteremia or septicemia.

Suppurative cholangitis: Reynold's pentad

In the presence of profound septicemia, the patient may develop hemodynamic instability and mental confusion. When added to Charcot's triad described above, hypotension and coma are collectively known as Reynold's pentad, which signifies a severe attack of suppurative cholangitis associated with significant mortality. As the condition can be rapidly fatal, vigorous resuscitation, intensive care support, and urgent biliary decompression should be provided in order to minimize mortality.

Clinical management

Of patients with clinical cholangitis, 80–90% may respond to conservative treatment; the remaining 5–10% with suppurative cholangitis will need urgent biliary decompression.

Initial conservative management

Patients with suspected acute cholangitis should be admitted to hospital for further management. It is imperative to control the sepsis as early as possible. Aggressive fluid resuscitation and high-dose intravenous broad spectrum antibiotics are the key initial measures. Close monitoring of the vital signs, including urine output, is necessary. With such initial treatment, control of sepsis is achieved in 90% of patients. Further intervention and drainage for the obstructing lesion can be performed on a semielective or elective basis in the next available session.

Urgent biliary decompression

Some 5–10% of patients, especially those with Reynold's pentad, may not respond to the initial resuscitation. Emergency decompression of the obstructed biliary system is mandatory. In the case of unstable patients with compromised hemodynamic status and respiratory function, intensive care monitoring, including the use of inotropes and/or ventilatory support, should be sought before biliary drainage.

Role of ERCP ES with stone extraction is considered to be the procedure of choice in patients with acute cholangitis. It is often performed when the initial treatment was to control the sepsis. However, in patients with severe cholangitis not responding to the initial medical therapy, the only possible option is decompression and drainage of the infected biliary system. In one of our earlier series, endoscopic drainage of the biliary tree was attempted in 105 patients with severe cholangitis [72]. The success rate was 97%, resulting in rapid resolution of fever and improvement in liver function tests in most of the patients. Mortality was found to be associated with a delay in drainage. In another subgroup of 40 patients with severe cholangitis managed by urgent ERCP, we have demonstrated that endoscopic drainage is an effective method of lowering bile and serum endotoxin levels and aborting the process of SIRS [73].

Endoscopic drainage vs. surgery In a retrospective series which compared surgery with endoscopic drainage for acute cholangitis, patients undergoing emergency exploration of the common duct had a significantly higher mortality (21%) than those who underwent ES alone (4.7%) [74]. The most concrete evidence favoring endoscopic intervention for acute cholangitis comes from a prospective randomized trial in which patients were treated either by endoscopic drainage or surgical decompression [75]. There were significantly fewer complications in patients treated endoscopically than in those treated with surgery (34% vs. 66%, $P < 0.05$). The hospital mortality rate was also significantly lower in those who underwent endoscopy (10% vs. 32%, $P < 0.03$).

ERCP vs. PTBD There are relatively few data in the literature comparing ERCP with PTBD drainage procedures for acute cholangitis. Presumably PTBD may be more suitable for patients who are hemodynamically unstable and not suitable to be transferred to the endoscopy suite. However, in a non-randomized study comparing different modes of drainage for elderly patients with acute cholangitis, endoscopic drainage yielded significantly lower morbidity (16.7%) and mortality (5.6%) than surgical (87.5% and 25.0%, respectively) and per-cutaneous (36.4% and 9.1%, respectively) drainage [76].

Nasobiliary catheter drainage vs. stenting in acute cholangitis

Although nasobiliary catheter drainage has become well established for use in emergency decompression of the biliary system in patients with severe cholang-itis, it is not without problems in real clinical practice. Confused patients may pull the nasobiliary drain (NBD) out shortly after it has been placed and repeat insertion may be required. It is often cumbersome and risky, especially in criti-cally ill patients. Inadvertent displacement or kinking of the NBD may happen from time to time during transfer of patients or other procedures. One way of avoiding these problems is to place an indwelling plastic stent in lieu of a naso-biliary catheter in such patients. A major drawback of an internal stent is that its

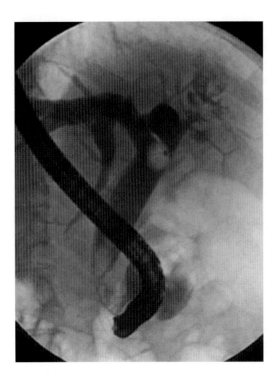

Fig. 5.13 Recurrent pyogenic cholangitis affecting mainly the right system.

patency and adequacy of drainage cannot be monitored. In a prospective randomized trial of 74 patients conducted in the authors' center, both approaches were shown to have similar efficacy on initial decompression for the biliary sepsis, with comparable mean procedure times [77]. Nasobiliary catheter displacement and kinking happened in five out of the 40 patients assigned to NBD, while stent blockage was found in one patient among the 34 with endoprosthesis placement. Patients' tolerance was much better in the stent group, but it had a higher mortality rate than the NBD group (12% vs. 2.5%), although the difference was not statistically significant. Currently, we still prefer NBD for decompression for patients with cholangitis.

Surgery to prevent recurrent cholangitis

Endoscopic or percutaneous transhepatic lithotripsy may not be feasible in some patients, when cholangitis affects the biliary tree at multiple sites with varying degrees of severity (Fig. 5.13). Surgery remains the last resort in removing the calculi and preventing stone recurrence in such patients.

Types of operation Although the details of various operative procedures are beyond the scope of this chapter, surgeons would like to achieve the following goals: (1) removal of the obstructing stones; (2) improved drainage of the biliary system; and (3) resection of non-functioning or atrophic liver segments. Transduodenal sphincteroplasty, supraduodenal choledochoduodenostomy, and end-to-side hepaticojejunostomy are the surgical procedures for improving bile drainage. Liver resection may be suitable for disease confined to a segment or to one side of the liver, especially if the affected parenchyma is atrophic with little residual function. It is performed not only to eradicate the source of symptoms and infections, but also to remove the underlying stricture which carries a malignant potential in the future.

Conclusion

Endoscopic treatment is now the first-line management option for choledocholithiasis. The success rate has increased with the recent advances in cannulation techniques and instrument design. Although endoscopic balloon dilatation has been proposed as a replacement for sphincterotomy for stone extraction, it is still restricted to selected cases with small calculi. It is advisable to refer patients with giant difficult stones to expert centers where advanced lithotripsy techniques are readily available. With the current endoscopic technology, very few patients with choledocholithiasis will require surgery. However, surgical resection still has a role for those with intractable intrahepatic stones and cholangitis localized to certain segments of the liver.

Outstanding issues and future trends

ERCP remains the gold standard for the diagnosis of CBD stones, although EUS has shown its very high sensitivity in identifying distal CBD stones. With improvements in resolution of the MRC technique, this may provide an alternative and non-invasive method of confirming the diagnosis before intervention. Randomized controlled studies have shown that endoscopic biliary drainage is the first line of urgent management for patients with suppurative cholangitis who have failed conservative treatment. Part of the reason for the failure of antibiotic therapy is the inability of most drugs to penetrate a completely obstructed biliary system with raised intrabiliary pressure. Drugs that can be excreted into bile against a pressure gradient would have considerable advantages in the management of these sick patients, but they are not a replacement for urgent biliary decompression in sick patients. For urgent biliary drainage, a prior sphincterotomy is not necessary for the placement of a nasobiliary catheter or an indwelling stent. The trick is to aspirate bile to decompress the bile ducts as soon as deep cannulation is achieved. Drainage without sphincterotomy also avoids the risk of pancreatitis and postsphincterotomy bleeding. In principle, a large 10 Fr stent provides better drainage for the thick infected bile than a 7 or 8 Fr stent. With improvements in scope design, we now have reasonably sized duodenoscopes fitted with larger therapeutic channels. This avoids the difficult manipulation of large therapeutic scopes in an emergency situation. Recognizing the significance of individual bacteria in biliary stone and sludge formation may open up a new avenue for the prevention of stone recurrence. Suppression of bacterial enzymatic activities through the use of enzyme blockers, or down-regulation of the genetic control of enzyme production, may offer an alternative approach to prevention.

References

1 Barbara L, Sama C, Morselli-Labate AM *et al*. 10-years incidence of gallstone disease: the Sirmione study. *J Hepatol* 1993; 18: S43.
2 Courvoisier OG (1890). *Kasuistisch-statistische Beitrage zur Pathologie und Chirurgie der Gallenwege*, pp. 57–8. Liepzig, FCW Vogel.
3 Kawai K, Akasaka Y, Murakami K. Endoscopic sphincterotomy of the ampulla of Vater. *Gastrointest Endosc* 1974; 20: 148.
4 Lygidakis NJ. Incidence of bile infection in patients with choledocholithiasis. *Am J Gastroenterol* 1982; 77: 12–17.
5 Leung JW, Sung JY, Costerton JW. Bacteriological and electron microscopy examination of brown pigment stones. *J Clin Microbiol* 1989; 27: 915–21.
6 Leung JW, Liu YL, Leung PS, Chan RC, Inciardi JF, Cheng AF. Expression of bacterial beta-gluconidase in human bile: an in-vitro study. *Gastrointest Endosc* 2001; 54: 346–50.
7 Bernhoft RA, Pellegrini CA, Motson RW *et al*. Composition and morphologic and clinical features of common duct stones. *Am J Surg* 1984; 148: 77–84.
8 Taylor TV, Armstrong CP. Migration of gallstones. *Br Med J* 1987; 294: 1320–2.
9 Calvo MM, Bujanda L, Calderon A *et al*. Role of magnetic resonance cholangiopancreatography in patients with suspected choledocholithiasis. *Mayo Clin Proc* 2002; 77: 422–8.
10 Amouyal P, Amouyal G, Levy P *et al*. Diagnosis of choledocholithiasis by endoscopic ultrasonography. *Gastroenterology* 1994; 106: 1062–7.
11 Prat F, Amouyal G, Pelletier V *et al*. Prospective controlled study of endoscopic ultrasonography and endoscopic retrograde cholangiography in patients with suspected common bile duct lithiasis. *Lancet* 1996; 346: 75–9.
12 Canto M, Chak A, Stellato T, Sivak MV Jr. Endoscopic ultrasonography versus cholangiography for the diagnosis of choledocholithiasis. *Gastrointest Endosc* 1998; 47: 439–48.
13 Kohut M, Nowakowska-Dulawa E, Marek T, Kaczor R, Nowak A. Accuracy of linear endoscopic ultrasonography in the evaluation of patients with suspected common bile duct stones. *Endoscopy* 2002; 34: 299–303.
14 Boender J, Nix GA, de Ridder MA. Endoscopic papillotomy for common bile duct stones: factors influencing the complication rate. *Endoscopy* 1994; 26: 209–16.
15 Chen YK, Foliente RL, Santoro MJ, Walter MH, Collen MJ. Endoscopic sphincterotomy-induced pancreatitis: increased risk associated with nondilated bile ducts and sphincter of Oddi dysfunction. *Am J Gastroenterol* 1994; 89: 327–33.
16 Freeman ML, Nelson DB, Sherman S *et al*. Complications of endoscopic biliary sphincterotomy. *N Engl J Med* 1996; 335: 909–18.
17 Loperfido S, Angelini G, Benedetti G *et al*. Major early complications from diagnostic and therapeutic ERCP: a prospective multicenter study. *Gastrointest Endosc* 1998; 48: 1–10.
18 Sherman S, Ruffolo TA, Hawes RH *et al*. Complications of endoscopic sphincterotomy: a prospective series with emphasis on the increased risk associated with sphincter of Oddi dysfunction and nondilated bile ducts. *Gastroenterology* 1991; 101: 1068–75.

19 Cotton PB, Lehmann GA, Vennes J *et al*. Endoscopic sphincterotomy complications and their management: an attempt at consensus. *Gastrointest Endosc* 1991; 37: 383–93.

20 Staritz M, Ewe K, Meyer zum Buschenfelde KH. Endoscopic papillary dilatation (EPD) for the treatment of common duct stones and papillary stenosis. *Endoscopy* 1983; 15: 197–8.

21 Minami A, Nakatsu T, Uchida N *et al*. Papillary dilation vs sphincterotomy in endoscopic removal of bile duct stones: a randomized trial with manometric function. *Dig Dis Sci* 1994; 40: 2250–4.

22 Yasuda I, Tomita E, Enya M, Kato T, Moriwaki H. Can endoscopic papillary balloon dilation really preserve sphincter of Oddi function? *Gut* 2001; 49: 686–91.

23 Bader M, Geenen JE, Hogan W *et al*. Endoscopic balloon dilatation of the sphincter of Oddi in patients with suspected biliary dyskinesia: results of a prospective randomized trial. *Gastrointest Endosc* 1986; 32: 158A.

24 Kozarek RA. Balloon dilatation of the sphincter of Oddi. *Endoscopy* 1988; 20: 207–10.

25 May GR, Cotton PB, Edmunds SE, Chong W. Removal of stones from the bile duct at ERCP without sphincterotomy. *Gastrointest Endosc* 1993; 39: 749–54.

26 MacMathuna P, White P, Clarke E *et al*. Endoscopic balloon sphincteroplasty (papillary dilation) for bile duct stones: efficacy, safety and follow-up in 100 patients. *Gastrointest Endosc* 1995; 42: 468–74.

27 Bergman JJ, Rauws EA, Fockens P *et al*. Randomised trial of endoscopic balloon dilation versus endoscopic sphincterotomy for removal of bile duct stones. *Lancet* 1997; 349: 1124–9.

28 Cotton PB, Geenen JE, Sherman S *et al*. Endoscopic sphincterotomy for stones by experts is safe, even in younger patients with normal ducts. *Ann Surg* 1998; 227: 201–4.

29 Costamagna G, Tringali A, Shah SK, Mutignani M, Zuccala G, Perri V. Long-term follow-up of patients after endoscopic sphincterotomy for choledocholithiasis, and risk factors for recurrence. *Endoscopy* 2002; 34: 273–9.

30 Bergman JJ, Tytgat GN, Huibregtse K. Endoscopic dilatation of the biliary sphincter for removal of bile duct stones: an overview of current indications and limitations. *Scand J Gastroenterol Suppl* 1998; 225: 59–65.

31 Stoker ME, Hebert JC, Bothe AJ. Common bile duct exploration in the era of laparoscopic surgery. *Arch Surg* 1995; 130: 265.

32 Lezoche E, Paganini AM, Carlei F *et al*. Laparoscopic treatment of gallbladder and common bile duct stones: a prospective study. *World J Surg* 1996; 20: 535.

33 Chan AC, Chung SC, Wyman A *et al*. Selective use of preoperative endoscopic retrograde cholangiopancreatography in laparoscopic cholecystectomy. *Gastrointest Endosc* 1996; 43: 212–15.

34 Santucci L, Natalini G, Sarpi L, Fiorucci S, Solinas A, Morelli A. Selective endoscopic retrograde cholangiography and preoperative bile duct stone removal in patients scheduled for laparoscopic cholecystectomy: a prospective study. *Am J Gastroenterol* 1996; 91: 1326–30.

35 Demartines N, Eisner L, Schnabel K, Fried R, Zuber M, Harder F. Evaluation of magnetic resonance cholangiography in the management of bile duct stones. *Arch Surg* 2000; 135: 148–52.

36 Zidi SH, Prat F, Le Guen O *et al*. Use of magnetic resonance cholangiography in the diagnosis of choledocholithiasis: prospective comparison with a reference imaging method. *Gut* 1999; 44: 118–22.

37 Laokpessi A, Bouillet P, Sautereau D *et al*. Value of magnetic resonance cholangiography in the preoperative diagnosis of common bile duct stones. *Am J Gastroenterol* 2001; 96: 2354–9.

38 Liu TH, Consorti ET, Kawashima A *et al*. Patient evaluation and management with selective use of magnetic resonance cholangiography and endoscopic retrograde cholangiopancreatography before laparoscopic cholecystectomy. *Ann Surg* 2001; 234: 33–40.

39 Binmoeller K, Seifert H, Gerke H *et al*. Papillary roof incision using the Erlangen-type pre-cut papillotome to achieve selective bile duct cannulation. *Gastrointest Endosc* 1996; 44: 689–95.

40 Kasmin F, Cohen D, Batra S *et al*. Needle-knife sphincterotomy in a tertiary referral center: efficacy and complications. *Gastrointest Endosc* 1996; 44: 48–53.

41 Gholson C, Favrot D. Needle knife papillotomy in a university referral practice: safety and efficacy of a modified technique. *J Clin Gastroenterol* 1996; 23: 177–80.

42 Calvo MM, Bujanda L, Ileras I *et al.* The rendezvous technique for the treatment of choledo-cholithiasis. *Gastrointest Endosc* 2001; 54: 511–13.

43 van der Velden JJ, Berger MY, Bonjer HJ, Brakel K, Lameris JS. Percutaneous treatment of bile duct stones in patients treated successfully with endoscopic retrograde procedures. *Gastrointest Endosc* 2000; 51: 418–22.

44 Riemann JF, Seuberth K, Demling L. Mechanical lithotripsy of common bile duct stones. *Gastrointest Endosc* 1985; 31: 207–10.

45 Higuchi T, Kon Y. Endoscopic mechanical lithotripsy for the treatment of common bile duct stones: experience with the improved double sheath basket catheter. *Endoscopy* 1987; 19: 216–17.

46 Chung SC, Leung JW, Leong HT, Li AKC. Mechanical lithotripsy of large common bile duct stones using a basket. *Br J Surg* 1991; 78: 1448–50.

47 Shaw MJ, Mackie RD, Moore JP *et al.* Results of a multicenter trial using a mechanical lithotriptor for the treatment of large bile duct stones. *Am J Gastroenterol* 1993; 88: 730–3.

48 Schneider MU, Matek W, Bauer R *et al.* Mechanical lithotripsy of bile duct stones in 209 patients: effect of technical advances. *Endoscopy* 1988; 20: 248–53.

49 Koch H, Stolte M, Walz V. Endoscopic lithotripsy in the common bile duct. *Endoscopy* 1977; 9: 95.

50 Binmoeller KF, Bruckner M, Thonke F, Soehendra N. Treatment of difficult bile duct stones using mechanical, electrohydraulic and extracorporeal shock wave lithotripsy. *Endoscopy* 1993; 25: 201.

51 Hixson LJ, Fennerty MB, Jaffee PE, Pulju JH, Palley SL. Peroral cholangioscopy with intra-corporeal electrohydraulic lithotripsy for choledocholithiasis. *Am J Gastroenterol* 1992; 87: 296.

52 Cotton PB, Kozarek RA, Schapiro RH *et al.* Endoscopic laser lithotripsy of large bile duct stones. *Gastroenterology* 1990; 99: 1128.

53 Prat F, Fritsch J, Choury AD, Frouge C, Marteau V, Etienne JP. Laser lithotripsy of difficult biliary stones. *Gastrointest Endosc* 1994; 40: 290.

54 Neuhaus H, Hoffmann W, Gottlieb K, Classen M. Endoscopic lithotripsy of bile duct stones using a new laser with automatic stone recognition. *Gastrointest Endosc* 1994; 40: 708.

55 Hochberger S, May A, Bayer J, Muhldorfer S, Hahn EG, Ell C. Laser lithotripsy of difficult bile duct stones: results in 50 patients using a rhodamine-6 G dye laser with automatic optical stone-tissue detection system. *Gastrointest Endosc* 1997; 45: 133A.

56 Chan AC, Ng EK, Chung SC *et al.* Common bile duct stones become smaller after endoscopic biliary stenting. *Endoscopy* 1998; 30: 356–9.

57 Maxton DG, Tweedle DE, Martin DF. Retained common bile duct stones after endoscopic sphincterotomy: temporary and long term treatment with biliary stenting. *Gut* 1995; 36: 446.

58 Jain SK, Stein R, Bhuva M, Goldberg MJ. Pigtail stents: an alternative in the treatment of difficult bile duct stones. *Gastrointest Endosc* 2000; 52: 490–3.

59 Chopra KB, Peters RA, O'Toole PA *et al.* Randomised study of endoscopic biliary endoprosthesis versus duct clearance for bile duct stones in high-risk patients. *Lancet* 1996; 21 (348): 791–3.

60 Schreiber F, Stern M. Fragmentation of bile duct stones by extracorporeal shock wave lithotripsy. *Gastroenterology* 1989; 146: 96.

61 Ellis RD, Jenkins AP, Thompson RP, Ede RJ. Clearance of refractory bile duct stones with extracorporeal shockwave lithotripsy. *Gut* 2000; 47: 728–31.

62 Chan AC, Chung SC. New wire-guided basket for intrahepatic stone extraction. *Gastrointest Endosc* 1999; 50: 401–4.

63 Park JH, Choi BI, Han MC, Sung KB, Choo IW, Kim CW. Percutaneous removal of residual intrahepatic stones. *Radiology* 1987; 163: 619–23.

64 Yeh YH, Huang MH, Yang JC, Mo LR, Lin J, Yueh SK. Percutaneous trans-hepatic cholangioscopy and lithotripsy in the treatment of intrahepatic stones: a study with 5 year follow-up. *Gastrointest Endosc* 1995; 42: 13–18.

65 January YY, Chen MF. Percutaneous trans-hepatic cholangioscopic lithotomy for hepatolithiasis: long-term results. *Gastrointest Endosc* 1995; 42: 1–5.

66 Lee SK, Seo DW, Myung SJ *et al.* Percutaneous transhepatic cholangioscopic treatment for hepatolithiasis: an evaluation of long-term results and risk factors for recurrence. *Gastrointest Endosc* 2001; 53: 318–23.

67 Cohen SA, Siegel JH, Kasmin FE. Complications of diagnostic and therapeutic ERCP. *Abdom Imaging* 1996; 21: 385–94.

68 Huibregtse K. Complications of endoscopic sphincterotomy and their prevention [Editorial]. *N Engl J Med* 1996; 335: 961–3.

69 Faylona JM, Qadir A, Chan AC, Lau JY, Chung SC. Small bowel perforations related to endoscopic retrograde cholangiopancreatography (ERCP) in patients with Billroth II gastrectomy. *Endoscopy* 1999; 31: 546–9.

70 Kim MH, Lee SK, Lee MH *et al.* Endoscopic retrograde cholangiopancreatography and needle-knife sphincterotomy in patients with Billroth II gastrectomy: a comparative study of the forward-viewing endoscope and the side-viewing duodenoscope. *Endoscopy* 1997; 29: 82–5.

71 Wang YG, Binmoeller KF, Seifert H, Maydeo A, Soehendra N. A new guide wire papillotome for patients with Billroth II gastrectomy. *Endoscopy* 1996; 28: 254.

72 Leung JW, Chung SC, Sung JJ *et al.* Urgent endoscopic drainage for acute suppurative cholangitis. *Lancet* 1989; 1: 1307–9.

73 Lau JY, Chung SC, Leung JW, Ling TK, Yung MY, Li AK. Endoscopic drainage aborts endotoxaemia in acute cholangitis. *Br J Surg* 1996; 83: 181–4.

74 Leese T, Neoptolemos JP, Baker AR *et al.* Management of acute cholangitis and the impact on endoscopic sphincterotomy. *Br J Surg* 1986; 73: 988–92.

75 Lai EC, Mok FP, Tan ES *et al.* Endoscopic biliary drainage for severe acute cholangitis. *N Engl J Med* 1992; 326: 1582–6.

76 Sugiyama M, Atomi Y. Treatment of acute cholangitis due to choledocholithiasis in elderly and younger patients. *Arch Surg* 1997; 132: 1129–33.

77 Lee DW, Chan AC, Lam YH *et al.* Biliary decompression by nasobiliary catheter or biliary stent in acute suppurative cholangitis: a prospective randomized trial. *Gastrointest Endosc* 2002; 56: 361–5.

CHAPTER 6

The Role of ERCP in Pancreatico-Biliary Malignancies

GULSHAN PARASHER AND JOHN G. LEE

Synopsis

Approximately 30 000 new cases of pancreatic cancer and 7000 biliary tract cancers are diagnosed annually in the United States [1]. The most common cause of malignant biliary obstruction is pancreatic adenocarcinoma, followed by cholangiocarcinoma, ampullary neoplasm, and extrinsic compression by metastatic lymphadenopathy in the liver hilum. The role of ERCP in pancreatico-biliary malignancies is to (1) confirm the diagnosis of obstructive jaundice in patients with suspected pancreatic carcinoma or biliary tumors; (2) obtain tissue for histopathologic diagnosis; (3) establish the exact site of obstruction, i.e. ampullary, pancreatic, or bile duct; (4) decompress the bile duct; and (5) facilitate palliative therapy such as intraluminal brachytherapy or intraductal photodynamic therapy. This chapter describes various current and emerging applications of ERCP in the management of pancreatico-biliary malignancies.

ERCP in diagnosis of pancreatico-biliary malignancies

Radiological diagnosis

Significance of 'double duct stricture' sign

The radiographic features of ERCP cannot reliably distinguish between benign and malignant diseases. Although the double duct sign with simultaneous narrowing of the common bile duct and the pancreatic duct has been regarded traditionally as predictive of pancreatic cancer (Fig. 6.1), recent studies showed that its specificity is much lower than previously thought, with 15–37% of such patients having benign disease on long-term follow-up [2,3]. Stricture length > 14 mm was highly predictive of malignancy in one study [4], while in another study the pancreatic duct stricture length measured on ERCP correlated with both size ($P < 0.001$) and staging ($P < 0.002$) of the pancreatic cancer [5]. The

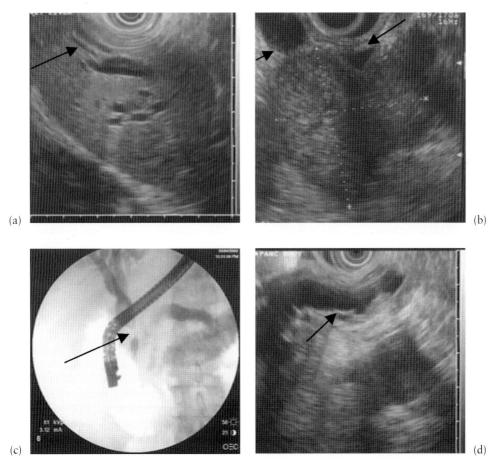

(a)   (b)   (c)   (d)

Fig. 6.1 A 76-year-old female was referred for evaluation of obstructive jaundice. CT showed dilated intrahepatic ducts, common duct, and pancreatic duct and fullness of the pancreatic head. ERCP was unsuccessful. (a) EUS shows dilated intrahepatic ducts (*arrow* showing tram track sign) in the left lobe of the liver. (b) EUS shows a 3.6 cm × 3.5 cm mass in the head of the pancreas compressing the bile duct (*arrows*). (c) ERCP shows stricture in the distal common duct (*arrow*) corresponding to the EUS images. (d) EUS shows a dilated pancreatic duct (*arrow*).

cholangiographic appearance was non-specific as benign-appearing strictures were usually found to be malignant on follow-up [4].

Tissue diagnosis

Histopathological confirmation of pancreatico-biliary malignancy permits more accurate decision-making with reference to comprehensive management including the potential use of radiation and/or chemotherapy.

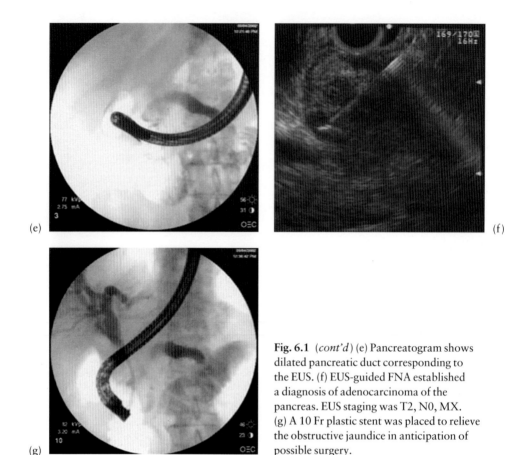

(e)

(f)

(g)

Fig. 6.1 (*cont'd*) (e) Pancreatogram shows dilated pancreatic duct corresponding to the EUS. (f) EUS-guided FNA established a diagnosis of adenocarcinoma of the pancreas. EUS staging was T2, N0, MX. (g) A 10 Fr plastic stent was placed to relieve the obstructive jaundice in anticipation of possible surgery.

Brush cytology, biopsy, and fine-needle aspiration (FNA)

Endoscopic wire-guided brush cytology and endoscopic needle aspiration or forceps biopsy can be successfully performed during ERCP for cytological diagnosis (Fig. 6.2). Wire-guided brushing cytology is performed initially by passing the cytology catheter sheath beyond the proximal margin of the stricture; the brush is then advanced out of the sheath. The brush and sheath are then withdrawn to the distal margin of the stricture and the brush is passed back and forth across the stricture.

Earlier studies of brush cytology (usually from the bile duct) showed a sensitivity of approximately 40% and a specificity of 100% for the diagnosis of malignancy [6,7]. Sampling of both ducts and dilating the bile duct stricture before brushing have been shown to improve the sensitivity of diagnosing pancreatic and biliary cancers to approximately 50–70% in several studies [8,9]. Pancreatic duct

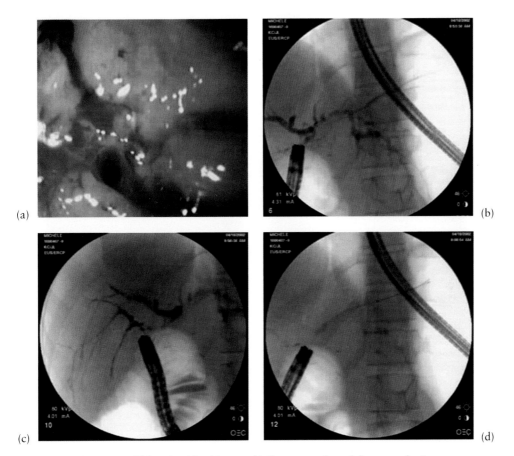

(a)　(b)　(c)　(d)

Fig. 6.2 A 34-year-old female with a history of inflammatory bowel disease and primary sclerosing cholangitis underwent resection of the common bile duct and hepatic duct for cholangiocarcinoma. The right and left hepatic ducts were anastomosed to the jejunum. The patient was referred for asymptomatic elevation of tumor markers. ERCP identified only part of the intrahepatic duct, possibly the left side, and EUS did not show an obvious mass. ERCP was repeated for cytology and stenting in anticipation of possible photodynamic therapy. (a) ERCP performed using a forward-viewing endoscope shows only one of the openings leading to the left intrahepatic system. A separate opening to the right intrahepatic system is located inferior to this opening, just outside of the visual field. (b) Cholangiography of the left hepatic duct shows changes of sclerosing cholangitis. (c) The right hepatic duct is imaged through a separate opening and shows changes of sclerosing cholangitis. (d) Brush cytology was selectively obtained from distal and proximal ducts of the right and left systems to identify local recurrence. Unfortunately, all cytological samples were positive for recurrent carcinoma.

brushing appears to be safe without an increased risk of pancreatitis in these studies.

Finally, combining the results of brush cytology, FNA, and/or forceps biopsy improves the overall sensitivity of ERCP in diagnosing pancreatic and biliary

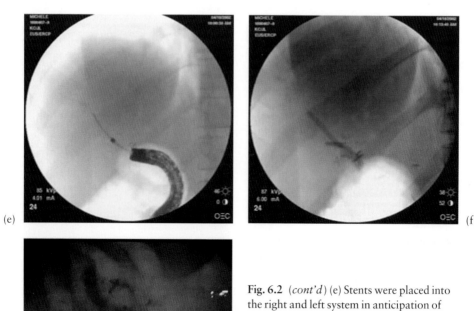

(e)

(f)

(g)

Fig. 6.2 (*cont'd*) (e) Stents were placed into the right and left system in anticipation of possible photodynamic therapy for local recurrence. (f) Two 7 Fr stents were placed into the right and left intrahepatic ducts. (g) This endoscopic view clearly shows the two separate orifices of the right and left hepatic ducts. Photodynamic therapy was not performed due to widespread disease and the stents were removed several weeks later.

cancers to 70–85%, which is higher than any single method of tissue sampling [10–12]. We recommend performing at least two different types of tissue sampling procedure to improve the diagnostic accuracy of ERCP in patients with suspected pancreatico-biliary cancers.

Tumor markers in bile or pancreatic juice

A number of molecular and genetic markers have been studied alone or in combination in bile or pancreatic juice for the diagnosis of pancreatico-biliary malignancies (Fig. 6.3). Molecular-based tests may be helpful in diagnosing pancreatic cancer and other biliary malignancy at an early stage when surgical cure is still possible. The addition of DNA image analysis to routine cytology has been reported to increase the diagnostic sensitivity as compared to results of cytology alone [13]. Other studies have focused their attention on mutations in codon 12 of the K-*ras* oncogene, because they are seen in up to 95% of pancreatic adenocarcinoma and in the premalignant conditions of the pancreas [14–16]. Bile

(a) 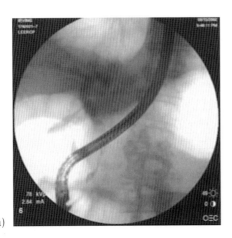 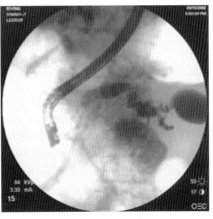 (b)

Fig. 6.3 An 84-year-old male presented with obstructive jaundice. EUS performed at another institution was interpreted as being normal except for a cyst in the tail of the pancreas. ERCP was unsuccessful. (a) Cholangiogram shows a stricture at the distal common bile duct. (b) Pancreatogram is grossly abnormal with diffuse dilation and cyst in the tail. Aspiration of the pancreatic duct revealed blood-tinged mucin with CEA > 13 000. A repeat EUS showed a grossly dilated pancreatic duct but no pancreatic mass. Pancreatic juice cytology showed atypical cells suggestive of malignancy.

obtained during ERCP can yield positive results in K-*ras* mutational analysis, even when results of conventional bile cytology are negative. One study reported a sensitivity of 33%, and specificity and positive predictive value of 100%, for the diagnosis of malignancy by K-*ras* mutational analysis in bile samples obtained during ERCP [15].

Most recent studies, however, suggest that K-*ras* mutational analysis is not specific for the diagnosis of pancreatic cancer as this mutation is also seen in a number of patients with chronic pancreatitis [16,17]. The specificity of K-*ras* mutational analysis may be increased by additional molecular genetic analysis. For example, the combination of K-*ras* mutation and telomerase activity or p53 immunostaining has been reported to increase the specificity for diagnosis of cancer to 100% [18,19]. Another study showed that detection of antigen 90K in pancreatic juice in combination with serum CA 19–9 correctly identified 84.2% of pancreatic cancers and 90% of chronic pancreatitis cases [20]. In conclusion, the presence of K-*ras* mutations in pancreatic juice (and other material obtained during ERCP) is not specific enough to justify its use in clinical practice. Although combining K-*ras* mutational analysis with other tumor markers such as p53 and telomerase may further increase its specificity, the sparse data available are preliminary and therefore such analysis should be considered investigational at this time.

Direct endoscopic examination of pancreatico-biliary malignancies

Choledochoscopy

Choledochoscopy using the mother and baby scope system is employed to visualize the bile duct, to obtain specimens, and to treat stones and tumors [21]. In a series of 61 patients who underwent choledochoscopy for various indications, three patients with suspected choledocholithiasis were diagnosed with benign epithelioid tumor, large cell lymphoma, and cholangiocarcinoma [22]. Of six patients with suspected cholangiocarcinoma, four had cholangiocarcinoma, one had ampullary cancer, and one had an eroding surgical suture. Choledochoscopy showed intraductal metastasis from colorectal cancer, bleeding hepatoma, cholangiocarcinoma, and angiodysplasia of the bile duct in four patients with hemobilia. Finally, choledochoscopy-guided Nd:YAG laser was used to debulk tumor ingrowth in several patients with blocked Wallstents [22].

Pancreatoscopy

Pancreatoscopy has been shown to be an effective tool in the diagnosis of cystadenoma and cystadenocarcinoma of the pancreas [23–25]. Pancreatoscopy was successful in 30 of 41 patients (73.2%) and showed villous or vegetative elevations in patients with dysplastic adenoma or adenocarcinoma. Pancreatoscopy led to partial resection in seven of 30 patients with non-malignant tumors resulting in favorable outcomes [26]. Pancreatoscopy was also useful for detecting and distinguishing benign from malignant intraductal papillary mucinous tumor (IPMT) and in determining the extent of tumor involvement of the main pancreatic duct in planning for resection [25–27].

Intraductal ultrasound

Intraductal ultrasound (IDUS) is performed by selectively cannulating the bile duct using a 6 Fr gauge, high-frequency (20 MHz) mini-probe during ERCP. This technique can visualize the extrahepatic and right and left intrahepatic ducts and is useful for performing tumor staging during the initial ERCP. IDUS can assess portal vein and right hepatic artery invasion at the liver hilum and is more accurate than conventional endoscopic ultrasound (EUS) in assessing pancreatic parenchymal invasion by bile duct cancer [28].

IDUS has been used in combination with other methods to increase the diagnostic yield for cancer. In one study, a combination of peroral pancreatoscopy and IDUS was helpful in differentiating malignant from benign IPMT and resulted in an improvement in postoperative survival [27]. Tamada *et al.* showed that the presence of sessile tumor, tumor size > 1 cm, and interrupted wall structures was helpful in predicting malignancy in 62 patients with malignant biliary strictures and prior negative biopsies [29].

Magnetic resonance cholangiopancreatography

Magnetic resonance cholangiopancreatography (MRCP) is an emerging application of magnetic resonance imaging (MRI) applied to the pancreatico-biliary tree. MRCP relies on heavily T2–weighted sequences. Fluid-containing structures have a much longer T2 than solid tissue, resulting in higher signal intensity. Stationary fluid in the biliary and pancreatic ducts serves as an intrinsic contrast medium and the ductal system appears white against a black background, similar to ERCP.

MRCP vs. ERCP

The major advantages of MRCP are that it does not require endoscopy, contrast injection, or exposure to radiation. MRCP has been reported to distinguish between benign and malignant bile duct obstruction, with a sensitivity between 50 and 86% and a specificity between 92 and 98% [30–32]. MRCP has been reported to be similar to ERCP in distinguishing between malignant and benign biliary obstruction with respect to sensitivity (86% vs. 89%), specificity (82% vs. 94%), and likelihood ratios for positive (4.9 vs. 15.1) and negative (0.2 vs. 0.1) tests respectively [32].

In another comparative study, the sensitivity of ERCP for diagnosing pancreatic cancer was lower (70% vs. 84%) because it missed 11 lesions < 3 cm, most of which were in the head of the pancreas [33]. ERCP was associated with several mild cases of pancreatitis, fever, and epigastric pain while MRCP was free of complications [33]. MRCP is also helpful in visualizing the main pancreatic duct in patients with IPMT, especially when ERCP fails because of copious intraductal mucin [34].

Finally, MRCP can be used to confirm the presence and location of a biliary stricture in a patient with obstructive jaundice before therapeutic ERCP, particularly in those with complex hilar lesions, thus minimizing the risk of contamination and infection. MRCP-guided endoscopic unilateral stent placement was associated with lower morbidity and mortality as compared with the standard method of stent insertion in 35 patients with Bismuth types III and IV hilar tumors [35].

In conclusion, MRCP is a safe, non-invasive, and accurate, but operator-dependent, technique for imaging the pancreatico-biliary system. MRCP should be used instead of purely diagnostic ERCP when available and before attempting stenting in patients with hilar strictures.

Palliation of inoperable pancreatico-biliary malignancies

ERCP is the preferred method of palliating patients with malignant obstructive jaundice. Successful biliary drainage by endoscopic stenting can be achieved in more than 90% of patients with low procedure-related morbidity and mortality [36,37]. Although only surgery offers potential for a cure, endoscopic palliation continues to remain the therapeutic goal in most patients, because the majority of pancreatico-biliary cancers present at an advanced stage in elderly patients, who are poor surgical candidates. Several randomized trials comparing surgical bypass to endoscopic stenting in patients with unresectable lesions showed similar success rates for biliary decompression and overall survival, but lower morbidity and 30-day mortality for the ERCP-treated patients [36–38].

ERCP also reduced the cost and shortened hospital stay ($P < 0.001$) compared to surgery [39] and improved the quality of life [40]. Although the percutaneous approach is another alternative to ERCP for biliary drainage, it should be reserved for patients with duodenal obstruction or failed ERCP, because a randomized comparative study showed it to be less successful and to cause more complications compared to ERCP [41]. Pancreatic duct stenting has been reported to be helpful in relieving 'obstructive' pain from pancreatic cancer in some patients [42]. In conclusion, endoscopic palliation is highly successful, has a lower morbidity and mortality, and costs less compared with other approaches to pancreatico-biliary malignancies.

Endoscopic stenting for malignant jaundice

Technique of endoscopic stent insertion

ERCP and endoscopic stent insertion require deep cannulation of the common bile duct with a catheter and guidewire. A diagnostic ERCP is mandatory prior to stent insertion to evaluate the pancreatico-biliary system. The length and the location of the stricture should be carefully determined and the proximal biliary tree should be assessed.

The procedure may prove to be technically difficult in cases where tumors distort the duodenal or the ampullary anatomy. The stent is usually placed through a therapeutic duodenoscope with an instrument channel of at least 4 mm. A prior sphincterotomy is usually only needed for placement of multiple large stents or to facilitate future stent exchanges in patients with difficult

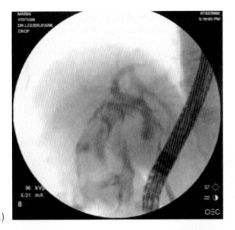

(a)

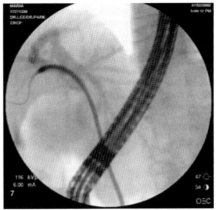

(b)

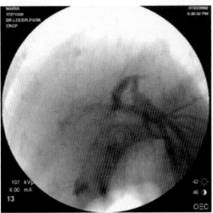

(c)

Fig. 6.4 A 64-year-old female was admitted for evaluation and treatment of mild cholangitis. (a) An abdominal ultrasound showed a probable mass in the gallbladder. ERCP was performed for treatment of cholangitis and showed multiple masses in the gallbladder with extrinsic compression of the common hepatic duct. (b) Dilation of the common hepatic duct stricture using a rotary dilator. (c) A 10 Fr plastic stent was placed for treatment of cholangitis and obstructive jaundice. CT scan showed unresectable widespread disease and the plastic stent was changed to a metal stent.

access. Difficult cannulation at times may require precutting of the ampulla using a needle-knife sphincterotome (needle-knife sphincterotomy) to gain access into the biliary system.

Dilatation prior to stent insertion is required only for extremely tight strictures, but we recommend routinely dilating hilar strictures prior to stenting (Fig. 6.4).

For insertion of a plastic stent, a basic three-layer coaxial system consisting of a 0.035-inch guidewire and a 6 Fr guiding catheter is used. These are placed sequentially across the stricture and the stent is deployed with the help of a pusher tube. A modified stenting system (OASIS, Wilson Cook) combines the pusher and inner catheter into one system to minimize the number of exchanges. In patients with bifurcation obstruction, two wires should be placed first into the right and left systems, before attempting double stenting into the right and left hepatic ducts.

Types of stent

Plastic stents Plastic stents are mostly made of polyethylene. Other materials used are polyurethane and Teflon. The mean patency of a plastic stent is approximately 2–4 months [43,44]. Important complications associated with plastic stents include stent occlusion, sepsis, stent migration, stent fracture, and, rarely, acute cholecystitis related to occlusion of the cystic duct [44].

The major disadvantage of plastic stents is occlusion from bacterial biofilm, which comprises protein, deconjugated bilirubin, microcolonies of bacteria, and amorphous debris [43]. Stent occlusion leads to recurrence of jaundice or cholangitis, necessitating stent exchanges in 30–60% of patients [43–45]. Unfortunately, attempts to improve the patency rates of plastic stents by alternative stent design and oral administration of bile acids, antibiotics, and aspirin have not been clinically successful [43–49].

Metal stents The self-expandable metal stent (SEMS) was developed to overcome the short patency of the plastic stent. SEMSs are made of either stainless steel alloy monofilaments (Wallstent, Boston Scientific, Natick, MA and Spiral Z-Stent, Wilson Cook, Winston Salem, NC) or nickel titanium alloy (Diamond Stent, Boston Scientific, Natick, MA and Za-Stent, Wilson Cook, Winston Salem, NC).

The comparative efficacy of each design is not well known and their use is guided more by physician preference. SEMSs can be compressed on to a 3-mm delivery system and expanded to 10 mm after deployment. The larger luminal diameter of these stents offers a prolonged patency of up to 10–12 months. However, the cost per device is significantly higher than for plastic stents ($1000–1500 vs. $50–100).

SEMSs can also occlude but through different mechanisms, including biliary sludge, dietary fiber, tumor ingrowth or overgrowth, epithelial hyperplasia, or a combination of these. Management of an occluded metal biliary stent includes mechanical dislodgement of the obstructing material, placement of a plastic stent within the metal stent, and placement of a second overlying or overlapping stent to improve drainage. Electrocoagulation or laser therapy to destroy the ingrowing tumor has not been effective [44].

Metal vs. plastic stents Metal stents have been compared with plastic stents in different studies. In 47 patients with pancreatic cancer with a mean survival of 6.2 months from the time of endoscopy, metal stents were shown to have a longer patency than plastic stents—8.2 months vs. 3.5 months ($P < 0.001$) [50].

A prospective randomized trial in France evaluated 97 patients with malignant strictures of the bile ducts (64% with pancreatic cancer), who were randomized to receive either an 11.5 Fr stent to be exchanged on demand or every 3 months, or a self-expanding metallic wall stent [51]. The mean duration of follow-up was 166 days. Cost effective analysis suggested that metal stents were advantageous for patients surviving longer than 6 months, whereas plastic stents were advantageous for patients surviving less than 6 months. This study showed initial metal stenting to be the most cost effective approach, provided that the patient survived for longer than 6 months.

The US Wallstent multicenter randomized trial evaluated the Wallstent compared with 10 Fr plastic stents for the palliation of malignant biliary obstruction [52]. Early stent occlusion was reported in 30% of the plastic group and in 0% of the Wallstent group. Sludge occlusion and stent migration were seen in 28% of plastic stents and 6% of Wallstents. The overall complication rate was significantly lower in the Wallstent group ($P < 0.05$) for both hilar and distal biliary strictures. Wallstents did not offer any survival advantage over the plastic stent but were less expensive because they required fewer repeat ERCPs and stent exchange.

A prospective study from Amsterdam compared Wallstents with plastic stents in distal malignant biliary obstruction and reported a lower occlusion rate (33% vs. 54%), longer stent patency (273 vs. 126 days), and 28% reduction in ERCPs per patient in the Wallstent group [53]. These studies show that Wallstents can be deployed successfully in most patients and occlude less frequently and less rapidly than the conventional 10 Fr and 11.5 Fr plastic stents.

Logically, therefore, Wallstent use reduces hospitalization and repeated interventions leading to a lower cost. In conclusion, the most cost effective approach to palliating malignant obstructive jaundice is to place a SEMS at the initial ERCP in patients with unresectable cancer who have a life expectancy of at least 6 months.

Covered and uncovered metal stents Metal stents partially covered with silicone or polyurethane membrane have been introduced to overcome the problem of tumor ingrowth and epithelial hyperplasia. Shim *et al.* compared endoscopically placed polyurethane-covered Z-Stent to non-coated Wallstent or Strecker stent [54]. The median patency of both covered and uncovered stents was comparable (267 vs. 233 days), but tumor ingrowth was seen in two patients with the covered stents compared to six in the non-covered stent group. Early and late complications were the same in both groups [54].

Reported complications associated with covered stents include tumor ingrowth or overgrowth, sludge accumulation, stent migration, pancreatitis, and gangrenous cholecystitis [44,54–56]. Finally, covered biliary metal stents have not uniformly shown a significant advantage in terms of greater patency rates [54,56].

Biodegradable stents Self-expanding mesh stents made of biodegradable materials behave similarly to their wire mesh counterparts, but disintegrate and disappear over time. Polylactic acid is used in one such bioabsorbable stent. Postimplantation, body heat and water degrade the polymer to lactic acid, then via the Krebs cycle to CO_2 and H_2O.

Animal studies of the canine bile duct using the bioabsorbable biliary mesh stent made from polylactic acid have shown that the stent becomes embedded within the bile duct epithelium within 1 month of implantation [57]. There was minimal inflammatory reaction after 6 months and the histology reverted to baseline, with complete disintegration of the stent after 2 years. These stents offer long-term palliation without precluding subsequent resection in patients with suspected but unproven malignant stricture, or for those in whom curative resection is unlikely but not ruled out. The exciting potential applications in the future for these devices include delivery of chemotherapeutic agents or cellular gene therapy and tissue remodeling.

Endoscopic stenting for hilar strictures

Most malignant hilar strictures are related to cholangiocarcinoma, metastatic lymphadenopathy, large pancreatic cancer, or gallbladder carcinoma [58–61]. Hilar lesions or Klatskin tumors are classified according to the degree of involvement of the intrahepatic ducts [58].

Bismuth classification for hilar obstruction Bismuth type I tumors involve the common hepatic duct, type II involve the right and left intrahepatic ducts, type III involve either the right (IIIA) or left (IIIB) secondary intrahepatic ducts, and type IV involve the secondary intrahepatic ducts bilaterally. Palliation of hilar strictures involving the bifurcation or its branches (Bismuth type II or type III) is technically difficult. Cholangitis can develop after ERCP in 0–40% of patients, depending on the complexity of the lesion and completeness of drainage [59].

Unilateral vs. bilateral drainage for hilar obstruction There is considerable debate in the literature about whether unilateral drainage is sufficient in patients with hilar strictures. Deverie *et al.* suggested draining both of the obstructed lobes in types II and III hilar lesions to maximize reduction in bilirubin and reduce the likelihood of developing cholangitis [60] (Fig. 6.5). They showed a decrease in biliary sepsis rate from 38% to 17% and an increase in the survival in type II and type III strictures from a mean of 119 days to 176 days by performing bilateral stenting [60].

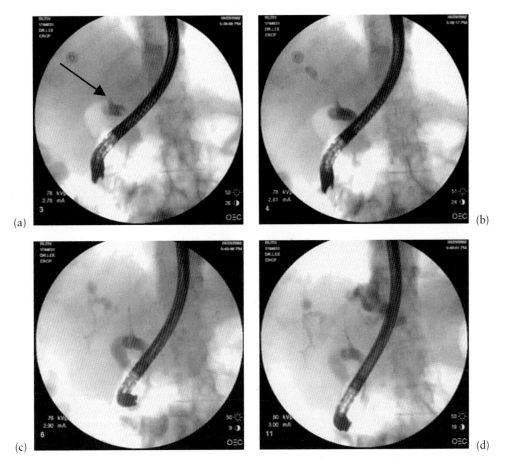

Fig. 6.5 A 74-year-old female presented with painless jaundice. ERCP showed a hilar stricture but stent insertion was not successful. The patient was referred for stenting 24 h after the initial study. She had a low-grade fever and leukocytosis suggestive of cholangitis and urgent ERCP was performed. (a) Initial cholangiogram shows a common hepatic duct stricture (*arrow*). (b) Selective cannulation of the right hepatic duct with filling of the right side. Filling of the left system is avoided initially, until deep access of the left side is performed, in order to ensure bilateral drainage in this patient with cholangitis resulting from prior unsuccessful ECRP. (c) Selective cannulation of the left intrahepatic system is obtained using a guidewire. (d) Selective deep cannulation of the left system followed by cholangiography showing a dilated left system.

Others recommend unilateral stenting as long as one-quarter to one-third of the liver volume is drained by the single endoprosthesis, leaving the option of a second stent for the 20% who do not respond favorably [61,62]. Polydorou *et al.* evaluated this selective approach in 190 consecutive patients with hilar malignancies [62]. A single prosthesis was placed in 89% of patients with successful drainage in 82%; 4% had additional stents due to insufficient response.

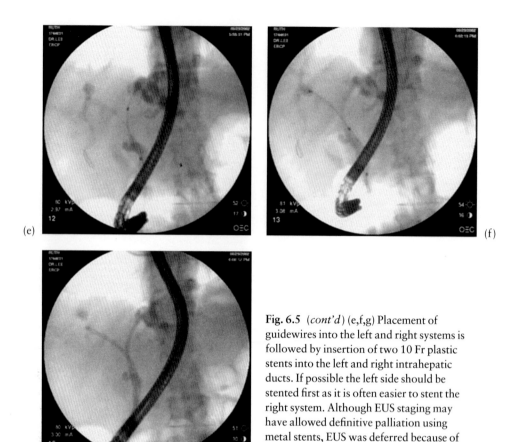

Fig. 6.5 (*cont'd*) (e,f,g) Placement of guidewires into the left and right systems is followed by insertion of two 10 Fr plastic stents into the left and right intrahepatic ducts. If possible the left side should be stented first as it is often easier to stent the right system. Although EUS staging may have allowed definitive palliation using metal stents, EUS was deferred because of cholangitis.

Seven per cent required a combined procedure with percutaneous transhepatic access. Stenting was technically successful in 93% of type I, 94% of type II, and 84% of type III patients, with successful drainage in 91%, 83%, and 73% of patients, respectively. Early complications were seen in 7%, 14%, and 31% of types I, II, and III patients, and the mortality rates for these groups were 14%, 15%, and 32%, respectively [62]. The authors concluded that a single prosthesis provides good palliation in 80% of patients, whereas a second stent should be reserved for stent failures. A small prospective randomized comparative trial showed significantly higher technical success and lower complication for patients treated by unilateral stenting [63].

Another study recommended bilobar drainage in patients in whom both of the lobes were filled during the ERCP, as patients with incomplete drainage had the worst survival among all patients with hilar tumors [64]. All things being equal, it probably makes more sense to drain the left system because the left hepatic duct has fewer side branches near the hilum, but this anatomical advantage has not been clearly proven to confer any clinical benefit [61].

In our opinion, the most elegant and physiological approach to stenting hilar tumor is to first map the lesion using MRCP and document its function using CT prior to determining which duct to stent. With these data in hand, it may be possible to selectively cannulate and stent the desired duct without contaminating the other ducts. Both plastic and SEMSs have been used for palliation of hilar malignancies with varying success and complication rates [61–64].

Metal stents in hilar strictures have the advantage over plastic stents of ease of insertion and drainage of side branches through the stent meshwork. If both lobes of the liver should be drained, two SEMSs can be placed either endoscopically or percutaneously, most often fashioned into a Y configuration or placed parallel to each other.

Other techniques of endoscopic palliation

Intraductal photodynamic therapy

Photodynamic therapy (PDT) involves intravenous administration of a photosensitizing compound, usually a hematoporphyrin derivative that preferentially accumulates within the tumor cells, followed by activation using laser lights. This releases reactive oxygen species leading to tumor necrosis. PDT has been studied in cholangiocarcinoma as the cancer cells have been shown to be sensitive to PDT. Photofrin 11 (Porfimer sodium) and 5-aminolevulinic acid (5-ALA) have been studied in humans [65,66]. These drugs are given intravenously and, 24 to 48 h later, endoscopic or percutaneous transhepatic cholangiography is performed and biliary catheters are advanced through the working channel of the duodenoscope and placed across the malignant stricture. Subsequently, flexible laser fibers are advanced through the biliary catheters. The tumor is treated sequentially from the proximal to distal margin. Laser light (630 nm) is delivered to activate the Photofrin with a total energy of 180 J/cm^2.

One study evaluated PDT for cholangiocarcinoma in patients with unresectable Bismuth types III and IV tumors, who had an inadequate decrease in bilirubin despite adequate biliary stent placement [65]. The patients received up to three monthly treatments. Patients had a significant decrease in serum bilirubin and improvement in the quality of life, including on the Karnofsky index, WHO index, and biliary obstruction scale, and improved survival. However, another recent study did not show any benefit to intraductal PDT using 5-ALA in patients with unresectable cholangiocarcinoma [66]. An important toxicity associated with PDT is photosensitization, which occurs in 20–40% of patients [67] despite avoidance of sunlight. Less common side-effects include infusion reaction and stricture, and fistula formation in the treated areas [68,69].

Brachytherapy

Brachytherapy involves the intracavitary placement of a radioactive source within a malignant stricture. ^{192}Ir has been studied in patients with cholangio-carcinoma to improve stent patency and survival. Intraluminal brachytherapy can be accomplished either endoscopically via a previously placed nasobiliary tube or by the percutaneous transhepatic route [70–73].

Radiation therapy is then applied to the area in calculated doses depending on the various radiation therapy protocols. Patients are hospitalized and given either low-dose brachytherapy using 30–45 Gy (3000–4500 rad) over 24–60 h or high-dose brachytherapy as an outpatient. In certain cases radiosensitizing chemotherapeutic agents such as 5-fluorouracil (5-FU) are also administered simultaneously [70]. Effective biliary drainage is maintained after treatment using plastic or metal stents. Important early complications include cholangitis and duodenal ulcers, and less common long-term complications include biliary enteric fistula and hematobilia [71,72]. Brachytherapy should be administered as part of an experimental protocol, because available data are preliminary and based on the treatment of very few patients, with only questionable benefit in survival [66,73].

ERCP in the management of ampullary neoplasms

Benign tumors

A number of benign tumors arise at the major papilla, including adenoma, lipoma, leiomyoma, lymphangioma, and hamartoma. Amongst these lesions adenoma is the most common benign but premalignant tumor. These tumors can cause symptoms of biliary colic, obstructive jaundice, recurrent pancreatitis, and, rarely, gastrointestinal bleeding [74–76]. Ampullary adenoma may be sporadic or occur as part of familial adenomatous polyposis (FAP) and Gardner's syndrome [75]. Ampullary adenoma may contain foci of adenocarcinoma [74–76] and can be excised surgically or endoscopically in many instances.

The surgical options include transduodenal local excision and pancreatico-duodenectomy [74].

Endoscopic treatment involves the combination of snare excision and thermal ablation. ERCP should be performed before ampullectomy to identify intra-ductal extension and to rule out other intraductal lesions. Tissue sampling after biliary sphincterotomy may increase the diagnostic yield for cancer [74,77]. There is accumulating evidence that endoscopic resection, ablation, or both, performed by an experienced endoscopist, is a safe and effective treatment for sporadic or FAP-associated periampullary adenoma [77,78].

Endoscopic snare papillectomy is indicated for tumor size < 4 cm without evidence of malignancy, as suggested by endoscopic and histological findings, and in the absence of intraductal extension on ERCP or EUS. Ampullectomy is performed by snare resection using a blended electrosurgical current either *en bloc* or in a piecemeal fashion [79].

Some suggest placing pancreatic stents in all patients after snare papillectomy; however, others advocate performing stenting only when the pancreatic duct fails to drain after papillectomy [77,78]. In general, extension of the adenoma into either duct warrants surgical excision, because of the increased likelihood of carcinoma and the difficulty of endoscopic excision.

Ampullary carcinoma

The role of endoscopic treatment of ampullary carcinoma is to adequately palliate those patients unsuitable for surgery using endoscopic sphincterotomy with stent insertion to relieve obstructive jaundice. In selected patients a large sphincterotomy may provide adequate drainage without a stent. Endoscopic palliation can then be achieved by a combination of snare excision and Nd:YAG laser ablation of the tumor tissue. ERCP-assisted ablation of ampullary neoplasm using ultra high-frequency ultrasound probes may be a promising alternative to thermal ablation in the future [80]. Finally, the application of new imaging methods during ERCP, such as optical coherence tomography (OCT), may lead to improved diagnostic accuracy of ampullary neoplasm. One recent study reported preliminary experience with this technique in five patients, with OCT identifying the characteristic epithelial morphology in two cases of papillary cholangiocarcinoma [81].

Outstanding issues and future trends

The management of pancreatico-biliary malignancies involves a multidisciplinary approach combining the expertise of gastroenterologists, radiologists, and surgeons. ERCP is an important diagnostic and therapeutic modality and plays a crucial role in the management of these patients. Emerging newer diagnostic modalities are helpful in defining the finite role of ERCP in the management of pancreatico-biliary malignancies.

At the present time ERCP is an effective, safe, and cost efficient treatment for the palliation of these tumors. ERCP in combination with EUS and FNA offers an effective means of tissue sampling. This, coupled with the new molecular technology, may improve the early diagnosis and staging of pancreatico-biliary malignancies. Although endoscopic stenting is an established palliation for malignant obstructive jaundice, major complications, including blockage of plastic stents by bacterial biofilm and biliary sludge, still limit its clinical benefits. Prolonged palliation of jaundice is achieved by the use of SEMSs but they too are limited by tissue and tumor ingrowth. Better innovations in technology and future studies will further widen the scope of this technique in the management of pancreatico-biliary malignancies.

References

1 American Cancer Society. Cancer Facts and Figures 2001.
2 Menges M, Lerch MM, Zeitz M. The double duct in patients with malignant and benign pancreatic lesions. *Gastrointest Endosc* 2000; 52: 74–7.
3 Ralls PW, Halls J, Renner I, Juttner H. Endoscopic retrograde cholangiopancreatography (ERCP) in pancreatic disease: a reassessment of the specificity of ductal abnormalities in differentiating benign from malignant disease. *Radiology* 1980; 134: 347–52.
4 Bain VG, Abraham N, Jhangri GS *et al*. Prospective study of biliary strictures to determine the predictors of malignancy. *Can J Gastroenterol* 2000; 14: 397–402.
5 Shah SA, Movson J, Ransil BJ, Waxman I. pancreatic duct stricture length at ERCP predicts tumor size and pathological stage of pancreatic cancer. *Am J Gastroenterol* 1997; 92 (6): 964–7.
6 Scudera PL, Koizumi J, Jacobson IM. Brush cytology evaluation of lesions encountered during ERCP. *Gastrointest Endosc* 1990; 36: 281–4.
7 Ryan ME. Cytologic brushings of ductal lesions during ERCP. *Gastrointest Endosc* 1991; 37: 139–42.
8 McGuire DE, Venu RP, Brown RD, Etzkorn KP, Glaws WR, Abu-Hammour A. Brush cytology for pancreatic carcinoma: an analysis of factors influencing results. *Gastrointest Endosc* 1996; 44: 300–4.
9 Vandervoort J, Soetikno RM, Montes H *et al*. Accuracy and complication rate of brush cytology from bile duct versus pancreatic duct. *Gastrointest Endosc* 1999; 49: 322–7.
10 Jailwala J, Fogel EL, Sherman S *et al*. Triple-tissue sampling at ERCP in malignant biliary obstruction. *Gastrointest Endosc* 2000; 51: 283–90.
11 Farrell RJ, Jain AK, Brandwein SL, Wang H, Chuttani R, Pleskow D. The combination of stricture dilation, endoscopic needle aspiration and biliary brushings significantly improves diagnostic yield from malignant bile duct strictures. *Gastrointest Endosc* 2001; 54: 587–94.
12 Schoefl R, Haefner M, Wrba F *et al*. Forceps biopsy and brush cytology during endoscopic retrograde cholangiopancreatography for the diagnosis of biliary stenoses. *Scand J Gastroenterol* 1997; 32: 363–8.
13 Krishnamurthy S, Katz RL, Shumate A *et al*. DNA image analysis combined with routine cytology improves diagnostic sensitivity of common bile duct brushings. *Cancer* 2001; 93: 229–35.
14 Ryan ME, Baldauf MC. Comparison of flow cytometry for DNA content and brush cytology for detection of malignancy in pancreaticobiliary strictures. *Gastrointest Endosc* 1994; 40: 133–9.
15 Lee JG, Leung JW, Cotton PB *et al*. Diagnostic utility of K-ras mutational analysis on bile obtained by endoscopic retrograde cholangiopancreatography. *Gastrointest Endosc* 1995; 42: 317–20.
16 Pugliese V, Pujic N, Saccomanno S *et al*. Pancreatic intraductal sampling during ERCP in patients with chronic pancreatitis and pancreatic cancer: cytologic studies and K-ras-2 codon 12 molecular analysis in 47 cases. *Gastrointest Endosc* 2001; 54: 595–9.

17 Boadas J, Mora J, Urgell E *et al*. Clinical usefulness of K-ras gene mutation detection and cyto-logy in pancreatic juice in the diagnosis and screening of pancreatic cancer. *Eur J Gastroenterol Hepatol* 2001; 13: 1153–9.

18 Myung SJ, Kim MH, Kim YS *et al*. Telomerase activity in pure pancreatic juice for the diagnosis of pancreatic cancer may be complimentary to K-ras mutation. *Gastrointest Endosc* 2000; 51: 708–13.

19 Itoi T, Shinohara Y, Takeda K *et al*. Detection of telomerase activity in biopsy specimens for diagnosis of biliary tract cancers. *Gastrointest Endosc* 2000; 52: 380–6.

20 Gentiloni N, Caradonna P, Costamagna G *et al*. Pancreatic juice 90K and serum CA 19–9 combined determination can discriminate between pancreatic cancer and chronic pancreatitis. *Am J Gastroenterol* 1995; 90: 1069–72.

21 Neuhaus H. Cholangioscopy. *Endoscopy* 1992; 24: 125–32.

22 Siddique I, Galati J, Ankoma-Sey V *et al*. The role of choledochoscopy in the diagnosis and management of biliary tract disease. *Gastrointest Endosc* 1999; 50: 67–73.

23 Tajiri H, Kobayashi M, Ohtsu A, Ryu M, Yoshida S. Peroral pancreatoscopy for the diagnosis of pancreatic disease. *Pancreas* 1998; 16: 408–12 .

24 Rieman JF, Kohler B. Endoscopy of the pancreatic duct: value of different endoscope types. *Gastrointest Endosc* 1993; 39: 367–70.

25 Seo DW, Kim MH, Lee SK *et al*. The value of pancreatoscopy in patients with mucinous ductal ectasia. *Endoscopy* 1997; 29: 315–18.

26 Yamaguchi T, Hara T, Tsuyuguchi T *et al*. Peroral pancreatoscopy in the diagnosis of mucin-producing tumors of the pancreas. *Gastrointest Endosc* 2000; 52: 67–73.

27 Hara T, Yamaguchi T, Ishihara T *et al*. Diagnosis and patient management of intraductal papillary mucinous tumor of the pancreas by using peroral pancreatoscopy and intraductal ultrasonography. *Gastroenterology* 2002; 122: 34–43.

28 Tamada K, Ueno N, Ichiyama M *et al*. Assessment of pancreatic parenchymal invasion by bile duct cancer using intraductal ultrasonography. *Endoscopy* 1996; 28: 492–6.

29 Tamada K, Tomiyama T, Wada S *et al*. Endoscopic transpapillary bile duct biopsy with the combination of intraductal ultrasonography in the diagnosis of biliary strictures. *Gut* 2002; 50: 326–31.

30 Hintze RE, Adler A, Veltzke EK *et al*. Clinical significance of magnetic resonance cholangio-pancreaticography (MRCP) compared to endoscopic retrograde cholangio-pancreaticography (ERCP). *Endoscopy* 1997; 29: 182–7.

31 Guibaud L, Bret PM, Reinhold C, Atri M, Barkun AN. Bile duct obstruction and choledo-cholithiasis: diagnosis with MR cholangiography. *Radiology* 1995; 197: 109–15.

32 Arslan A, Geitung JT, Viktil E, Abdelnoor M, Osnes M. Pancreaticobiliary diseases. Com-parisons of 2D single-shot turbo spin-echo MR cholangiopancreatography with endoscopic retrograde cholangiopancreatography. *Acta Radiol* 2000; 41: 621–6.

33 Adamek HE, Albert J, Breer H, Weitz M, Schilling D, Riemann JF. Pancreatic cancer detection with magnetic resonance cholangiopancreatography and endoscopic retrograde cholangiopan-creatography: a prospective controlled study. *Lancet* 2000; 356: 190–3.

34 Sugiyama M, Atomi Y, Hachiya J. Intraductal papillary tumors of the pancreas: evaluation with magnetic resonance cholangiopancreatography. *Am J Gastroenterol* 1998; 93: 156–9.

35 Hintze RE, Abou-Rebyeh H, Adler A, Velzke-Schlieker W, Felix R, Wiedenmann B. Magnetic resonance cholangiopancreatography-guided unilateral endoscopic stent placement for Klatskin tumors. *Gastrointest Endosc* 2001; 53: 40–6.

36 Andersen JR, Sorensen SM, Kruse A, Rokkjaer M, Matzen P. Randomized trial of endoprosthe-sis versus operative bypass and malignant obstructive jaundice. *Gut* 1989; 30: 1132–5.

37 Shepherd HA, Diba A, Ross AP, Arthur M, Ryle G, Collin-Jones D. Endoscopic biliary prosthesis and the palliation of malignant biliary obstruction: a randomized trial. *Br J Surg* 1988; 75: 1166–8.

38 Smith AC, Dowset JF, Russell RCG, Hatfield ARW, Cotton PB. Randomized trial of endoscopic stenting versus surgical bypass in malignant low bile duct obstruction. *Lancet* 1994; 344: 1655–60.

39 Raikar G, Melin M, Ress A *et al*. Cost-effective analysis of surgical palliation versus endoscopic stenting in the management of unresectable pancreatic cancer. *Ann Surg Oncol* 1996; 3: 470–5.

40 Luman W, Cull A, Palmer K. Quality of life in patient's stented malignant biliary obstruction. *Eur J Gastroenterol Hepatol* 1997; 9: 481–4.

41 Speer AG, Cotton PB, Russell RCG *et al.* Randomized trial of endoscopic versus percutaneous stent insertion in malignant obstructive jaundice. *Lancet* 1987; 2: 57–62.

42 Tham TC, Lichtenstein DR, Vandervoort J *et al.* Pancreatic duct stents for 'obstructive type' pain in pancreatic malignancy. *Am J Gastroenterol* 2000; 95: 956–60.

43 Libby ED, Leung JW. Prevention of biliary stent clogging: a clinical review. *Am J Gastroenterol* 1996; 91: 1301–8.

44 Conio M, Demarquay JF, De Luca L, Marchi S, Dumas R. Endoscopic treatment of pancreatico-biliary malignancies. *Crit Rev Oncol Hematol* 2001; 37: 127–35.

45 Smit JM, Out MM, Groen AK *et al.* A placebo-controlled study on the efficacy of aspirin and doxycycline in preventing clogging of biliary endoprosthesis. *Gastrointest Endosc* 1989; 35: 485–9.

46 Ghosh S, Palmer KR. Prevention of biliary stent occlusion using cyclical antibiotics and ursodeoxycholic acid. *Gut* 1994; 26: 478–82.

47 Catalano MF, Geenen JE, Lehman GA *et al.* 'Tannenbaum' Teflon stents versus traditional polyethylene stents for treatment of malignant biliary strictures. *Gastrointest Endosc* 2002; 55: 354–8.

48 Speer AG, Cotton PB, Macrae KD. Endoscopic management of malignant biliary obstruction: stents of 10 French gauge are preferable to stents of 8 French gauge. *Gastrointest Endosc* 1988; 34: 412–17.

49 Pereira-Lima JC, Jakobs R, Maier M, Benz C, Kohler B, Rieman JF. Endoscopic biliary stenting for the palliation of pancreatic cancer: results, survival predictive factors and comparisons of 10-French with 11.5-French gauge stents. *Am J Gastroenterol* 1996; 91: 2179–84.

50 Born P, Rosch T, Triptrap A *et al.* Long term results of endoscopic treatment of biliary duct obstruction due to pancreatic disease. *Hepatogastroenterology* 1998; 45: 833–9.

51 Prat F, Chapat O, Ducot B *et al.* A randomized trial of endoscopic drainage methods for inoperable malignant stricture of the common bile duct. *Gastrointest Endosc* 1998; 47: 1–7.

52 Carr-Locke DL, Ball TJ, Connors PJ *et al.* Multicenter randomized trial of Wallstent biliary endoprosthesis versus plastic stents. *Gastrointest Endosc* 1993; 39: A310.

53 Davids PHP, Groen AK, Rauws EA, Tytgat GN, Huibregtse K. Randomized trial of self-expanding metal stents versus polyethylene stents for distal malignant biliary obstruction. *Lancet* 1992; 340: 1488–92.

54 Shim CS, Lee YH, Cho YD *et al.* Preliminary results of a new covered biliary metal stent for malignant biliary obstruction. *Endoscopy* 1998; 30: 345–50.

55 Isayama H, Komatsu Y, Tsujino T *et al.* Polyurethane-covered metal stent for management of distal malignant biliary obstruction. *Gastrointest Endosc* 2002; 55: 366–70.

56 Hauseggar K, Thurnher S, Bodendorfer G, Zollikofer C. Treatment of malignant biliary obstruction with polyurethane covered Wallstents. *Am J Roentgenol* 1998; 170: 403–8.

57 Freeman ML. Bioabsorbable stents for gastrointestinal endoscopy. *Tech Gastrointest Endosc* 2001; 3: 120–5.

58 Bismuth H, Castaign D, Trayner O. Resection or palliation: priority of surgery in the treatment of hilar cancer. *World J Surg* 1988; 12: 39–47.

59 Ducreux M, Liguory C, Lefebvre JF *et al.* Management of malignant hilar biliary obstruction by endoscopy: results and prognostic factors. *Dig Dis Sci* 1992; 37: 778–83.

60 Deverie J, Baize M, De Touef J, Cremer M. Long-term follow-up of patients with hilar malignant stricture treated by endoscopic internal biliary drainage. *Gastrointest Endosc* 1998; 34: 95–101.

61 Polydorou AA, Chisholm EM, Romanos AA *et al.* A comparison of right versus left hepatic duct endoprosthesis insertion in malignant hilar biliary obstruction. *Endoscopy* 1989; 21: 266–71.

62 Polydorou AA, Cairns SR, Dowsett JF *et al.* Palliation of proximal malignant biliary obstruction by endoprosthesis insertion. *Gut* 1991; 32: 685–9.

63 De Palma G, Galloro G, Siciliano S, Iovino P, Catanzano C. Unilateral versus bilateral endoscopic hepatic drainage in patients with malignant hilar biliary obstruction. *Gastrointest Endosc* 2001; 53: 547–53.

64 Chang WH, Kortan P, Haber G. Outcome in patients with bifurcation tumors who undergo unilateral vs. bilateral hepatic duct drainage. *Gastrointest Endosc* 1996; 43: 376.
65 Rumalla A, Baron TH, Wang KK, Gores GJ, Stadheim LM, de Groen PC. Endoscopic application of photodynamic therapy for cholangiocarcinoma. *Gastrointest Endosc* 2001; 53: 500–4.
66 Zoepf T, Jakobs R, Rosenbaum A, Apel D, Arnold JC, Rieman JF. Photodynamic therapy with 5-aminolevulinic acid is not effective in bile duct cancer. *Gastrointest Endosc* 2001; 54: 763–6.
67 Dougherty T, Cooper M, Mang T. Cutaneous phototoxic occurrences in patients receiving photofrin. *Lasers Surg Med* 1990; 10: 485–8.
68 Koehler IK. Acute immediate urticaria like reaction to i.v. injected photofrin. *Lasers Surg Med* 1997; 29: 97–8.
69 Luketich J, Westkaemper J, Sommer K. Bronchoesophagopleural fistula after photodynamic therapy for malignant mesothelioma. *Ann Thorac Surg* 1996; 62: 283–4.
70 Whittington R, Neuberg D, Tester WJ, Benson AB, Haller DG. Protracted intravenous fluorouracil infusion with radiation therapy in the management of localized pancreaticobiliary carcinoma: a phase 1 Eastern Cooperative Oncology Group Trial. *J Clin Oncol* 1995; 13: 227–32.
71 Leung J, Kuan R. Intraluminal brachytherapy in the treatment of bile duct carcinomas. *Australas Radiol* 1997; 41: 151–4.
72 Kuvshinoff B, Armstrong J, Fong Y *et al.* Palliation of irresectable hilar cholangiocarcinoma with biliary drainage and radiotherapy. *Br J Surg* 1995; 82: 1522–5.
73 Bowling TE, Galbraith SM, Hatfield AR, Solano J, Spittle MF. A retrospective comparison of endoscopic stenting alone with stenting and radiotherapy in non-resectable cholangiocarcinoma. *Gut* 1996; 39: 852–5.
74 Sivak MV Jr. Clinical and endoscopic aspects of tumor of the major duodenal papilla. *Endoscopy* 1988; 20: 211–17.
75 Alexander JR, Andrews JM, Buchi KN, Lee RG, Becker JM, Burt RW. High prevalence of adenomatous polyps of the duodenal papilla in familial adenomatous polyposis. *Dig Dis Sci* 1989; 34: 167–70.
76 Sakorafas GH, Freiss H, Dervenis CG. Villous tumors of the duodenum: biologic characters and clinical implications. *Scand J Gastroenterol* 2000; 35: 337–44.
77 Norton ID, Geller A, Petersen BT, Sorbi D, Gostout CJ. Endoscopic surveillance and ablative therapy for peripapillary adenomas. *Am J Gastroenterol* 2001; 96: 101–6.
78 Bertoni G, Sassatelli R, Nigrisoli B, Bedogni G. Endoscopic snare polypectomy in patients with familial adenomatous polyposis and papillary adenoma. *Endoscopy* 1997; 29: 685–8.
79 Hirasawa R, Lishi H, Tatsuta M, Ishiguro S. Clinicopathologic features and endoscopic resection of duodenal adenocarcinomas and adenomas with the submucosal saline injection technique. *Gastrointest Endosc* 1997; 46: 507–13.
80 Prat F, Lafon C, Theilliere JY *et al.* Destruction of a bile duct carcinoma by intraductal high intensity ultrasound during ERCP. *Gastrointest Endosc* 2001; 53: 797–800.
81 Poneros JM, Tearney GJ, Shiskov M *et al.* Optical coherence tomography of the biliary tree during ERCP. *Gastrointest Endosc* 2001; 54: 595–9.

CHAPTER 7

Management of Postsurgical Bile Leaks and Bile Duct Strictures

JACQUES J. G. H. M. BERGMAN

Synopsis

Although most centers performing laparoscopic cholecystectomy may now be well beyond the 'learning-curve' phase, the incidence of postsurgical bile duct injuries will probably stay higher than in the era before laparoscopic cholecystectomy. In addition, with surgeons embarking on more complex laparoscopic biliary interventions, such as laparoscopic duct exploration, a further increase in the incidence of surgical bile duct injuries may be expected in the near future. Adequate management of these injuries requires an early postoperative diagnosis with a low threshold for performing an ERCP.

Patients with a complete ductal transection require an elective surgical repair, 6–8 weeks after diagnosis and drainage. Most of the other bile duct injuries (minor leaks from the cystic stump or peripheral hepatic radicles, major bile duct leaks, and isolated bile duct strictures) can in general be managed endoscopically.

Patients who require long-term stenting for bile duct strictures should be treated with at least two 10 Fr plastic stents that are electively exchanged every 3 months. If possible, more than two stents should be inserted. There is currently no place for self-expandable metal stents for this indication.

Optimal management of patients with bile duct injuries requires a multidisciplinary team approach of interventional radiology, therapeutic endoscopy, and reconstructive surgery.

Introduction

The majority of surgical bile duct injuries occur during cholecystectomy, but any surgical procedure involving the liver and/or bile ducts may cause these lesions. Over the last decade laparoscopic cholecystectomy has gained widespread acceptance among surgeons and the public and has replaced conventional 'open' cholecystectomy as the treatment of choice for symptomatic cholecystolithiasis. Compared with 'open' cholecystectomy, laparoscopic cholecystectomy is associated with less postoperative pain, shorter stay in hospital and recovery, earlier return to work, and a better cosmetic outcome [1]. Laparoscopic chole-cystectomy does, however, carry an increased risk for biliary tract injury [2]. These injuries occur in 0.2–0.5% of patients undergoing open cholecystectomy and in 0.5–2.7% after laparoscopic cholecystectomy [3–6]. The injury often results from poorly defined anatomy or from attempts to stop hilar bleeding by means of clipping or thermal devices. Besides direct injury due to clipping and diathermy, delayed injury may arise from ischemia of the bile ducts [7]. The presence of acute cholecystitis, and a low case volume of the surgeon, are accepted risk factors for bile duct injury during laparoscopic cholecystectomy [8,9]. Intraoperative cholangiography does not seem to reduce the frequency of these complications [9]. Management of patients with postsurgical bile duct injuries requires a multidisciplinary approach of radiologists, endoscopists, and surgeons. In general, multiple invasive procedures are required and, although the functional outcome is usually good, postsurgical bile duct injuries have a marked influence on the patients' physical and mental quality of life, even at long-term follow-up [10].

Classification of bile duct injuries

In general, four types of bile duct injury can be recognized.

Type A   Cystic duct leaks or leakage from aberrant or peripheral hepatic rad-icles (Figs 7.1 and 7.2).

Type B   Major bile duct leaks with or without concomitant biliary strictures (Figs 7.3 and 7.4).

Type C   Bile duct strictures without bile leakage (Figs 7.4 and 7.5).

Type D   Complete transections of the duct with or without excision of some portion of the biliary tree (Fig. 7.6) [11].

Presentation

The majority of bile duct lesions during cholecystectomy are not recognized during the procedure. The postoperative clinical presentation varies widely and is mainly influenced by the type of injury [11]. The diagnosis is usually straight-forward in patients with an isolated ductal stricture (type C). These lesions pre-sent with jaundice, cholestatic liver function tests, and dilated bile ducts on ultrasound and have a relatively long symptom-free interval after the cholecys-tectomy (median of 2 months in our series) [11]. In contrast to isolated stric-tures, bile leaks due to minor bile duct lacerations (type A lesions), major bile duct lacerations (type B lesions), or complete transections (type D lesions) pre-sent in a less uniform way. Here, symptoms are frequently absent or non-specific

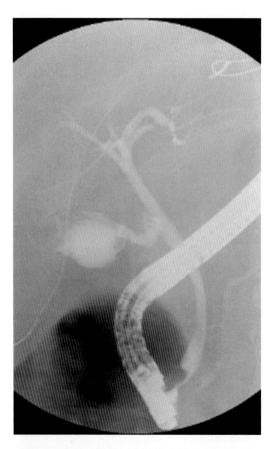

Fig. 7.1 Type A bile duct lesion after laparoscopic cholecystectomy showing leakage originating from the cystic stump.

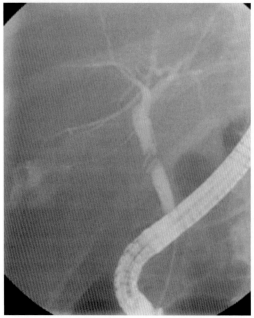

Fig. 7.2 Type A bile duct lesion after cholecystectomy. Here the bile leakage originates from a peripheral branch of the right hepatic system. A subhilar obstruction, due to misplacement of clips, prevents the leak from sealing spontaneously. Note that part of the right hepatic system is missing!

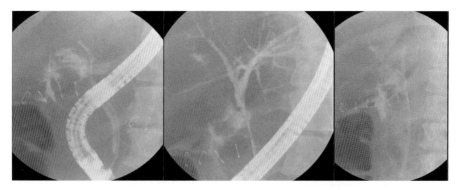

Fig. 7.3 *Left*: major bile duct leak after cholecystectomy (type B). *Middle*: passage of the diagnostic catheter into the proximal hepatic system. *Right*: after placement of a 14 cm 10 Fr stent, bypassing the defect.

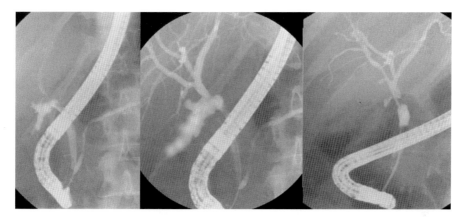

Fig. 7.4 *Left*: major bile duct leak after laparoscopic cholecystectomy (type B). *Middle*: passage of the diagnostic catheter into the proximal hepatic system. *Right*: situation 6 weeks after stent insertion: the leak has sealed but there is a subhilar stenosis (type C) that will require prolonged stent therapy.

in the early postoperative phase (general malaise, low-grade fever, marginally increased liver function tests). However, the patient's clinical condition may rapidly deteriorate after 3–5 days when ileus, peritonitis, and sepsis develop. Early aggressive investigation in patients with diffuse abdominal pain, fever, malaise, or liver function abnormalities after laparoscopic cholecystectomy is therefore mandatory [12,13].

Diagnostic protocol

The first step is to perform an abdominal ultrasound to investigate the presence of ductal dilatation or fluid collections [14]. Biliary dilatation is often absent (in our series in 71% of cases) [11] because the biliary system is decompressed by

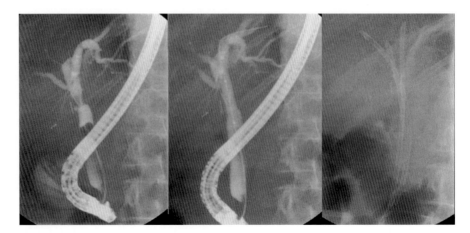

Fig. 7.5 *Left*: balloon occlusion cholangiogram showing a subhilar stenosis after cholecystectomy (type C). *Middle*: balloon dilation using an 8 mm dilation balloon passed over a guidewire. *Right*: placement of three 14 cm 10 Fr endoprostheses.

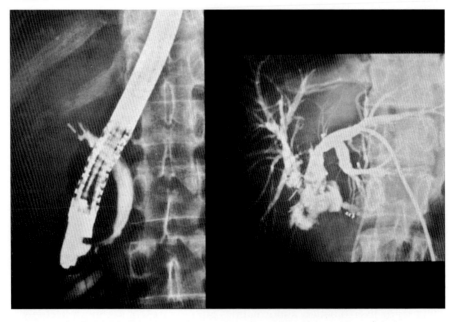

Fig. 7.6 *Left*: ERCP showing a total obstruction in the middle of the common bile duct. *Right*: PTC via the left hepatic system: there is communication between the left and right system and leakage at the site of the hilum. Part of the extrahepatic system has been accidentally resected during the laparoscopic cholecystectomy.

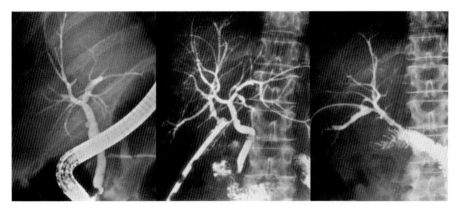

Fig. 7.7 Example of an isolated lesion of a segmental right hepatic duct. The patient had signs of bile leakage after cholecystectomy: an abdominal ultrasound showed a fluid collection and percutaneous drainage yielded bile. *Left*: ERCP showing an intact hepatic system without signs of leakage but the right hepatic system is not complete. *Middle*: fistulography through the percutaneous subhepatic drain showing two segments of the right hepatic system that are not in continuity with the remainder of the biliary system. *Right*: PTC of these two segments after construction of a surgical hepaticojejunostomy.

the leak. In the event of fluid collections, percutaneous needle aspiration may differentiate an abscess from a biloma [15]. When ductal dilatation is present or needle aspiration yields bile, an ERCP should be the next diagnostic procedure [11]. At ERCP, care should be taken that the whole biliary system is visualized. Bile leaks associated with the anatomical variant of a low-inserting right segmental hepatic duct can be particularly difficult to diagnose and ERCP results are often interpreted falsely as 'normal', with no leaks demonstrated (Fig. 7.7).

Management of bile duct leakage after cholecystectomy

Spontaneous resolution of bile leakage has been described in patients with external drains [16]. Some have therefore advocated a 'wait-and-see' policy in these patients and this seems justified in clinically stable patients without evidence of sepsis or peritonitis. However, if percutaneous bile leakage persists or the patient's clinical condition deteriorates, an ERCP is indicated. This will establish the diagnosis in all patients with types A, B, and C lesions and will allow for effective therapeutic intervention in most of them [11].

Type A injury (peripheral leaks)

Patients with bile leakage from the cystic duct or peripheral hepatic radicles are treated by insertion of a short biliary stent to lower the pressure of the biliary

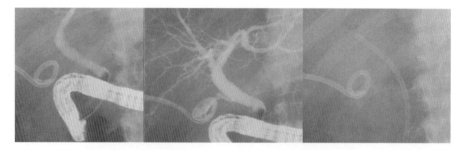

Fig. 7.8 Type A bile duct lesion after laparoscopic cholecystectomy treated with temporary stenting. *Left*: bile leakage originating from the cystic duct. *Middle*: insertion of a 6 cm 10 Fr stent to lower the pressure in the biliary system. A percutaneous drain can be seen on the left-hand side of the image. *Right*: situation after 6 weeks: no more leakage from the cystic stump.

system by bypassing the biliary sphincter (Fig. 7.8). The stent is preferably inserted without endoscopic sphincterotomy unless this is necessary to extract bile duct stones or gain biliary access. Endoscopic treatment is effective in 90% of patients with type A lesions, although 15–20% will require additional percutaneous drainage of a biloma [11]. Insertion of a stent gives the patient the burden of a second endoscopic intervention for removal of the stent but prevents a sphincterotomy that may cause acute and late complications. Placement of a nasobiliary tube is another option in treating leakage from minor bile ducts: closure of the leak can be monitored by repeating cholangiography, low pressure suction can be applied, and drain removal does not require an additional endoscopy [17,18]. However, nasobiliary tubes are not well tolerated by patients and long-term drainage may require recirculation of bile to prevent electrolyte disturbances [19].

Type B injury (main duct leaks)

Bile leakage from major bile ducts may be more challenging to treat endoscopically. Extensive duct damage and leakage can make it difficult to pass a guidewire into the proximal biliary system (Fig. 7.9). The presence of clips and stenoses (due to inflammatory reactions in the hepatoduodenal ligament) may also hamper passage into the proximal hepatic system or insertion of a stent. When ERCP fails, PTC and a rendezvous procedure should be the next step (Fig. 7.10). Endoscopic treatment is successful in approximately 75% of patients with leakage from major bile ducts [8,11,20]. An important late complication of bile leakage from major bile ducts is a secondary stenosis at the site of the leak (Fig. 7.4). Insertion of a stent not only adequately seals the bile leakage but also allows for prevention or treatment of secondary ductal stenosis.

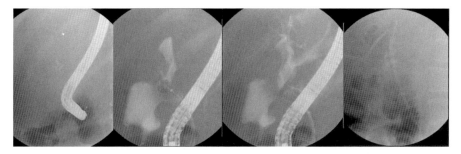

Fig. 7.9 Leakage from the common bile duct (CBD) after laparoscopic cholecystectomy (type B bile duct injury). *Far left*: ERCP showing presence of clips after laparoscopic cholecystectomy. *Middle left and right*: ERCP showing extensive leakage at the mid-CBD. An occlusion balloon is used to seal off the defect in the CBD and a guidewire is passed through a second catheter to access the proximal hepatic system. *Far right*: situation after insertion of a 14 cm 10 Fr stent.

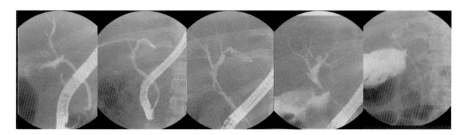

Fig. 7.10 Leakage from the common bile duct after laparoscopic cholecystectomy (type B bile duct injury). *Far left*: ERCP showing leakage of contrast 2 cm below the hepatic hilum. No access to the proximal hepatic system could be obtained and a PTCD via the right hepatic system was performed. *Middle left*: ERCP–PTC rendezvous procedure. Through the PTC-drain a guidewire is advanced into the duodenum where it is captured with a dormia and pulled into the duodenoscope. *Middle*: after removal of the PTC-drain, the guidewire is *in situ*. *Middle right*: a diagnostic catheter is advanced retrograde over the wire into the proximal hepatic system. *Far right*: situation after insertion of a 14 cm 10 Fr stent.

Type C injury (postoperative biliary strictures)

Most postoperative bile duct strictures are short (less than 10 mm in length) and situated distal to the confluence of the right and left hepatic ducts. Postoperative strictures are usually classified according to Bismuth by their position relative to the hepatic confluence [21].

Options for therapy include surgery, percutaneous balloon dilation and stenting, and endoscopic stenting, if necessary combined with balloon dilation. The different treatment options are discussed below.

Type D injury (transections)

Patients with complete transection of the bile duct are not amenable to endoscopic treatment because the distal and proximal biliary systems are not in continuity (Fig. 7.6). These patients should undergo reconstructive surgery: Roux-en-Y hepaticojejunostomy is the procedure of choice. The outcome of surgical management of these lesions is influenced by a variety of factors including proximal extent of the injury, type of reconstructive procedure performed, experience of the performing surgeon, timing of intervention, presence of proximal dilation and local inflammation at the time of the procedure, condition of the patient, and the length of follow-up. The timing of the procedure is a key factor determining the outcome of reconstructive surgery.

Delayed reconstruction

We observed that early complications and late anastomotic stenoses occurred in 80% of patients treated with early reconstructive surgery, whereas these complications were observed in only 17% of patients who underwent elective surgery after 8–12 weeks [11]. Reconstructive surgery in the acute postoperative phase, often started as a diagnostic procedure in a patient with peritonitis, ileus, or sepsis, is at risk for leakage and stenosis because of the absence of proximal dilatation and the presence of severe inflammatory changes of the tissue. Adequate drainage for 8–12 weeks through percutaneously placed drains allows for the acute local inflammatory reaction to subside and enables the surgeon to establish the exact proximal extent of the injury before surgery [22]. In most patients, a percutaneous transhepatic cholangiography and drainage (PTCD) is performed for this purpose and to delineate the proximal anatomy prior to the reconstruction [23]. The biliary system in these patients is often not dilated because it is decompressed by leak. A PTC may therefore be technically difficult and one may choose to drain the biloma by subhepatic and/or abdominal drains and to use MRCP and/or fistulography through these drains to delineate the proximal extent of the injury (Fig. 7.7).

Surgical treatment of postoperative biliary strictures

The outcome of surgery for benign biliary strictures is good in 75–93% of patients [22,24,25]. The treatment of choice is usually a Roux-en-Y hepaticojejunostomy. Anastomotic strictures develop later in approximately 20% of patients [24,26], and when a subsequent repair is undertaken, a further recurrence develops in 26% [27,28]. The majority of anastomotic stenoses develop within 7 years of surgery [28]. Reported surgical mortality rates are in the range of 3.2–27%, the higher rate being related to patients with coexisting pathology such as portal hypertension [24,25,27]. Factors that are associated with a favorable outcome include greater distance from the hepatic confluence, early referral, no previous repair, and the quality of the proximal duct.

It is important to note that there are only a few reports on the surgical treatment of patients with postoperative biliary strictures, and that most reports describe surgical treatment of more than a decade ago. Since then, surgeons have benefited from the improvement in endoscopic and invasive radiographic techniques. Nowadays, ultrasound, CT scanning, ERCP, and PTC provide surgeons with accurate preoperative information and allow for the optimal timing of the reconstructive procedure. Combined with improved surgical techniques, this may have resulted in an improved outcome of surgical treatment. Lillemoe *et al.* [23] have reported on a series of 156 patients undergoing surgical reconstruction for postoperative bile duct strictures. Two patients died of unrelated disease before completion of treatment; 12 patients had biliary stents in place at the time of the report. Of the 142 patients who completed treatment (mean follow-up 58 months), 91% were considered to have a successful outcome without the need for further interventional procedures.

Percutaneous treatment of postoperative strictures

Percutaneous dilation via transhepatic puncture or T-tube has an associated morbidity of less than 7% [29], but the reported success rates vary widely from 33 to 100% [29,30]. In general, percutaneous therapy requires several sessions to obtain a satisfactory outcome. In our hospital, patients undergo a PTC on the first day to obtain a diagnostic cholangiogram and to decompress the biliary system. The next day a percutaneous balloon dilation (8–10 mm balloon) is performed and an internal–external PTC-drain is inserted through the anastomosis. This drain is left *in situ* for 6 weeks and then removed after a second balloon dilatation procedure. Misra *et al.* recently reported their results in 51 patients. The success rate of percutaneous management without the need for subsequent interventions was 59% [31].

The major concerns with the transhepatic approach are the attendant risks of hemorrhage and bile leakage associated with liver puncture. Additionally, two-thirds of patients may have a non-dilated biliary tract, making ductal puncture technically difficult [32]. A further disadvantage is the requirement for long-term transhepatic intubation. In our unit, the percutaneous approach is mainly reserved for patients with postsurgical anastomotic stenoses (usually after hepaticojejunostomy) and as part of a rendezvous procedure with ERCP after a failed prior endoscopic approach (Fig. 7.10).

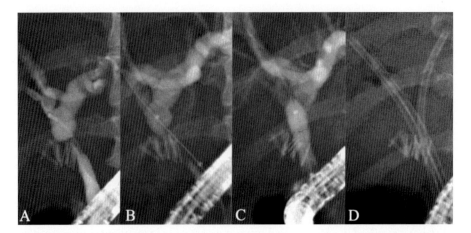

Fig. 7.11 Subhilar stenosis after laparoscopic cholecystectomy (type C lesion). (a) passage of the diagnostic catheter proximal to the stenosis. (b) a 3-cm 8-mm dilation balloon, indicated by two radiopaque markers, is passed over a guidewire. (c) inflation to 8 atmospheres pressure, showing nearly complete resolution of the stenosis at the site of the clips. (d) after insertion of three 10 Fr stents.

Endoscopic treatment of postoperative biliary strictures

Endoscopic management of patients with postoperative biliary strictures comprises endoscopic balloon dilation, placement of biliary stents, or a combination of the two.

Endoscopic balloon dilation can be performed with 4–8 mm diameter balloons that are passed over a prepositioned guidewire (Fig. 7.11). In the case of very tight strictures, dilating catheters can be used to facilitate advancement of the balloon catheter. Under fluoroscopic control the balloons are then inflated to 4–10 atmospheric pressures. The optimum duration of the maximum insufflation and the number of dilation cycles during one procedure are not well established. Usually balloon dilation does not result in complete disappearance of the waist in the balloon at the first procedure and thus multiple procedures are necessary for radiological resolution. Some preliminary data for endoscopic balloon dilation alone appeared favorable, but this was not confirmed in other studies [33].

Reported results

Many reports have been published on the outcome of endoscopic treatment in patients with postoperative strictures, but it is difficult to extrapolate general figures for success and complication rates and to determine what factors influence these outcome parameters. Virtually all series are retrospective single-

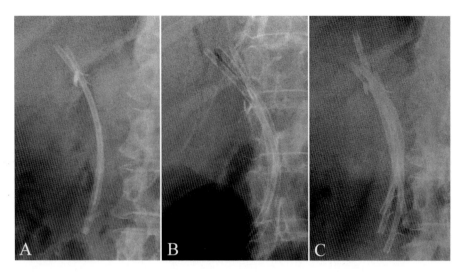

Fig. 7.12 Progressive increase in the number of inserted stents. (a) two stents inserted at the initial ERCP. (b) three stents inserted after 3 months. (c) four stents inserted after 6 months.

center reports on the treatment of a heterogeneous group of patients: isolated strictures and leaks, different mixtures of Bismuth localizations, with or without secondary cirrhosis at the time of treatment, with or without prior treatment before referral to expert centers, etc. Most series have included patients during a period of many years in which endoscopic protocols have changed. Many studies, therefore, describe study populations that have not been uniformly treated. Series with a relatively short follow-up period may reliably report early success and complication rates but will lack the rate of restenosis after stent removal. For this, long-term follow-up studies are required but these may suffer from the same drawbacks as the aforementioned antiquated surgical reports (e.g. the rate of early complications may be an overestimation of the current practice). In Fig. 7.14 (see p.155), the different phases of endoscopic management of postoperative bile duct stenoses are shown, as well as the outcome parameters of interest. This flow-chart should preferably be used as guidance for further reports on the endoscopic management of patients with postoperative bile duct stenoses.

An early study by our group found that a combination of balloon dilation and insertion of a 10 Fr polyethylene stent yielded satisfactory results in 21 of 27 patients during a follow-up period of 18 months [34]. Other investigators obtained similar results with this combination therapy [33,35–38]. The standard endoscopic technique nowadays involves placement of usually two stents during a maximum treatment period of 12 months (Figs 7.12 and 7.13). To prevent cholangitis due to clogging, stents are exchanged at 3-month intervals. The

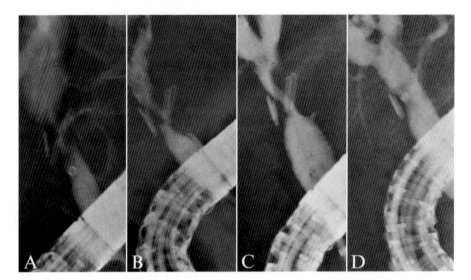

Fig. 7.13 Gradual resolution of a postsurgical bile duct stricture during stent therapy. (a) Situation at the initial ERCP. (b) After 3 months of stenting. (c) After 6 months. (d) After 12 months of stent therapy. (Reprinted from *Gastrointestinal Endoscopy*. Vol. 54(2). Bergman *et al*. Long-term follow-up after biliary stent placement for postoperative surgical stenosis, 2001: 154–61, with permission from American Society for Gastrointestinal Endoscopy.)

treatment protocol therefore consists of three phases: a *stent insertion phase*, a *stenting phase* with stents *in situ* and trimonthly stent exchange, and a *follow-up phase* after removal of the stents (Fig. 7.14).

One of the most comprehensive studies comes from Dumonceau and colleagues, who treated 48 patients with postoperative biliary strictures [39]. Endoscopic dilation of the strictures by means of dilating catheters or balloons was successful in 47 (98%). Four patients had self-expandable metal stents inserted and 43 received plastic stents that were electively exchanged every 6 months. Complications occurred in 6/48 patients (13%) after the initial ERCP. Stenting was maintained for a mean of 8.3 months (0.3–32 months) during which complications occurred in 20% of patients (mainly cholangitis or mild fever after elective stent exchange). Five patients discontinued the stenting phase but in only one patient was this due to complications. In 38 patients, the endoscopic treatment was completed: 36 had stricture dilation judged to be satisfactory during a stent exchange and had no new stents inserted. In two patients, plastic stents were replaced by Wallstents. After removal of the stents, the 36 patients were followed up for a mean period of 44 months (1–130 months). In seven patients (19%), the strictures recurred, with all but one of these occurring within 1 year of stent removal.

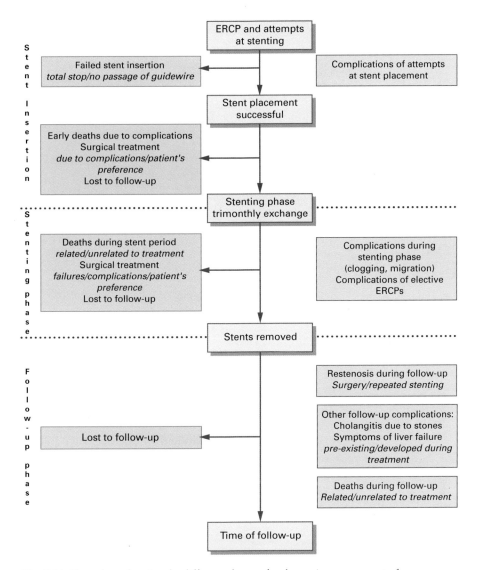

Fig. 7.14 Flow-chart showing the different phases of endoscopic management of postoperative bile duct strictures and the outcome parameters of interest. This flow-chart should preferably be used as guidance for further reports on the endoscopic management of patients with postoperative bile duct strictures.

Our group has performed a retrospective analysis of 63 patients with incomplete biliary strictures [40]. Stent insertion was successful in 59 (94%). After the initial ERCP, early complications occurred in 13 patients (20%), whereas 19 patients (33%) suffered from complications during the stenting phase (mainly cholangitis). Stents were eventually removed in 44 patients after a median

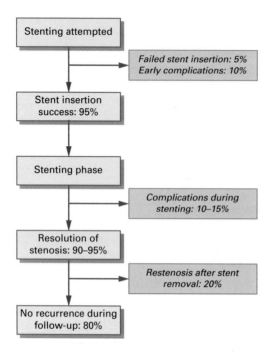

Fig. 7.15 In this flow-chart, the results of endoscopic treatment of postoperative biliary strictures are summarized.

period of 12 months (3–37 months). During a median follow-up period of 109 months (2–180 months), restenosis occurred in nine patients (20%) and all cases of restenosis occurred within 2 years of follow-up.

In Fig. 7.15, the results of endoscopic treatment of postoperative biliary strictures are summarized.

Phases of endoscopic treatment

Stent insertion phase

Stent insertion is successful in about 95% of patients with incomplete ductal strictures [39,40]. In patients with a total ductal obstruction, endoscopic treatment is not possible. Since an ERCP is required to make this diagnosis, these patients are inevitably failures of endoscopic treatment. In a strict sense these patients do not have a true stenosis and most studies have therefore limited the inclusion to patients with *incomplete* ductal stenosis [39,41]. Early complications are mainly sphincterotomy-related or reflect the patient's condition (e.g. pre-existent fever in the case of bile leakage). Dumonceau *et al.* [39] reported early complications in six of their 48 patients (12.5%), whereas Costamagna *et al.* observed four complications in 45 patients (9%) [41]. In our series, an early complication rate as high as 19% was observed. This study, however, was performed to evaluate the long-term outcome of endoscopic treatment, and patients were treated 10–15 years ago [40]. With the current endoscopic standards, early complications should not be observed in more than 10% of patients.

Stenting phase

Since the stenting phase covers a period of up to 1 year, complications are not uncommon (33% and 20% in the aforementioned studies, respectively). Dumonceau *et al.* used an interval of 6 months between elective ERCPs and this may be too long given the average time to stent occlusion reported in other studies [39]. In our retrospective study, complications during the stenting period mainly occurred in cases in which the patients and/or referring physicians did not adhere to the treatment protocol [40]. Many years have passed since then, and the endoscopic treatment of patients with benign biliary strictures has become more accepted. Currently, in patients in whom elective trimonthly ERCPs are performed, complications due to stent dysfunction are mild and occur at a maximum of 10–15% during a stenting period of 1 year. With this regimen, 90–95% of patients will have their stenosis adequately dilated within 1 year.

Follow-up phase

Studies have reported a recurrence rate of 20% after removal of the stents [39,40]. In the series of Dumonceau *et al.*, 36 patients were followed for a mean period of 44 months after removal of the stents, whereas our group followed 44 patients for a median period of 9.1 years after stent removal. It is important to note that almost all cases of restenosis occurred relatively early after removal of the stents: only one patient was diagnosed with recurrent stenosis after more than 6 months and all cases occurred within 2 years of stent removal. This suggests that endoscopic treatment of postsurgical stenoses is not associated with a high rate of *long-term* restenosis after stent removal, as suggested by antagonists of this treatment regimen. This is in contrast to the anastomotic recurrences after hepaticojejunostomy, which may occur after many years [28]. It also implies that strict follow-up after stent removal is necessary, especially during the first 6–12 months, in order to diagnose restenosis at an early stage.

It is important to note that, apart from recurrence of the initial stenosis, other late complications may also occur after stent removal, e.g. cholangitis from bile duct stones or symptoms associated with (pre-existing) liver failure [40,41]. Bile duct stones may develop because of impeded bile flow due to a relative stenosis; however, since all patients initially underwent biliary surgery for stone disease, the underlying stone disease may also be held responsible [42].

Table 7.1 Retrospective comparison of surgery with endoscopy in the management of postoperative biliary strictures.

	Surgery	Endoscopy
No. of patients	35	66
Early complications	26	8
Thirty-day mortality	0	1
Complications in 1 year	0	27
Outcome assessment[b] (no. of patients)	35	46[a]
Excellent	25	33
Good	4	5
Poor	6	8

[a]Stents were eventually removed in 46 patients in the endoscopy group.
[b]Excellent results were defined as asymptomatic and normal or stable liver function tests; good results as occurrence of only one episode of cholangitis; poor results as recurrent cholangitis or stricture.

Postoperative biliary strictures: surgery or endoscopy [43]?

Prospective randomized studies comparing surgical and endoscopic treatment of postoperative biliary strictures are not available. We have performed a retrospective study comparing surgical with endoscopic therapy (Table 7.1) [26]. Both approaches were found to have a similar long-term success rate, with recurrences being seen in 17% of patients.

Since there appear to be no clear differences in the primary outcomes between surgical and endoscopic management, the choice between the two is determined by other factors: the two most important ones are the different characteristics of restenosis and patients' preference.

Recurrent strictures after surgery

The diagnosis of anastomotic stenosis after hepaticojejunostomy may be difficult since most patients already have mild liver function abnormalities and dilatation of the biliary tree on ultrasound is often absent [44]. After Roux-en-Y hepaticojejunostomy, endoscopic approach to the biliary tree is usually not possible. Most physicians are reluctant to perform a PTC in these patients because of the risk of hemorrhage and bile leakage, especially in cases of non-dilated bile ducts [32]. In patients with prior endoscopic treatment of bile duct strictures, diagnosis of recurrent stenosis is easier, safer, and therefore associated with less medical delay (which may cause secondary biliary cirrhosis). Furthermore, restenosis after endoscopic treatment occurs relatively early after stent removal (less than 1–2 years) [40,45], whereas anastomotic recurrences after surgery may develop after more than 10 years [28].

Treatment of recurrent stenosis after hepaticojejunostomy involves either percutaneous balloon dilation, often supplemented with internal–external stenting, or repeated surgery. Nowadays, most patients with anastomotic stenosis are initially managed by percutaneous treatment, but multiple sessions are often required and the cumulative morbidity due to bleeding and bile leakage may be as high as 30%. Repeat surgery will eventually be required in 20–30% of these patients. Compared to primary hepaticojejunostomy, repeated reconstructive surgery is associated with a higher complication and failure rate [27,28].

Whereas endoscopic treatment is impossible once a Roux-en-Y loop has been constructed, prior endoscopic treatment does not preclude further surgical treatment. In addition, recurrent strictures after prior endoscopic therapy can also be successfully treated by repeated stenting. Finally, although endoscopic treatment requires multiple ERCPs, many patients and their referring doctors prefer endoscopic treatment to surgery.

Therefore, we feel that surgery should be reserved for patients with failed endoscopic therapy or for patients who refuse endoscopic therapy.

Metal stents for benign strictures

The use of metal expandable stents in benign biliary disease remains controversial. Initially, several groups reported favorable results in the management of postoperative strictures. Gianturco–Rösch Z-Stents were placed percutaneously in 43 such patients by Coons [46]. All patients had previously undergone an unsuccessful balloon cholangioplasty. The 1-year reocclusion rate was 13%. Maccioni et al. reported long-term patency in 100% of patients with a CBD stricture [47]. Foerster et al., reporting on endoscopic Wallstent placement in four patients, identified no stent-related complications and no cases of occlusion during a follow-up period of 53 weeks [48]. More recent follow-up studies, however, have obtained less satisfactory results. Hausegger et al. reported that the patency rate rapidly decreased to 19% at 57 months of follow-up [49]. Dumonceau et al. reported a 100% occlusion rate of Wallstents inserted in six patients with postoperative strictures within 48 months of follow-up [45]. Lopez et al. reported a good clinical result, arbitrarily defined as the need for two or fewer invasive interventions, in only five out of 15 patients. The remaining 10 patients underwent multiple interventions, including surgery in five with a poor general outcome [50].

Studies in dogs have demonstrated marked bile duct narrowing related to extensive fibrosis after insertion of Wallstents but only minimal changes after

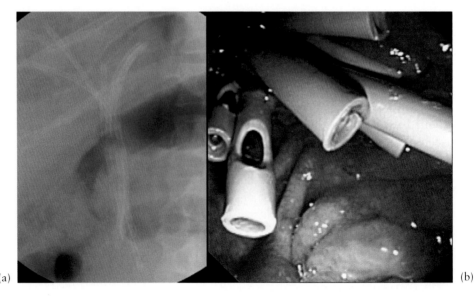

(a)
(b)

Fig. 7.16 Multiple stents inserted for treatment of a postoperative biliary stricture.
(a) Plain X-ray after ERCP. (b) View from the duodenum after insertion of seven 10 Fr
biliary stents.

insertion of plastic or covered metal stents [51]. An important disadvantage of metallic stents is that they cannot be removed once they become obstructed. Because of these results, we do not advise inserting metallic stents in this context. The advent of removable expandable stents may, however, alter this situation in the future [52].

A more aggressive treatment protocol?

Currently, the standard protocol for patients with benign strictures involves placement of two stents during a maximum treatment period of 12 months. Recently, a more aggressive treatment protocol has been suggested in which there is no maximum period of stenting and as many stents as possible are inserted in order to obtain maximum dilatation. Costamagna and colleagues treated 45 patients with such an aggressive protocol [41]. They inserted as many stents as possible according to the downstream duct diameter (Fig. 7.16). Endoscopic treatment was discontinued only if the stricture was considered to be adequately dilated on fluoroscopy. A mean number of 3.2 stents were inserted (range 1–6 stents) for a mean duration of 12 months (range 2–24 months). Forty-two patients completed the treatment protocol; all stenoses resolved and none of the 42 patients suffered from restenosis during a median period of follow-up of 29 months (range 24 months to 11.3 years). These impressive results suggest that a more prolonged and aggressive endoscopic approach may be justified in more difficult cases.

Conclusions

Although most centers performing laparoscopic cholecystectomy may now be well beyond the 'learning-curve' phase, the incidence of postsurgical bile duct injuries will probably stay higher than in the era before laparoscopic cholecystectomy. In addition, with surgeons embarking on more complex laparoscopic biliary interventions, such as laparoscopic duct exploration, a further increase in the incidence of surgical bile duct injuries may be expected in the near future. Adequate management of these injuries requires an early postoperative diagnosis with a low threshold for performing an ERCP. Patients with type D lesions (complete ductal transection) require an elective surgical repair, 6–8 weeks after diagnosis and drainage. Most of the other bile duct injuries (minor leaks from the cystic stump or peripheral hepatic radicles, major bile duct leaks, and isolated bile duct strictures) can in general be managed endoscopically.

Patients who require long-term stenting for bile duct strictures should be treated with at least two 10 Fr plastic stents that are electively exchanged every 3 months. If possible, more than two stents should be inserted. There is currently no place for self-expandable metal stents for this indication.

Optimal management of patients with bile duct injuries requires a multidisciplinary team approach of interventional radiology, therapeutic endoscopy, and reconstructive surgery.

Outstanding issues and future trends

Most controversies connected to the management of postsurgical bile duct lesions relate to the treatment of biliary stenoses. There are still many questions concerning the optimal endoscopic management of these patients. Should stent placement always be preceded by balloon dilation? How many stents should be inserted? What is the optimal period of stenting? Some groups treat patients only for a relatively short time (e.g. 6 months) before deciding on success or failure. Others do not have a maximum period of stenting and attempt to insert as many stents as possible in order to obtain maximum dilatation.

With such an aggressive endoscopic treatment protocol, however, the question arises of what are the long-term effects of stenting on the biliary system. Studies using intraductal ultrasonography have shown that stenting induces profound thickening and fibrosis of the bile duct wall that occurs as soon as 2 weeks after insertion of a single plastic endoprosthesis [53]. Placing multiple stents for a period of over 1 year might thus reduce the chances of a successful surgical reconstruction if endoscopic treatment should fail. In the near future, the use of biodegradable self-expandable stents that gradually dissolve after 1–2 years, or the insertion of covered self-expandable stents that can be removed, might be options.

Which subset of patients will most likely benefit from endoscopic management? The impression exists that patients in whom the stricture is diagnosed relatively early after surgery have a better prognosis than patients who present a long time after surgery, but this has not been substantiated in follow-up studies. Patients with more proximal lesions are more difficult to treat and some experts have advised primary surgical treatment in patients with hilar strictures [54]. Multivariate analysis of large cohorts of patients will be necessary to solve these issues.

References

1 McMahon AJ, Russell IT, Baxter JN et al. Laparoscopic versus minilaparotomy cholecystectomy: a randomised trial [see comments]. Lancet 1994; 343 (8890): 135–8.
2 Gouma DJ, Go PM. Bile duct injury during laparoscopic and conventional cholecystectomy. J Am Coll Surg 1994; 178 (3): 229–33.
3 Glenn F. Iatrogenic injuries to the biliary ductal system. Surg Gynecol Obstet 1978; 146 (3): 430–4.
4 Way LW, Bernhoft RA, Thomas MJ. Biliary stricture. Surg Clin North Am 1981; 61 (4): 963–72.
5 The Southern Surgeons Club. A prospective analysis of 1518 laparoscopic cholecystectomies. N Eng J Med 1991; 324 (16): 1073–8.
6 Deziel DJ, Millikan KW, Economou SG et al. Complications of laparoscopic cholecystectomy: a national survey of 4292 hospitals and an analysis of 77 604 cases. Am J Surg 1993; 165 (1): 9–14.
7 Terblanche J, Allison HF, Northover JM. An ischemic basis for biliary strictures. Surgery 1983; 94 (1): 52–7.
8 Woods MS, Traverso LW, Kozarek RA et al. Characteristics of biliary tract complications during laparoscopic cholecystectomy: a multi-institutional study. Am J Surg 1994; 167 (1): 27–33.
9 Schol FP, Go PM, Gouma DJ. Risk factors for bile duct injury in laparoscopic cholecystectomy, analysis of 49 cases [see comments]. Br J Surg 1994; 81 (12): 1786–8.
10 Boerma D, Rauws EA, Keulemans YC et al. Impaired quality of life 5 years after bile duct injury during laparoscopic cholecystectomy: a prospective analysis. Ann Surg 2001; 234 (6): 750–7.
11 Bergman JJ, van den Brink GR, Rauws EA et al. Treatment of bile duct lesions after laparoscopic cholecystectomy. Gut 1996; 38 (1): 141–7.
12 Rossi RL, Schirmer WJ, Braasch JW et al. Laparoscopic bile duct injuries: risk factors, recognition, and repair. Arch Surg 1992; 127 (5): 596–601.
13 Davidoff AM, Pappas TN, Murray EA et al. Mechanisms of major biliary injury during laparoscopic cholecystectomy [see comments]. Ann Surg 1992; 215 (3): 196–202.
14 Ress AM, Sarr MG, Nagorney DM et al. Spectrum and management of major complications of laparoscopic cholecystectomy. Am J Surg 1993; 165 (6): 655–62.
15 Mueller PR, Ferrucci JTJ, Simeone JF et al. Detection and drainage of bilomas: special considerations. AJR Am J Roentgenol 1983; 140 (4): 715–20.
16 Albasini JL, Aledo VS, Dexter SP et al. Bile leakage following laparoscopic cholecystectomy. Surg Endosc 1995; 9 (12): 1274–8.

17 Chow S, Bosco JJ, Heiss FW *et al.* Successful treatment of post-cholecystectomy bile leaks using nasobiliary tube drainage and sphincterotomy. *Am J Gastroenterol* 1997; 92 (10): 1839–43.

18 Saab S, Martin P, Soliman GY *et al.* Endoscopic management of biliary leaks after T-tube removal in liver transplant recipients: nasobiliary drainage versus biliary stenting. *Liver Transpl Surg* 2000; 6 (5): 627–32.

19 Wills VL, Gibson K, Karihaloot C *et al.* Complications of biliary T-tubes after choledochotomy. *Aust NZ J Surg* 2002; 72 (3): 177–80.

20 Traverso LW, Kozarek RA, Ball TJ *et al.* Endoscopic retrograde cholangiopancreatography after laparoscopic cholecystectomy. *Am J Surg* 1993; 165 (5): 581–6.

21 Bismuth H. (1982) Postoperative strictures of the bile duct. In: *The Biliary Tract* (ed. Blumgart, LH), pp. 209–18. Churchill Livingstone, Edinburgh.

22 Nealon WH, Urrutia F. Long-term follow-up after bilioenteric anastomosis for benign bile duct stricture. *Ann Surg* 1996; 223 (6): 639–45.

23 Lillemoe KD, Melton GB, Cameron JL *et al.* Postoperative bile duct strictures: management and outcome in the 1990s. *Ann Surg* 2000; 232 (3): 430–41.

24 Raute M, Podlech P, Jaschke W *et al.* Management of bile duct injuries and strictures following cholecystectomy. *World J Surg* 1993; 17 (4): 553–62.

25 Chapman WC, Halevy A, Blumgart LH *et al.* Postcholecystectomy bile duct strictures: management and outcome in 130 patients. *Arch Surg* 1995; 130 (6): 597–602.

26 Davids PH, Tanka AK, Rauws EA *et al.* Benign biliary strictures. Surgery or endoscopy? *Ann Surg* 1993; 217 (3): 237–43.

27 Genest JF, Nanos E, Grundfest-Broniatowski S *et al.* Benign biliary strictures: an analytic review (1970–84). *Surgery* 1986; 99 (4): 409–13.

28 Pitt HA, Miyamoto T, Parapatis SK *et al.* Factors influencing outcome in patients with postoperative biliary strictures. *Am J Surg* 1982; 144 (1): 14–21.

29 Mueller PR, vanSonnenberg E, Ferrucci JTJ *et al.* Biliary stricture dilatation: multicenter review of clinical management in 73 patients. *Radiology* 1986; 160 (1): 17–22.

30 Citron SJ, Martin LG. Benign biliary strictures: treatment with percutaneous cholangioplasty. *Radiology* 1991; 178 (2): 339–41.

31 Misra S, Melton GB, Geschwind JF *et al.* Percutaneous management of bile duct strictures and injuries associated with laparoscopic cholecystectomy: a decade of experience. *J Am Coll Surg* 2004; 198 (2): 218–26.

32 Speer AG, Cotton PB, Russell RC *et al.* Randomised trial of endoscopic versus percutaneous stent insertion in malignant obstructive jaundice. *Lancet* 1987; 2 (8550): 57–62.

33 Geenen DJ, Geenen JE, Hogan WJ *et al.* Endoscopic therapy for benign bile duct strictures. *Gastrointest Endosc* 1989; 35 (5): 367–71.

34 Huibregtse K, Katon RM, Tytgat GN. Endoscopic treatment of postoperative biliary strictures. *Endoscopy* 1986; 18 (4): 133–7.

35 Berkelhammer C, Kortan P, Haber GB. Endoscopic biliary prostheses as treatment for benign postoperative bile duct strictures. *Gastrointest Endosc* 1989; 35 (2): 95–101.

36 Davids PH, Rauws EA, Coene PP *et al.* Endoscopic stenting for post-operative biliary strictures. *Gastrointest Endosc* 1992; 38 (1): 12–8.

37 Cunningham JT, Draganov PV, Rawls E *et al.* Long term outcomes in patients with benign biliary stricture treated endoscopically with multiple stents. *Gastrointest Endosc* 1998; 47 (4): AB112.

38 Weber J, Adamek HE, Riemann JF. Endoscopic stent placement and clip removal for common bile duct stricture after laparoscopic cholecystectomy. *Gastrointest Endosc* 1992; 38 (2): 181–2.

39 Dumonceau JM, Deviere J, Delhaye M *et al.* Plastic and metal stents for postoperative benign bile duct strictures: the best and the worst [see comments]. *Gastrointest Endosc* 1998; 47 (1): 8–17.

40 Bergman JJ, Burgemeister L, Bruno MJ *et al.* Long-term follow-up after biliary stent placement for postoperative bile duct stenosis. *Gastrointest Endosc* 2001; 54 (2): 154–61.

41 Costamagna G, Pandolfi M, Mutignani M *et al.* Long-term results of endoscopic management of postoperative bile duct strictures with increasing numbers of stents. *Gastrointest Endosc* 2001; 54 (2): 162–8.

42 Bergman JJ, van der Mey S, Rauws EA *et al.* Long-term follow-up after endoscopic sphinctero-tomy for bile duct stones in patients younger than 60 years of age [see comments]. *Gastrointest Endosc* 1996; 44 (6): 643–9.

43 De Palma GD, Galloro G, Romano G *et al.* Long-term follow-up after endoscopic biliary stent placement for bile duct strictures from laparoscopic cholecystectomy. *Hepatogastroenterology* 2003; 50 (53): 1229–31.

44 Plaisier PW, van der Hul RL, Lameris JS *et al.* Routine testing of liver function after biliary-enteric anastomosis has no clinical relevance. *Hepatogastroenterology* 2001; 48 (39): 622–4.

45 Dumonceau JM, Deviere J, Delhaye M *et al.* Plastic and metal stents for postoperative benign bile duct strictures: the best and the worst. *Gastrointest Endosc* 1998; 47 (1): 8–17.

46 Coons H. Metallic stents for the treatment of biliary obstruction: a report of 100 cases. *Cardiovasc Intervent Radiol* 1992; 15 (6): 367–74.

47 Maccioni F, Bezzi M, Gandini R *et al.* [Metallic stents in benign biliary stenosis: a four-year follow-up]. [Italian]. *Radiol Med (Torino)* 1993; 86 (3): 294–301.

48 Foerster EC, Hoepffner N, Domschke W. Bridging of benign choledochal stenoses by endo-scopic retrograde implantation of mesh stents. *Endoscopy* 1991; 23 (3): 133–5.

49 Hausegger KA, Kugler C, Uggowitzer M *et al.* Benign biliary obstruction: is treatment with the Wallstent advisable? *Radiology* 1996; 200 (2): 437–41.

50 Lopez RR Jr, Cosenza CA, Lois J *et al.* Long-term results of metallic stents for benign biliary strictures. *Arch Surg* 2001; 136 (6): 664–9.

51 Silvis SE, Sievert CEJ, Vennes JA *et al.* Comparison of covered versus uncovered wire mesh stents in the canine biliary tract. *Gastrointest Endosc* 1994; 40 (1): 17–21.

52 Goldin E, Beyar M, Safra T *et al.* A new self-expandable and removable metal stent for biliary obstruction: a preliminary report. *Endoscopy* 1993; 25 (9): 597–9.

53 Tamada K, Tomiyama T, Ichiyama M *et al.* Influence of biliary drainage catheter on bile duct wall thickness as measured by intraductal ultrasonography. *Gastrointest Endosc* 1998; 47 (1): 28–32.

54 Draganov P, Hoffman B, Marsh W *et al.* Long-term outcome in patients with benign biliary strictures treated endoscopically with multiple stents. *Gastrointest Endosc* 2002; 55 (6): 680–6.

CHAPTER 8

Sphincter of Oddi Dysfunction

EVAN L. FOGEL AND STUART SHERMAN

Synopsis

Sphincter of Oddi dysfunction (SOD) refers to a motor abnormality of the sphincter of Oddi, typically resulting in a hypertonic sphincter, and may be manifested clinically by chronic abdominal pain, pancreatitis, or abnormal liver function tests. In this chapter, we discuss the classification systems typically used in SOD, as well as the epidemiology of this controversial disease. The diagnostic criteria for SOD and appropriate evaluation of patients are reviewed. Both non-invasive and invasive diagnostic methods are discussed. Sphincter of Oddi manometry (SOM) is the only available method to measure motor activity directly, and is considered currently to be the diagnostic gold standard. Indications, performance, and complications of this technique are reviewed. Therapy for SOD is discussed, using an evidence-based approach.

Introduction

Since its original description by Ruggero Oddi in 1887, the sphincter of Oddi (SO) has been the subject of much study and controversy. Its very existence as a distinct anatomical or physiological entity has been disputed. Hence, it is not surprising that the clinical syndrome of sphincter of Oddi dysfunction (SOD) and its therapy are controversial areas [1]. Nevertheless, SOD is commonly diagnosed and treated by physicians, most often (but not exclusively) amongst patients who have residual or recurrent symptoms after cholecystectomy, and in whom more common organic causes have been excluded [2]. This chapter reviews the epidemiology and clinical presentation of SOD, as well as currently available diagnostic and therapeutic modalities.

Definitions

A distinction is sometimes made between SOD and true sphincter stenosis.

Sphincter of Oddi dysfunction

SOD refers to an abnormality of SO contractility. It is a benign, non-calculus obstruction to flow of bile or pancreatic juice through the pancreatico-biliary junction, i.e. the SO. SOD may be manifested clinically by 'pancreatico-biliary' pain, pancreatitis, or abnormal liver function tests. SO dyskinesia refers to a motor abnormality of the SO, which may result in a hypotonic sphincter but, more commonly, causes a hypertonic sphincter.

Sphincter of Oddi stenosis

In contrast, SO stenosis refers to a structural alteration of the sphincter, probably from an inflammatory process, with subsequent fibrosis.

Classification of SOD

Since it is often impossible to distinguish patients with SO dyskinesia from those with SO stenosis, the term SOD has been used to incorporate both groups of patients. A variety of less accurate terms—such as papillary stenosis, ampullary stenosis, biliary dyskinesia, and postcholecystectomy syndrome—are listed in the medical literature to describe this entity. The latter term is somewhat of a misnomer, as SOD may clearly occur with an intact gallbladder.

In an attempt to deal with this confusion, and also to determine the appropriate utilization of SO manometry (SOM), a biliary clinical classification system has been developed for patients with suspected SOD (Hogan–Geenen SOD classification system; Table 8.1) based on clinical history, laboratory results, and endoscopic retrograde cholangiopancreatography (ERCP) findings [3]. A pancreatic classification has also been developed, but is less commonly utilized [4] (Table 8.2). Both the biliary and pancreatic classification systems have been modified [5], making them more applicable for clinical use, as biliary and pancreatic drainage times have been abandoned.

Epidemiology

SOD may occur in pediatric or adult patients of any age; however, patients with SOD are typically middle-aged females [6]. Although SOD most commonly occurs after cholecystectomy, it may be present with the gallbladder *in situ*. In a survey on functional gastrointestinal disorders, SOD appeared to have a significant impact on the quality of life, as it was highly associated with work absenteeism, disability, and health care use [7].

Table 8.1 Hogan–Geenen biliary sphincter of Oddi classification system (post-cholecystectomy) related to the frequency of abnormal sphincter of Oddi manometry and pain relief by biliary sphincterotomy.

| Patient group classifications | Approximate frequency of abnormal sphincter manometry | Probability of pain relief by sphincterotomy if manometry: | | Manometry before sphincter ablation |
		Abnormal	Normal	
Biliary Type I Patients with biliary-type pain, abnormal SGOT or alkaline phosphatase > 2 × normal documented on two or more occasions, delayed drainage of ERCP contrast from the biliary tree > 45 min, and dilated CBD > 12 mm diameter	75–95%	90–95%	90–95%	Unnecessary
Biliary Type II Patients with biliary-type pain but only one or two of the above criteria	55–65%	85%	35%	Highly recommended
Biliary Type III Patients with only biliary-type pain and no other abnormalities	25–60%	55–65%	< 10%	Mandatory

Table 8.2 Pancreatic sphincter of Oddi classification system.

Patient group classification

Pancreatic Type I
Patients with pancreatic-type pain, abnormal amylase or lipase 1.5 × normal on any occasion, delayed drainage of ERCP contrast from the pancreatic duct > 9 min, and dilated PD > 6 mm diameter in the head or 5 mm in the body

Pancreatic Type II
Patients with pancreatic-type pain but only one or two of the above criteria

Pancreatic Type III
Patients with only pancreatic-type pain and no other abnormalities

SOD in patients with gallbladder disease

The frequency of manometrically documented SOD in patients prior to cholecystectomy has received limited study. Guelrud and colleagues [8] evaluated 121 patients with symptomatic gallstones and a normal common bile duct diameter (by transcutaneous ultrasound) by SOM prior to cholecystectomy. An elevated basal sphincter pressure was found in 14 patients (11.6%). SOD was diagnosed in 4.1% of patients with a normal serum alkaline phosphatase (4 of 96) and in 40% with an elevated serum alkaline phosphatase (10 of 25). Ruffolo and associates evaluated 81 patients with symptoms suggestive of biliary disease, but normal ERCP and no gallbladder stones on transcutaneous ultrasound, by scintigraphic gallbladder ejection fraction and endoscopic SOM [9]. Fifty-three per cent of patients had SOD and 49% had an abnormal gallbladder ejection fraction. SOD occurred with a similar frequency in patients with an abnormal gallbladder ejection fraction (50%) and a normal ejection fraction (57%).

SOD after cholecystectomy

The frequency of diagnosing SOD in reported series varies considerably with the patient selection criteria, the definition of SOD, and the diagnostic tools employed. In a British report, SOD was diagnosed in 41 (9%) of 451 consecutive patients being evaluated for postcholecystectomy pain [10]. Roberts-Thomson and Toouli evaluated 431 similar patients and found SOD in 47 (11%). In a subpopulation of such patients with a normal ERCP (except dilated ducts in 28%) and recurrent pain of more than 3 months' duration, SOD was diagnosed in 68% [11]. Sherman and colleagues used SOM to evaluate 115 patients with pancreaticobiliary pain with and without liver function test abnormalities [4]. Patients with bile duct stones and tumors were excluded from the analysis. Fifty-nine of 115 patients (51%) showed abnormal basal SO pressure greater than 40 mmHg. These patients were further categorized by the Hogan–Geenen SOD classification system (Table 8.1). The frequency of abnormal manometry of a single sphincter segment was 86%, 55%, and 28%, for Type I, II, and III patients, respectively. These abnormal manometric frequencies were very similar to those reported by others for Type I and Type II patients [12,13]. In biliary Type III patients, the finding of an abnormal basal sphincter pressure has varied from 12% to 55% [14]. As noted, patient selection factors may be one explanation for this great variability.

SOD in the biliary or pancreatic sphincter, or both

SOD can involve abnormalities in the biliary sphincter, pancreatic sphincter, or both. The true frequency of SOD therefore depends on whether one or both sphincters are studied. Eversman and colleagues performed manometry of the biliary and pancreatic sphincter segments in 360 patients with pancreatico-biliary pain and intact sphincters [5]. In this large series, 19% had abnormal pancreatic basal sphincter pressure alone, 11% had abnormal biliary basal sphincter pressure alone, and, in 31%, the basal sphincter pressure was abnormal in both segments (overall frequency of sphincter dysfunction was 61%). Among the 214 patients labeled as Type III, 17%, 11%, and 31% had elevated basal sphincter pressure in the pancreatic sphincter alone, biliary sphincter alone, or both segments, respectively (overall frequency of SOD 59%). In the 123 Type II patients, SOD was diagnosed in 65%: 22%, 11%, and 32% had elevated basal sphincter pressure in the pancreatic sphincter only, biliary sphincter only, or both sphincter segments, respectively. Similar findings were reported by Aymerich and colleagues [15]. In a series of 73 patients with suspected SOD, basal pressures were normal in both segments in 19%, abnormal in both segments in 40%, and abnormal in one segment but normal in the other in 41%. The negative predictive value of normal biliary basal sphincter pressure in excluding SOD was 0.42; when the pancreatic basal sphincter pressure was normal, the negative predictive value was 0.58. These two studies clearly suggest that both the bile duct and pancreatic duct must be evaluated when assessing the sphincter by SOM.

SOD and pancreatitis

Dysfunction may occur in the pancreatic duct portion of the SO and cause recurrent pancreatitis. As noted earlier, a pancreatic SOD classification system has been developed (Table 8.2), but has not been widely utilized [5]. Manometrically documented SOD has been reported in 15% to 72% of patients with recurrent pancreatitis, previously labeled as idiopathic [5,12,16].

Clinical presentation

Abdominal pain is the most common presenting symptom of patients with SOD. The pain is usually epigastric or right upper quadrant, may be disabling, and lasts from 30 min to several hours. In some patients the pain is continuous with episodic exacerbations. It may radiate to the back or shoulder and be accompanied by nausea and vomiting. Food or narcotics may precipitate the pain. The pain may begin several years after a cholecystectomy was performed for a gallbladder dysmotility or stone disease and is similar in character to the pain leading to the cholecystectomy. Alternatively, patients may have continued pain that was not relieved by a cholecystectomy. Jaundice, fever, or chills are rarely observed.

The Rome criteria

Recently, a symposium on functional disorders of the pancreas and biliary tree established the Rome II diagnostic criteria [6] for SOD. These include episodes of severe abdominal pain located in the epigastrium and/or right upper quadrant, and all of the following: (1) symptom episodes lasting 30 min or more with pain-free intervals; (2) symptoms have occurred on one or more occasions in the previous 12 months; (3) the pain is steady and interrupts daily activities or requires consultation with a physician; and (4) there is no evidence of structural abnormalities to explain the symptoms. Physical examination is typically characterized only by mild epigastric or right upper quadrant tenderness. The pain is not relieved by trial medications for acid peptic disease or irritable bowel syndrome. Laboratory abnormalities consisting of transient elevation of liver function tests, typically during episodes of pain, are present in less than 50% of patients. After initial evaluation, patients are commonly categorized according to the Hogan–Geenen SOD classification system (Table 8.1). Patients with SOD may present with typical pancreatic pain (epigastric or left upper quadrant radiating to the back) and recurrent pancreatitis.

SOD may exist in the presence of an intact gallbladder [17]. As the symptoms of SOD and gallbladder dysfunction cannot be reliably separated, the diagnosis of SOD is commonly made after cholecystectomy or less frequently after gallbladder abnormalities have been excluded [6].

Initial evaluation

The diagnostic approach to suspected SOD may be influenced by the presence of key clinical features. However, the clinical manifestations of functional abnormalities of the SO may not always be easily distinguishable from those caused by organic conditions (e.g. common bile duct stones) or other functional non-pancreatico-biliary disorders (e.g. irritable bowel syndrome). Standard evaluation and treatment of other more common upper gastrointestinal conditions, such as peptic ulcer disease and gastroesophageal reflux, should be performed simultaneously. In the absence of mass lesions, stones, or response to acid suppression therapeutic trials, the suspicion for sphincter disease is increased.

Serum chemistries

The evaluation of patients with suspected SOD (i.e. patients with upper abdominal pain with characteristics suggestive of a pancreatico-biliary origin) should be initiated with standard serum liver chemistries, serum amylase, or lipase. The serum enzyme studies should be drawn during bouts of pain, if possible. Mild elevations (< 2 × upper limits of normal) are frequent in SOD, whereas greater abnormalities are more suggestive of stones, tumors, and liver parenchymal disease. Although the diagnostic sensitivity and specificity of abnormal serum liver chemistries are low [18], recent evidence suggests that the presence of abnormal liver tests in Type II biliary SOD patients may predict a favorable response to endoscopic sphincterotomy [19].

Standard imaging

CT scans and abdominal ultrasounds are usually normal but occasionally a dilated bile duct or pancreatic duct may be found (particularly in patients with Type I SOD).

Non-invasive diagnostic methods for SOD

Because SOM (considered by most authorities to be the gold standard for diagnosing SOD) is difficult to perform, invasive, not widely available, and associated with a relatively high complication rate, several non-invasive and provocative tests have been designed in an attempt to identify patients with SOD.

Morphine–prostigmin provocative test (Nardi test)

Morphine has been shown to cause SO contraction, as assessed manometrically. Prostigmin (neostigmine), 1 mg subcutaneously, is added as a vigorous cholinergic secretory stimulant to morphine (10 mg subcutaneously) to make this challenge test. The morphine–prostigmin test, historically, had been used extensively to diagnose SOD. Reproduction of the patient's typical pain, associated with a fourfold increase in AST, ALT, alkaline phosphatase, amylase, or lipase levels, constitutes a positive response. The usefulness of this test is limited by its low sensitivity and specificity in predicting the presence of SOD and its poor correlation with outcome after sphincter ablation [20]. This test has largely been replaced by tests believed to be more sensitive.

Radiographic assessment of extrahepatic bile duct and main pancreatic duct diameter after secretory stimulation

Ultrasound provocation testing

After a lipid-rich meal or cholecystokinin administration, the gallbladder contracts, bile flow from the hepatocytes increases, and the SO relaxes, resulting in bile entry into the duodenum. Similarly, after a lipid-rich meal or secretin administration, pancreatic exocrine juice flow is stimulated and the SO relaxes. If the SO is dysfunctional and causes obstruction to flow, the common bile duct or main pancreatic duct may dilate under secretory pressure. This can be monitored by transcutaneous ultrasonography. Sphincter and terminal duct obstruction from other causes (stones, tumors, strictures) may similarly cause ductal dilation and need to be excluded. Pain provocation should also be noted if present. Limited studies comparing these non-invasive tests with SOM or outcome after sphincter ablation [21–26] show only modest correlation. Due to overlying intestinal gas, the pancreatic duct may not be visualized on standard transcutaneous ultrasound.

Endoscopic ultrasound monitoring

Despite the superiority of endoscopic ultrasound (EUS) in visualizing the pancreas, Catalano *et al*. [27] reported the sensitivity of secretin-stimulated EUS in detecting SOD to be only 57%.

MRCP monitoring

Magnetic resonance cholangiopancreatography (MRCP) can also be performed to non-invasively monitor the pancreatic duct after secretin stimulation. However, recent preliminary data from Devereaux and colleagues [28] revealed that secretin-stimulated MRCP demonstrated a diminished, rather than exaggerated, ductal dilation response in 28 patients with SOD.

Quantitative hepatobiliary scintigraphy

Hepatobiliary scintigraphy (HBS) assesses bile flow through the biliary tract. Impairment to bile flow from sphincter disease, tumors, or stones (as well as parenchymal liver disease) results in i42mpaired radionuclide flow. The precise criteria to define a positive (abnormal) study remain controversial, but a duodenal arrival time greater than 20 min and hilum to duodenum time greater than 10 min are most widely used [29–31].

Results

Four studies [29,32–34] have shown a correlation between HBS and ERCP with SOM. Taking these four studies as a whole, totaling 105 patients, the overall sensitivity of HBS using SOM as the gold standard was 78% (range 44–100%), specificity 90% (range 80–100%), positive predictive value 92% (range 82–

100%), and negative predictive value 81% (range 62–100%). However, these promising results have not been reproduced by others. Overall, it appears that patients with dilated bile ducts and high-grade obstruction are likely to have a positive scintigraphic study. Esber and colleagues [35] found that patients with lower grade obstruction (Hogan–Geenen classification Types II and III) generally have normal scintigraphy, even if performed after cholecystokinin provocation.

Adding morphine provocation

The value of adding morphine provocation to HBS was recently reported [34]. Thirty-four patients with a clinical diagnosis of Type II and Type III SOD underwent scintigraphy with and without morphine and subsequent biliary manometry. The standard scan did not distinguish between patients with normal and abnormal SOM. However, following provocation with morphine, there were significant differences in the time to maximal activity and the percentage of excretion at 45 and 60 min. Using a cut-off value of 15% excretion at 60 min, the use of morphine during HBS increased the sensitivity and specificity for SOD detection to 83% and 81%, respectively.

Comparing non-invasive tests

The Milwaukee group recently reported their retrospective review of fatty-meal sonography (FMS) and HBS as potential predictors of SOD [36]. In this study, 304 postcholecystectomy patients suspected of having SOD were evaluated by SOM, FMS, and HBS. A diagnosis of SOD was made in 73 patients (24%) by using SOM as the reference standard. The sensitivity of FMS was 21% and HBS 49%, whereas the specificities were 97% and 78%, respectively. FMS, HBS, or both were abnormal in 90%, 50%, and 44% of patients with Hogan–Geenen SOD Types I, II, and III, respectively. Of the 73 patients who underwent biliary sphincterotomy, 40 had a long-term response. Among these SOD patients, 11/13 patients (85%) with an abnormal HBS and FMS had a good long-term response. This study suggested that while non-invasive tests are not able to predict an abnormal SOM, they may be of assistance in predicting response to sphincter ablation in SOD patients.

Current status of non-invasive methods

In the absence of more definitive data, we conclude that the use of HBS as a screening tool for SOD should not be recommended for general clinical use. Abnormal results may be found in asymptomatic controls [37]. Furthermore,

HBS does not address the pancreatic sphincter. The use of HBS and other non-invasive methods should be reserved for situations in which more definitive testing (manometry) is unsuccessful or unavailable.

Invasive diagnostic methods for SOD

Because of their associated risks, invasive testing with ERCP and manometry should be reserved for patients with clinically significant or disabling symptoms. In general, invasive assessment of patients for SOD is not recommended unless definitive therapy (sphincter ablation) is planned if abnormal sphincter function is found.

Cholangiography

Cholangiography is essential to rule out stones, tumors, or other obstructing processes of the biliary tree that may cause symptoms identical to those of SOD. Once such lesions are ruled out by a good quality cholangiographic study, ducts that are dilated or drain slowly suggest obstruction at the level of the sphincter. A variety of methods to obtain a cholangiogram are available. For non-invasive imaging, magnetic resonance cholangiography (MRC) is most promising, but the quality varies greatly from center to center. Software development continues and the quality of images continues to evolve. Direct cholangiography can be obtained by percutaneous methods, intraoperative methods, or more conventionally at ERCP. Although some controversy exists, extrahepatic ducts that are greater than 12 mm in diameter (postcholecystectomy), when corrected for magnification, are considered dilated. Drugs that affect the rate of bile flow and relaxation or contraction of the SO influence drainage of contrast. Such drugs must be avoided to obtain accurate drainage times. Since the extrahepatic bile duct angulates from anterior (the hilum) to posterior (the papilla), the patient must be supine to assess gravitational drainage through the sphincter. Although definitive normal supine drainage times have not been well defined [38], a postcholecystectomy biliary tree that fails to empty all contrast medium by 45 min is generally considered abnormal.

Endoscopy

Endoscopic evaluation of the papilla and peripapillary area can yield important information that can influence the diagnosis and treatment of patients with suspected SOD. Occasionally, ampullary cancer may simulate SOD. The endoscopist should perform tissue sampling of the papilla (preferably after sphincterotomy) in suspicious cases [39].

Pancreatography

Radiographic features of the pancreatic duct are also important to assess in the patient with suspected SOD. Dilation of the pancreatic duct (> 6 mm in the pancreatic head, and > 5 mm in the body) and delayed contrast drainage time (9 min in the prone position) may give indirect evidence for the presence of SOD.

Intraductal ultrasonography (IDUS)

IDUS makes it possible to assess SO morphology during endoscopy. The sphincter appears as a thin hypoechoic circular structure on IDUS [40]. Limited studies thus far reveal no correlation between the basal sphincter pressures (as detected at SOM) and the thickness of the hypoechoic layer [41]. While IDUS may provide additional information at the level of the sphincter, it cannot be used as a substitute for SOM.

Sphincter of Oddi manometry

The most definitive development in our understanding of the pressure dynamics of the SO came with the advent of SOM. SOM is the only available method to measure SO motor activity directly. Although SOM can be performed intra-operatively and percutaneously, it is most commonly carried out in the ERCP setting. SOM is considered by most authorities to be the gold standard for evaluating patients for sphincter dysfunction [42,43]. The use of manometry to detect motility disorders of the SO is similar to its use in other parts of the gastrointestinal tract. However, performance of SOM is more technically demanding and hazardous, with complication rates (pancreatitis in particular) reported to be as high as 30%. Questions remain as to whether these short-term observations (two 10-min recordings per pull-through) reflect the 24-h pathophysiology of the sphincter. Despite some problems, SOM is gaining more widespread clinical application.

SOM: technique and indications

SOM is usually performed at the time of ERCP.

Drug interactions

All drugs that relax (anticholinergics, nitrates, calcium channel blockers, glucagon) or stimulate (narcotics, cholinergic agents) the sphincter should be avoided for at least 8–12 h prior to manometry and during the manometric session. Current data indicate that benzodiazepines do not affect the sphincter pressure and therefore are acceptable sedatives for SOM. Meperidine, at a dose of ≤ 1 mg/kg, does not affect the basal sphincter pressure but does alter phasic wave characteristics [44]. Since the basal sphincter pressure is generally the only manometric criterion used to diagnose SOD and determine therapy, it was suggested that meperidine could be used to facilitate conscious sedation for manometry. Droperidol [45] and propofol [46] are being increasingly utilized for SOM, and it appears that these agents also do not affect the basal sphincter pressure. However, further study is required before their routine use in SOM is recommended. If glucagon must be used to achieve cannulation, an 8–15-min waiting period is required to restore the sphincter to its basal condition.

Manometry catheters

Five French catheters should be used, since virtually all standards have been established with these catheters. Triple lumen catheters are state of the art and are available from several manufacturers. A variety of catheter types can be used. Catheters with a long intraductal tip may help secure the catheter within the bile duct, but such a long nose is commonly a hindrance if pancreatic manometry is desired. Over-the-wire (monorail) catheters can be passed after first securing one's position within the duct with a guidewire. Whether this guidewire influences the basal sphincter pressure is unknown. Some triple lumen catheters will accommodate a 0.018-inch diameter guidewire passed through the entire length of the catheter and can be used to facilitate cannulation or maintain position in the duct. However, a recent study in our unit found that stiffer-shafted nitinol core guidewires used for this purpose commonly increase the basal sphincter pressure by 50–100%. To avoid such artifacts, such wires need to be avoided or very soft core guidewires must be used. Guidewire-tipped catheters are being evaluated. Aspiration catheters in which one recording port is sacrificed to permit both end- and side-hole aspiration of intraductal juice are highly recommended for pancreatic manometry (Fig. 8.1). Most centers prefer to perfuse the catheters at 0.25 ml/channel using a low-compliance pump. Lower perfusion rates will give accurate basal sphincter pressures, but will not give accurate phasic wave information. A new water-perfused sleeve system, similar to that used in the lower esophageal sphincter, awaits more definitive trial in the SO [47]. The perfusate is generally distilled water, although physiological saline needs further evaluation. The latter may crystallize in the capillary tubing of perfusion pumps and must be flushed out frequently.

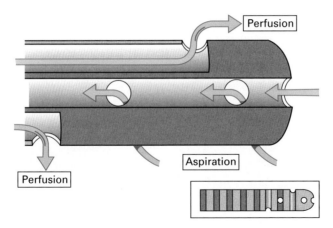

Fig. 8.1 A modified triple lumen aspirating catheter.

Cannulation techniques

SOM requires selective cannulation of the bile duct or pancreatic duct. The duct entered can be identified by gently aspirating on any port (Fig. 8.2). The appearance of yellow-colored fluid in the endoscopic view indicates entry into the bile duct. Clear aspirate indicates that the pancreatic duct was entered. It is preferable to obtain a cholangiogram and/or pancreatogram prior to performing SOM as certain findings (e.g. common bile duct stone) may obviate the need for SOM. This can be simply done by injecting contrast through one of the perfusion ports. Blaut and colleagues [48] have recently shown that injection of contrast into the biliary tree prior to SOM does not significantly alter sphincter pressure characteristics. Similar evaluation of the pancreatic sphincter after contrast injection has not been reported. One must be certain that the catheter is not impacted against the wall of the duct to ensure accurate pressure measurements. Once deep cannulation is achieved and the patient is acceptably sedated, the catheter is withdrawn across the sphincter at 1–2-mm intervals by standard station pull-through technique.

Study both sphincters   Ideally, both the pancreatic and bile ducts should be studied. Data indicate that an abnormal basal sphincter pressure may be confined to one side of the sphincter in 35% to 65% of patients with abnormal manometry [5,15,49–52]. Thus, one sphincter may be dysfunctional whereas the other is normal. Raddawi and colleagues [49] reported that an abnormal basal sphincter was more likely to be confined to the pancreatic duct segment in patients with pancreatitis and to the bile duct segment in patients with biliary-type pain and elevated liver function tests.

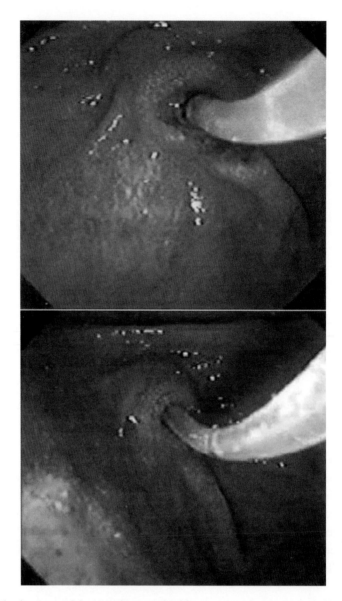

Fig. 8.2 The duct entered during sphincter of Oddi manometry can be identified by aspirating the catheter. Dark-colored yellow fluid signifies entry into the bile duct, whereas clear fluid indicates pancreatic duct entry.

Abnormalities of the basal sphincter pressure should ideally be observed for at least 30 s in each lead and be seen on two or more separate pull-throughs. From a practical clinical standpoint, we settle for one pull-through (from each duct) if the readings are clearly normal or abnormal. During standard station pull-through technique, it is necessary to establish good communication between the endoscopist and the manometrist who is reading the tracing as it rolls off the recorder or appears on the computer screen. This permits optimal positioning of the catheter to achieve interpretable tracings. Alternatively, electronic manometry systems with a television screen can be mounted near the endoscopic image screen to permit the endoscopist to view the manometry tracing during endoscopy. Once the baseline study is done, agents to relax or stimulate the sphincter can be given (e.g. cholecystokinin) and manometric or pain response monitored. The value of these provocative maneuvers for everyday use needs further study before widespread application is recommended.

Interpretation of manometry tracings

Criteria for the interpretation of an SO tracing are relatively standard; however, they may vary somewhat from center to center. Some areas where there may be disagreement in interpretation include the required duration of basal SO pressure elevation, the number of leads in which basal pressure elevation is required, and the role of averaging pressures from the three (or two in an aspirating catheter) recording ports [3]. Our recommended method for reading the manometry tracings is first to define the zero duodenal baseline before and after the pull-through. Alternatively, the intraduodenal pressure can be continuously recorded from a separate intraduodenal catheter attached to the endoscope. The highest basal pressure (Fig. 8.3) that is sustained for at least 30 s is then identified. From the four lowest amplitude points in this zone, the mean of these readings is taken as the basal sphincter pressure for that lead for that pull-through. The basal sphincter pressure for all interpretable observations is then averaged; this is the final basal sphincter pressure. The amplitude of phasic wave contractions is measured from the beginning of the slope of the pressure increase from the basal pressure to the peak of the contraction wave. Four representative waves are taken for each lead and the mean pressure determined. The number of phasic waves per minute and the duration of the phasic waves can also be determined. Most authorities read only the basal sphincter pressure as an indicator of

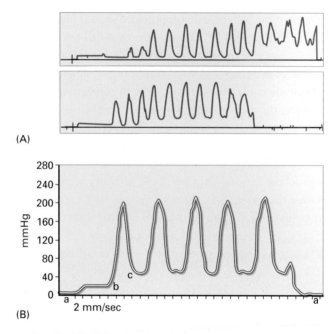

(A)

(B)

Fig. 8.3 (A) An abnormal station pull-through at sphincter of Oddi manometry. The study has been abbreviated to fit onto one page. (B) Schematic representation of one lead of the above tracing. (a) Baseline duodenal 0 reference. (b) Intraductal (pancreatic) pressure of 20 mmHg (abnormal). (c) Basal pancreatic sphincter pressure of 45 mmHg (abnormal). Phasic waves are 155–175 mmHg amplitude and 6 s duration (normal).

pathology of the SO. However, data from Kalloo and colleagues [53] suggest that the intraductal biliary pressure, which is easier to measure than SO pressure, correlates with SO basal pressure. In this study, intrabiliary pressure was significantly higher in patients with SOD than those with normal SO pressure (20 vs. 10 mmHg; $P < 0.01$). This study needs to be confirmed but supports the theory that increased intrabiliary pressure is a cause of pain in SOD.

Normal values

The best study establishing normal values for SOM was reported by Guelrud and associates [54]. Fifty asymptomatic control patients were evaluated and SOM was repeated on two occasions in 10 subjects. This study established normal values for intraductal pressure, basal sphincter pressure, and phasic wave parameters (Table 8.3). Moreover, the reproducibility of SOM was confirmed. Various authorities interchangeably use 35 mmHg or 40 mmHg as the upper limits of normal for mean basal SO pressure.

Table 8.3 Suggested standard for abnormal values for endoscopic sphincter of Oddi manometry obtained from 50 volunteers without abdominal symptoms.

Basal sphincter pressure[a]	> 35 mmHg
Basal ductal pressure	> 13 mmHg
Phasic contractions	
−3 Amplitude	> 220 mmHg
−4 Duration	> 8 s
−5 Frequency	> 10/min

Note: Values were obtained by adding three standard deviations to the mean (means were obtained by averaging the results of 2–3 station pull-throughs). Data combine pancreatic and biliary studies.
[a]Basal pressures determined by: (1) reading the peak basal pressure (i.e. the highest single lead as obtained using a triple lumen catheter); (2) obtaining the mean of these peak pressures from multiple station pull-throughs. [Adapted from reference 54.]

Complications of SOM

Several studies have demonstrated that pancreatitis is the most common major complication after SOM [55–57]. Using standard perfused catheters, pancreatitis rates as high as 31% have been reported. Such high complication rates have initially limited more widespread use of SOM. These data also emphasize that manometric evaluation of the pancreatic duct is associated with a high complication rate. Rolny and associates [56] found that patients with chronic pancreatitis were at higher risk of postprocedure pancreatitis following pancreatic duct manometry. They reported an 11% incidence of pancreatitis following manometric evaluation of the pancreatic duct. Twenty-six per cent of chronic pancreatitis patients undergoing SOM developed pancreatitis.

Methods to reduce complications

A variety of methods to decrease the incidence of postmanometry pancreatitis have been proposed:
• use of an aspiration catheter
• gravity drainage of the pancreatic duct after manometry
• decrease the perfusion rate to 0.05–0.1 ml/lumen/min
• limit pancreatic duct manometry time to less than 2 min (or avoid pancreatic manometry)
• use the microtransducer (non-perfused) system [13]
• placement of pancreatic stent after manometry and/or sphincterotomy [58].

Aspirating catheter system

In a prospective randomized study, Sherman and colleagues found that the aspirating catheter (this catheter allows for aspiration of the perfused fluid from end- and side-holes while accurately recording pressure from the two remaining side-ports) reduced the frequency of pancreatic duct manometry-induced pancreatitis from 31% to 4% [55]. The reduction in pancreatitis with the use of this catheter in the pancreatic duct, and the very low incidence of pancreatitis after bile duct manometry, lend support to the notion that increased pancreatic duct hydrostatic pressure is a major cause of this complication. Thus, when the pancreatic duct sphincter is studied by SOM, aspiration of pancreatic juice and the perfusate is strongly recommended.

Prophylactic stenting

In a prospective randomized trial, Tarnasky and colleagues showed that stenting the pancreatic duct decreased post-ERCP pancreatitis from 26% to 6% in a group of patients with pancreatic sphincter hypertension undergoing biliary sphincterotomy alone [58].

SOM: conclusion

SOM is recommended in patients with idiopathic pancreatitis or unexplained disabling pancreatico-biliary pain with or without hepatic enzyme abnormalities. An attempt is made to study both sphincters, but clinical decisions can be made when the first sphincter evaluated is abnormal. An ERCP is usually performed (if an adequate study is not available) immediately before SOM to exclude other potential causes for the patient's symptoms. Indications for the use of SOM have also been developed according to the Hogan–Geenen SOD classification system (Table 8.1).

Type I patients

In Type I patients, there is a general consensus that a structural disorder of the sphincter (i.e. sphincter stenosis) exists. Although SOM may be useful in documenting SOD, it is not an essential diagnostic study prior to endoscopic or surgical sphincter ablation. Such patients uniformly benefit from sphincter ablation regardless of the SOM results.

Type II patients

Type II patients demonstrate SO motor dysfunction in 50–65% of cases. In this group of patients, SOM is highly recommended as the results of the study predict outcome from sphincter ablation.

Type III patients

Type III patients have pancreatico-biliary pain without other objective evidence of sphincter outflow obstruction. SOM is mandatory to confirm the presence of SOD. Although not well studied, it appears that the results of SOM may predict outcome from sphincter ablation in these patients.

Therapy for SOD

The therapeutic approach in patients with SOD is aimed at reducing the resistance caused by the SO to the flow of bile and/or pancreatic juice [6]. Historically, emphasis has been placed on definitive intervention, i.e. surgical sphincteroplasty or endoscopic sphincterotomy. This appears appropriate for patients with high-grade obstruction (Type I as per Hogan–Geenen criteria). In patients with lesser degrees of obstruction, the clinician must carefully weigh the risks and benefits before recommending invasive therapy. Most reports indicate that SOD patients have a complication rate from endoscopic sphincterotomy of at least twice that of patients with ductal stones [59,60].

Medical therapy

Medical therapy for documented or suspected SOD has received only limited study. As the SO is a smooth muscle structure, it is reasonable to assume that drugs that relax smooth muscle might be an effective treatment for SOD. Sublingual nifedipine and nitrates have been shown to reduce the basal sphincter pressures in asymptomatic volunteers and symptomatic patients with SOD [1,61].

Nifedipine

Khuroo and colleagues [62] evaluated the clinical benefit of nifedipine in a placebo-controlled crossover trial. Twenty-one of 28 patients (75%) with manometrically documented SOD had a reduction in pain scores, emergency room visits, and use of oral analgesics during short-term follow-up. In a similar study, Sand and associates [63] found that nine of 12 (75%) Type II SOD (suspected; SOM was not performed) patients improved with nifedipine. Although medical therapy may be an attractive initial approach in patients with SOD, several drawbacks exist [1]. First, medication side-effects may be seen in up to one-third of patients. Second, smooth muscle relaxants are unlikely to be of any benefit in patients with the structural form of SOD (i.e. SO stenosis), and the response is incomplete in patients with a primary motor abnormality of the SO (i.e. SO dyskinesia). Finally, long-term outcome from medical therapy has not been reported. Nevertheless, because of the relative safety of medical therapy and the benign (although painful) character of SOD, this approach should be considered in all Type III and less severely symptomatic Type II SOD patients before considering more aggressive sphincter ablation therapy.

Electrical nerve stimulation

Guelrud and colleagues have demonstrated that transcutaneous electrical nerve stimulation (TENS) lowers the basal sphincter pressure in SOD patients by a mean of 38%, but, unfortunately, generally not into the normal range [64]. This stimulation was associated with an increase in serum VIP levels. Electro-acupuncture applied at acupoint GB 34 (a specific acupoint that affects the hepatobiliary system) was shown to relax the SO in association with increased plasma CCK levels [65]. Its role in the management of SOD has not been investigated.

Surgical therapy

Historically, surgery was the traditional therapy of SOD. The surgical approach, most commonly, is a transduodenal biliary sphincteroplasty with a transampullary septoplasty (pancreatic septoplasty). Sixty to 70% of patients were reported to have benefited from this therapy during a 1- to 10-year follow-up [66,67]. Patients with an elevated basal sphincter pressure, determined by intra-operative SOM, were more likely to improve from surgical sphincter ablation than those with a normal basal pressure [67]. Some reports have suggested that patients with biliary-type pain have a better outcome than patients with idiopathic pancreatitis, whereas others have suggested no difference [66,67]. However, most studies found that symptom improvement following surgical sphincter ablation alone was relatively uncommon in patients with established chronic pancreatitis [67].

The surgical approach for SOD has largely been replaced by endoscopic therapy. Patient tolerance, cost of care, morbidity, mortality, and cosmetic results are some of the factors that favor an initial endoscopic approach. At present, surgical therapy is reserved for patients with restenosis following endoscopic sphincterotomy and when endoscopic evaluation or therapy is not available or technically feasible (e.g. Roux-en-Y gastrojejunostomy). In many centers, however, operative therapy continues to be the standard treatment of pancreatic sphincter hypertension [6,68].

Endoscopic balloon dilation and biliary stent trials

Balloon dilation of strictures in the gastrointestinal tract has become commonplace. In an attempt to be less invasive and possibly to preserve sphincter function, adaptation of this technique to treat SOD has been described. Unfortunately, because of the unacceptably high complication rates, primarily pancreatitis, this technology has little role in the management of SOD [69].

Placement of a pancreatic or biliary stent on a trial basis in the hope of achieving pain relief and of predicting the response to more definitive therapy (i.e. sphincter ablation) has received only limited evaluation. Pancreatic stent trials, especially in patients with normal pancreatic ducts, are strongly discouraged as serious ductal and parenchymal injury may occur if stents are left in place for more than a few days [70,71]. Goff reported a biliary stent trial in 21 Type II and III SOD patients with normal biliary manometry [72]. Stents (7 Fr) were left in place for at least 2 months if symptoms resolved and removed sooner if they were judged ineffective. Relief of pain with the stent was predictive of long-term pain relief after biliary sphincterotomy. Unfortunately, 38% of the patients developed pancreatitis (14% were graded severe) following stent placement. Due to this high complication rate, biliary stent trials are strongly discouraged. Rolny also reported a series of bile duct stent placement as a predictor of outcome following biliary sphincterotomy in 23 postcholecystectomy patients (seven Type II and 16 Type III) [73]. Similar to the study by Goff [72], resolution of pain during at least 12 weeks of stenting predicted a favorable outcome from sphincterotomy irrespective of SO pressure. In this series, there were no complications related to stent placement.

Endoscopic sphincterotomy

Endoscopic sphincterotomy is the standard therapy for patients with SOD. Most data on endoscopic sphincterotomy relate to biliary sphincter ablation alone. Clinical improvement following therapy has been reported to occur in 55% to 95% of patients (Table 8.1). These variable outcomes are reflective of the different criteria used to document SOD, the degree of obstruction (Type I biliary patients appear to have a better outcome than Type II and III), the methods of data collection (retrospective vs. prospective), and the techniques used to determine benefit. Rolny and colleagues [74] studied 17 Type I postcholecystectomy biliary patients by SOM (Table 8.4). In this series, 65% had an abnormal SOM (although not specifically stated, it appears that the biliary sphincter was studied alone). Nevertheless, during a mean follow-up interval of 2.3 years, all patients benefited from biliary sphincterotomy. The results of this study suggested that since Type I biliary patients invariably benefit from biliary

Table 8.4 Biliary sphincter ablation in Type I SOD (28-month follow-up)[a].

Basal sphincter of Oddi pressure	No.	Asymptomatic/ improved after ES/SS
< 40 mmHg	6 (35%)	6 (100%)
≥ 40 mmHg	11 (65%)	11 (100%)

15 endoscopic (ES), 2 surgical (SS) sphincterotomies.
[a]From reference [74].

Table 8.5 Biliary sphincterotomy for sphincter of Oddi dysfunction documented by sphincter of Oddi manometry: results of four non-randomized controlled trials.

	Clinical benefit	
Reference	Type II	Type III
Choudhry et al. [17]	10/18 (56%)	9/16 (56%)
Botoman et al. [13]	13/19 (68%)	9/16 (56%)
Bozkurt et al. [75]	14/19 (78%)	5/5 (100%)
Wehrmann et al. [76]	12/20 (60%)	1/13 (8%)

[a]Six had cholecystectomy.

sphincterotomy, SOM in this patient group is not only unnecessary, but may also be misleading. The results of this study, however, have never been validated at another center. In contrast, results of several non-randomized controlled trials [13,17,75,76] suggest that performance of SOM is highly recommended in biliary Type II and Type III patients, as clinical benefit is less certain (Table 8.5).

Although most of the studies reporting the efficacy of endoscopic therapy in SOD have been retrospective, three notable randomized trials have been reported.

Randomized controlled trials of endoscopic sphincterotomy for SOD

In a landmark study by Geenen and associates [77], 47 postcholecystectomy Type II biliary patients were randomized to biliary sphincterotomy or sham sphincterotomy. SOM was performed in all patients but was not used as a criterion for randomization. During a 4-year follow-up, 95% of patients with an elevated basal sphincter pressure benefited from sphincterotomy. In contrast, only 30% to 40% of patients with an elevated sphincter pressure treated by sham sphincterotomy, or with a normal sphincter pressure treated by endoscopic sphincterotomy or sham sphincterotomy, benefited from this therapy. The two important findings of this study were that SOM predicted the outcome from endoscopic sphincterotomy and that endoscopic sphincterotomy offered long-term benefit in Type II biliary patients with SOD. Confirmatory data were seen in a 2-year follow-up study by Toouli et al. [78,79]. In this study,

Table 8.6a Change in the mean pain score (using a 0-none to 10-most severe linear pain scale) and number of hospital days per month required for pain in patients with manometrically documented sphincter of Oddi dysfunction randomized to endoscopic sphincterotomy (ES), sham sphincterotomy (S-ES), and surgical sphincteroplasty with or without cholecystectomy (SSp ± CCx).

Therapy	Follow-up (years)	Mean pain score		Hospital days/ month		Patients improved (%)
		Pre-Rx	Post-Rx	Pre-Rx	Post-Rx	
ES (n = 19)	3.3	9.2	3.9[a]	0.85	0.23[b]	68[c]
S-ES (n = 17)	2.2	9.4	7.2	0.87	0.89	24
SSp ± CCx (n = 16)	3.4	9.4	3.3[a]	0.94	0.27[b]	69[c]

[a]$P < 0.04$.
[b]$P = 0.002$.
[c]$P = 0.009$.
ES and SSp ± CCx vs. S-ES.

Table 8.6b Clinical benefit correlated with sphincter of Oddi dysfunction (SOD) type.

SOD type[a]	Patients improved / total patients		
	ES	S-ES	SSp ± CCx
Type II	5/6 (83%)[b]	1/7 (14%)	8/10 (80%)[b]
Type III	8/13 (62%)	3/10 (30%)	3/6 (50%)

[a]SOD type based on Hogan–Geenen SOD classification system.
[b]$P < 0.02$; ES and SSp ± CCx vs. S-ES.
[Adapted from reference 80.]

postcholecystectomy patients with biliary-type pain (mostly Type II) were prospectively randomized to endoscopic sphincterotomy or sham following stratification according to SOM. Eighty-five per cent (11 of 13) of patients with elevated basal pressure improved at 2 years after endoscopic sphincterotomy, while 38% (five of 13) of patients improved after a sham procedure ($P = 0.041$). Patients with normal SOM were also randomized to sphincterotomy or sham. The outcome was similar for the two groups (eight of 13 improved after sphincterotomy and eight of 19 improved after sham; $P = 0.47$).

Sherman and associates [80] reported their preliminary results of a randomized study comparing endoscopic sphincterotomy and surgical biliary sphincteroplasty with pancreatic septoplasty (with or without cholecystectomy) to sham sphincterotomy for Type II and III biliary patients with manometrically documented SOD. The results are shown in Table 8.6. During a 3-year follow-up period, 69% of patients undergoing endoscopic or surgical sphincter ablation improved compared to 24% in the sham sphincterotomy group ($P = 0.009$). There was a trend for Type II patients to benefit more frequently from sphincter ablation than Type III patients (13/16, 81%, vs. 11/19, 58%; $P = 0.14$).

Is pancreatic sphincterotomy necessary?

Evidence is now accumulating that the addition of a pancreatic sphincterotomy to an endoscopic biliary sphincterotomy in such patients may improve the outcome, as preliminarily reported by Guelrud *et al.* [81]. Soffer and Johlin reported that 25 of 26 patients (mostly Type II), who failed to respond to biliary sphincterotomy, had elevated pancreatic sphincter pressure [82]. Pancreatic sphincter therapy was performed with overall symptomatic improvement in two-thirds of patients. Eversman and colleagues found that 90% of patients with persistent pain or pancreatitis after biliary sphincterotomy had residual abnormal pancreatic basal pressure [83]. Five-year follow-up data revealed that patients with untreated pancreatic sphincter hypertension were much less likely to improve after biliary sphincterotomy than patients with isolated biliary sphincter hypertension (Fig. 8.4). Elton *et al.* [84] performed pancreatic sphincterotomy on 43 Type I and Type II SOD patients who failed to benefit from biliary sphincterotomy alone. During the follow-up period, 72% were symptom-free and 19% were partially or transiently improved. Kaw and colleagues [85] presented preliminary data demonstrating that response to sphincterotomy also depends on treating the diseased sphincter segment. Patients with pancreatic sphincter hypertension who fail to respond to biliary sphincterotomy can be 'rescued' by undergoing pancreatic sphincterotomy (Table 8.7). Recent preliminary data from our unit examined the outcome of endoscopic therapy in

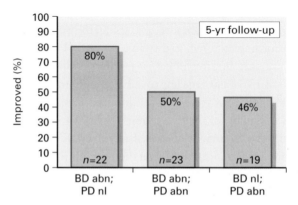

Fig. 8.4 Long-term outcome after biliary sphincterotomy alone depends on pancreatic SO pressure. (BD = bile duct; PD = pancreatic duct; nl = normal; abn = abnormal.)

Table 8.7 Response to sphincterotomy in relation to sphincter segment treated (follow-up 17 months).

SO dysfunction	Biliary sphincterotomy		Pancreatic sphincterotomy	
	Total	Response	Total	Response
Biliary	10	8 (80%)	0	0 (0%)
Pancreatic	13	2 (15%)	11	8 (72%)
Combined	10	5 (50%)	5	3 (60%)
Total	33	15 (45%)	16	11 (69%)

Overall benefit 26/33 (79%). [Adapted from reference 85.]

SOD patients with initial pancreatic sphincter hypertension (with or without biliary sphincter hypertension). Patients were followed for a mean of 45.3 months (range 11–77 months); re-intervention was offered for sustained or recurrent symptoms at a mean of 14.3 months following initial therapy. Performance of an initial dual pancreatico-biliary sphincterotomy was associated with a lower re-intervention rate (69/284, 24.3%) than biliary sphincterotomy alone (31/95, 33%; $P < 0.05$). Confirmatory outcome studies, preferably in randomized trials, are awaited.

Risks and benefits of endoscopic treatment for SOD

These results clearly indicate that the response rate and enthusiasm for sphincter ablation must be correlated with patient presentation and results of manometry and balanced against the high complication rates reported for endoscopic therapy of SOD. Most studies indicate that patients undergoing endoscopic sphincterotomy for SOD have complication rates two to five times higher than patients undergoing endoscopic sphincterotomy for ductal stones [59,60]. Pancreatitis is the most common complication, occurring in up to 30% of patients in some series. A recent prospective, multicenter study examining risk factors for post-ERCP pancreatitis identified suspected SOD as an independent factor by multivariate analysis [86]. A suspicion of SOD tripled the risk of postprocedure pancreatitis to a frequency (23%) that was comparable to that found in other recent prospective studies [58,60,81–89]. Endoscopic techniques are being developed (e.g. pancreatic duct stenting prior to combined pancreatico-biliary sphincterotomy) to limit such complications [58,90].

Botulinum toxin injection

Botulinum toxin (Botox), a potent inhibitor of acetylcholine release from nerve endings, has been successfully applied to smooth muscle disorders of the gastrointestinal tract such as achalasia. In a preliminary clinical trial, toxin injection into the SO resulted in a 50% reduction in the basal biliary sphincter pressure and improved bile flow [91]. This reduction in pressure may be accompanied by symptom improvement in some patients. Although further study is warranted, Botox may serve as a therapeutic trial for SOD with responders undergoing permanent sphincter ablation. In a small series [92], 22 postcholecystectomy Type III patients with manometric evidence of SOD underwent Botox injection into the intraduodenal sphincter segment. Eleven of the 12 patients who responded to botulinum toxin injection later benefited from endoscopic sphincterotomy, while only two of 10 patients who did not benefit from Botox injection later responded to sphincter ablation. Such an approach, however, does require two endoscopies to achieve symptom relief. Further studies are needed before recommending this technique.

SOD in recurrent pancreatitis

Disorders of the pancreatic sphincter may give rise to unexplained (idiopathic) pancreatitis or episodic pain suggestive of a pancreatic origin [68]. SOD has been manometrically documented in 15% to 72% of patients with recurrent pancreatitis, previously labeled as idiopathic [5,14,16,93]. Biliary sphincterotomy alone has been reported to prevent further pancreatitis episodes in more than 50% of such patients. From a scientific, but not practical viewpoint, care must be taken to separate out subtle biliary pancreatitis [94] that will similarly respond to biliary sphincterotomy.

Endoscopic sphincterotomy for SOD in pancreatitis

Lans and colleagues

The value of ERCP, SOM, and sphincter ablation therapy was studied in 51 patients with idiopathic pancreatitis [43]. Twenty-four (47.1%) had an elevated basal sphincter pressure. Thirty were treated by biliary sphincterotomy ($n = 20$) or surgical sphincteroplasty with septoplasty ($n = 10$). Fifteen of 18 patients (83%) with an elevated basal sphincter pressure had long-term benefit (mean follow-up, 38 months) from sphincter ablation therapy (including 10 of 11 treated by biliary sphincterotomy) in contrast to only four of 12 (33.3%; $P < 0.05$) with a normal basal sphincter pressure (including four of nine treated by biliary sphincterotomy).

Table 8.8 Pancreatic sphincter dysfunction and recurrent pancreatitis: response to sphincter therapy.

Treatment	Patients improved/ total patients
Biliary sphincterotomy alone	5/18 (28%)
Biliary sphincterotomy followed by pancreatic sphincter balloon dilation	13/24 (54%)
Biliary sphincterotomy plus pancreatic sphincterotomy at later session	10/13 (77%)[a]
Biliary sphincterotomy and pancreatic sphincterotomy at same session	12/14 (86%)[a]

[a]$P < 0.005$ vs. biliary sphincterotomy alone. [Adapted from reference 81.]

Guelrud and colleagues

Guelrud and colleagues [81], by contrast, found that severance of the pancreatic sphincter was necessary to resolve the pancreatitis (Table 8.8). In this series, 69 patients with idiopathic pancreatitis due to SOD underwent treatment by standard biliary sphincterotomy ($n = 18$), biliary sphincterotomy with pancreatic sphincter balloon dilation ($n = 24$), biliary sphincterotomy followed by pancreatic sphincterotomy in separate sessions ($n = 13$), or combined pancreatic and biliary sphincterotomy in the same session ($n = 14$). Eighty-one per cent of patients undergoing pancreatic and biliary sphincterotomy had resolution of their pancreatitis compared to 28% of patients undergoing biliary sphincterotomy alone ($P < 0.005$). These data are consistent with the theory that many such patients who benefit from biliary sphincterotomy alone have subtle gallstone pancreatitis. The results of Guelrud and colleagues [81] also support the anatomic findings of separate biliary and pancreatic sphincters, and the manometry findings of residual pancreatic sphincter hypertension in more than 50% of persistently symptomatic patients who undergo biliary sphincterotomy alone.

Kaw and Brodmerkel

Kaw and Brodmerkel [95] recently reported that, among patients with idiopathic pancreatitis secondary to SOD, 78% had persistent manometric evidence of pancreatic sphincter hypertension despite a biliary sphincterotomy.

Toouli and colleagues

Toouli and colleagues [96] also demonstrated the importance of pancreatic and biliary sphincter ablation in patients with idiopathic pancreatitis. In this series,

23 of 26 patients (88%) undergoing surgical ablation of both the biliary and pancreatic sphincter were either asymptomatic or had minimal symptoms at a median follow-up of 24 months (range 9–105 months).

Okolo and colleagues

Okolo and colleagues [97] retrospectively evaluated the long-term results of endoscopic pancreatic sphincterotomy in 55 patients with manometrically documented or presumed pancreatic sphincter hypertension (presumption based on recurrent pancreatitis with pancreatic duct dilation and contrast medium drainage time from the pancreatic duct of greater than 10 min). During a median follow-up of 16 months (range 3–52 months), 34 patients (62%) reported significant pain improvement. Patients with normal pancreatograms were more likely to respond to therapy than those with pancreatographic evidence of chronic pancreatitis (73% vs. 58%).

Endoscopic sphincterotomy as a cause of pancreatic sphincter stenosis

Jacob and colleagues [98] postulated that SOD might cause recurrent episodes of pancreatitis, even though SOM was normal, and pancreatic stent placement might prevent further attacks. In a randomized study, 34 patients with unexplained recurrent pancreatitis and normal pancreatic SOM were treated with pancreatic stents ($n = 19$; 5–7 Fr gauge, with stents exchanged three times over a 1-year period) or conservative therapy. During a 3-year follow-up, pancreatitis recurred in 53% of the patients in the control group and only 11% of the stented patients ($P < 0.02$). This study suggests that SOM may be an imperfect test, as patients may have SOD but not be detected at the time of SOM. However, long-term studies are needed to evaluate the outcome after removal of stents, and concern remains regarding stent-induced ductal and parenchymal changes [70,71,99].

Endoscopic Botox injection

Wehrmann and colleagues [100] recently evaluated the feasibility and effectiveness of botulinum toxin injection in patients with recurrent pancreatitis due to pancreatic sphincter hypertension. No side-effects of the injection were noted in any of the 15 treated patients. Twelve patients (80%) remained asymptomatic at 3-month follow-up, but 11 developed a relapse at a follow-up period of 6 ± 2 months. These 11 patients underwent pancreatic or combined pancreaticobiliary sphincterotomy with subsequent remission after a median follow-up of 15 months. This study showed that injection of botulinum toxin is safe and may be effective short term, but the need for definitive sphincter ablation in the majority of patients limits its clinical use.

SOD in recurrent pancreatitis: conclusion

Currently, establishing the best method of treating residual pancreatic sphincter stenosis (after biliary sphincterotomy) awaits further study. Patients with idiopathic pancreatitis who fail to respond to biliary sphincterotomy alone should have their pancreatic sphincter re-evaluated and be considered for sphincter ablation if residual high pressure is found.

Conclusion

Our knowledge of SOD, and manometric techniques to assist in this diagnosis, is evolving. Successful endoscopic SOM requires good general ERCP skills and careful attention to the main details listed above. If SOD is suspected in a Type III or mild to moderate pain level Type II patient, medical therapy should generally be tried. If medical therapy fails or is bypassed, ERCP and manometric evaluation are recommended. The role of less invasive studies remains uncertain owing to undefined sensitivity and specificity. Sphincter ablation is generally warranted in symptomatic Type I patients and Type II and III patients with abnormal manometry. The symptom relief rate varies from 55% to 95%, depending on the patient presentation and selection. Initial non-responders require thorough pancreatic sphincter and pancreatic parenchymal evaluation. SOD patients have relatively high complication rates after invasive studies or therapy. Thorough review of the risk–benefit ratio with individual patients is mandatory.

Outstanding issues and future trends

Our hopes for the future in this evolving field are to:
- Define the role, if any, of non-invasive imaging studies as a screening test and predictor of outcome from sphincter ablation
- Develop techniques to improve the safety of the procedures used to evaluate and treat patients with pancreatico-biliary pain
- Develop a device for longer term SOM such as a 24-h SOM probe
- Define predictors of good and poor outcome from therapy to better select patients for 'risky' interventions
- Further investigate the role of pancreatic sphincterotomy for improving outcomes

- Develop more long-term outcome studies, particularly in Type II and III patients
- Explore better medical therapy alternatives for less disabled patients.

References

1 Kalloo AN, Pasricha PJ. Therapy of sphincter of Oddi dysfunction. *Gastrointest Endosc Clin N Am* 1996; 6: 117–25.

2 Black NA, Thompson E, Sanderson CFB. Symptoms and health status before and six weeks after open cholecystectomy: a European cohort study. ECHSS Group. European Collaborative Health Services Study Group. *Gut* 1994; 35: 1301–5.

3 Hogan W, Sherman S, Pasricha P, Carr-Locke DL. Sphincter of Oddi manometry. *Gastrointest Endosc* 1997; 45: 342–8.

4 Sherman S, Troiano FP, Hawes RH, O'Connor KW, Lehman GA. Frequency of abnormal sphincter of Oddi manometry compared with the clinical suspicion of sphincter of Oddi dysfunction. *Am J Gastroenterol* 1991; 86: 586–90.

5 Eversman D, Fogel EL, Rusche M, Sherman S, Lehman GA. Frequency of abnormal pancreatic and biliary sphincter manometry compared with clinical suspicion of sphincter of Oddi dysfunction. *Gastrointest Endosc* 1999; 50: 637–41.

6 Corazziari E, Shaffer EA, Hogan W, Sherman S, Toouli J. Functional disorders of the biliary tract and pancreas. *Gut* 1999; 45 (Suppl 2): 48–54.

7 Anderson TM, Pitt HA, Longmire WP Jr. Experience with sphincteroplasty and sphincterotomy in pancreatobiliary surgery. *Ann Surg* 1985; 201: 399–406.

8 Guelrud M, Mendoza S, Mujica V, Uzcategui A. Sphincter of Oddi (SO) motor function in patients with symptomatic gallstones. *Gastroenterology* 1993; 104: A361.

9 Ruffolo TA, Sherman S, Lehman GA, Hawes RH. Gallbladder ejection fraction and its relationship to sphincter of Oddi dysfunction. *Dig Dis Sci* 1994; 39: 289–92.

10 Neoptolemos JP, Bailey IS, Carr-Locke DL. Sphincter of Oddi dysfunction: results of treatment by endoscopic sphincterotomy. *Br J Surg* 1988; 75: 454–9.

11 Roberts-Thomson IC, Toouli J. Is endoscopic sphincterotomy for disabling biliary-type pain after cholecystectomy effective? *Gastrointest Endosc* 1985; 31: 370–3.

12 Meshkinpoor H, Mollot M. Sphincter of Oddi dysfunction and unexplained abdominal pain: clinical and manometric study. *Dig Dis Sci* 1992; 37: 257–61.

13 Botoman VA, Kozarek RA, Novell LA, Patterson DJ, Ball TJ, Wechter DG *et al.* Long term outcome after endoscopic sphincterotomy in patients with biliary colic and suspected sphincter of Oddi dysfunction. *Gastrointest Endosc* 1994; 40: 165–70.

14 Lehman GA, Sherman S. Sphincter of Oddi dysfunction. *Int J Pancreatol* 1996; 20: 11–25.

15 Aymerich RR, Prakash C, Aliperti G. Sphincter of Oddi manometry: is it necessary to measure both biliary and pancreatic sphincter pressure? *Gastrointest Endosc* 2000; 52: 183–6.

16 Geenen JE, Nash JA. The role of sphincter of Oddi manometry and biliary microscopy in evaluating idiopathic recurrent pancreatitis. *Endoscopy* 1998; 30 (9): A237–41.

17 Choudhry U, Ruffolo T, Jamidar P, Hawes R, Lehman G. Sphincter of Oddi dysfunction in patients with intact gallbladder: therapeutic response to endoscopic sphincterotomy. *Gastrointest Endosc* 1993; 39: 492–5.

18 Steinberg WM. Sphincter of Oddi dysfunction: a clinical controversy. *Gastroenterology* 1988; 95: 1409–15.

19 Lin OS, Soetikno RM, Young HS. The utility of liver function test abnormalities concomitant with biliary symptoms in predicting a favorable response to endoscopic sphincterotomy in patients with presumed sphincter of Oddi dysfunction. *Am J Gastroenterol* 1998; 93: 1833–6.

20 Steinberg WM, Salvato RF, Toskes PP. The morphine-prostigmin provocative test: is it useful for making clinical decisions? *Gastroenterology* 1980; 78: 728–31.

21 Darweesh RM, Dodds WJ, Hogan WJ, Geenen JE, Collier BD, Shaker R *et al.* Efficacy of quantitative hepatobiliary scintigraphy and fatty-meal sonography for evaluating patients with suspected partial common duct obstruction. *Gastroenterology* 1988; 94: 779–86.

22 Simeone JF, Mueller PR, Ferrucci JT Jr, vanSonnenberg E, Hall DA, Wittenberg J *et al.* Sonography of the bile ducts after a fatty meal: an aid in detection of obstruction. *Radiology* 1982; 143: 211–15.

23 Troiano F, O'Connor K, Lehman GA, Madura J, Kopecky K, Bogan M. Comparison of secretin-stimulated ultrasound and sphincter of Oddi manometry in evaluating sphincter of Oddi dysfunction. *Gastrointest Endosc* 1989; 35: A166.

24 Warshaw AL, Simeone J, Schapiro RH, Hedberg SE, Mueller PE, Ferrucci JT Jr. Objective evaluation of ampullary stenosis with ultrasonography and pancreatic stimulation. *Am J Surg* 1985; 149: 65–72.

25 DiFrancesco V, Brunori MR, Rigo L, Toouli J, Angelini G, Frulloni L *et al.* Comparison of ultrasound-secretin test and sphincter of Oddi manometry in patients with recurrent acute pancreatitis. *Dig Dis Sci* 1999; 44: 336–40.

26 Silverman WB, Johlin FC, Crowe G. Does secretin stimulated ultrasound (SSUS) predict results: sphincter of Oddi manometry (SOM) basal sphincter pressure (BSP) in patients suspected of having sphincter of Oddi dysfunction (SOD)? *Gastrointest Endosc* 2001; 53: A100.

27 Catalano MF, Lahoti S, Alcocer E, Geenen JE, Hogan WJ. Dynamic imaging of the pancreas using real-time endoscopic ultrasonography with secretin stimulation. *Gastrointest Endosc* 1998; 48: 580–7.

28 Devereaux BM, Fogel EL, Aisen A, Stockberger S, Ness R, Lehman GA *et al.* Secretin-stimulated functional MRCP: correlation with sphincter of Oddi manometry. *Gastrointest Endosc* 2000; 51: A197.

29 Sostre S, Kalloo AN, Spiegler EJ, Camargo EE, Wagner HN Jr. A noninvasive test of sphincter of Oddi dysfunction in postcholecystectomy patients: the scintigraphic score. *J Nucl Med* 1992; 33: 1216–22.

30 Kalloo AN, Sostre S, Pasricha PJ. The Hopkins scintigraphic score: a noninvasive, highly accurate screening test for sphincter of Oddi dysfunction. *Gastroenterology* 1994; 106: A342.

31 Cicala M, Scopinaro F, Corazziari E, Vignoni A, Viscardi A, Habib FI *et al.* Quantitative cholescintigraphy in the assessment of choledochoduodenal bile flow. *Gastroenterology* 1991; 100: 1106–13.

32 Corazziari E, Cicala M, Habib FI, Scopinaro F, Fiocca F, Pallotta N *et al.* Hepatoduodenal bile transit in cholecystomized subjects. Relationship with sphincter of Oddi dysfunction and diagnostic value. *Dig Dis Sci* 1994; 39: 1985–93.

33 Peng NJ, Lai KH, Tsay DG, Liu RS, Su KL, Yeh SH. Efficacy of quantitative cholescintigraphy in the diagnosis of sphincter of Oddi dysfunction. *Nucl Med Commun* 1994; 15: 899–904.

34 Thomas PD, Turner JG, Dobbs BR, Burt MJ, Chapman BA. Use of 99m Tc-DISIDA biliary scanning with morphine provocation in the detection of elevated sphincter of Oddi basal pressure. *Gut* 2000; 46: 838–41.

35 Esber E, Ruffolo TA, Park H, Siddiqui A, Earle D, Pezzi J *et al.* Prospective assessment of biliary scintigraphy in patients with suspected sphincter of Oddi dysfunction. *Gastrointest Endosc* 1995; 41: A396.

36 Rosenblatt ML, Catalano MF, Alcocer E, Geenen JE. Comparison of sphincter of Oddi manometry, fatty meal sonography, and hepatobiliary scintigraphy in the diagnosis of sphincter of Oddi dysfunction. *Gastrointest Endosc* 2001; 54: 697–704.

37 Pineau BC, Knapple WL, Spicer KM, Gordon L, Wallace M, Hennessy WS *et al.* Cholecystokinin-stimulated mebrofenin (^{99m}Tc-Choletec) hepatobiliary scintigraphy in asymptomatic postcholecystectomy individuals: assessment of specificity, interobserver reliability, and reproducibility. *Am J Gastroenterol* 2001; 96: 3106–9.

38 Elta GH, Barnett JL, Ellis JH, Ackermann R, Wahl R. Delayed biliary drainage is common in asymptomatic post-cholecystectomy volunteers. *Gastrointest Endosc* 1992; 38: 435–9.

39 Ponchon T, Aucia N, Mitchell R, Chavaillon A, Bory R, Hedelius F. Biopsies of the ampullary region in patients suspected to have sphincter of Oddi dysfunction. *Gastrointest Endosc* 1995; 42: 296–300.

40 Itoh A, Tsukamoto Y, Naitoh Y, Hirooka Y, Furukawa T, Kato T *et al.* Intraductal ultrasonography for the examination of duodenal papillary region. *J Ultrasound Med* 1994; 13: 679–84.

41 Wehrmann T, Stergiou N, Riphaus A, Lembcke B. Correlation between sphincter of Oddi manometry and intraductal ultrasound morphology in patients with suspected sphincter of Oddi dysfunction. *Endoscopy* 2001; 33: 773–7.

42 Lehman GA. Endoscopic sphincter of Oddi manometry: a clinical practice and research tool. *Gastrointest Endosc* 1991; 37: 490–2.

43 Lans JL, Parikh NP, Geenen JE. Application of sphincter of Oddi manometry in routine clinical investigations. *Endoscopy* 1991; 23: 139–43.

44 Sherman S, Gottlieb K, Uzer MF, Smith MT, Khusro QE, Earle DT *et al.* Effects of meperidine on the pancreatic and biliary sphincter. *Gastrointest Endosc* 1996; 44: 239–42.

45 Fogel EL, Sherman S, Bucksot L, Philips SD, Lehman GA. Sphincter of Oddi manometry (SOM): effects of droperidol on the biliary and pancreatic sphincter. *Gastrointest Endosc* 2001; 53: A89.

46 Goff JS. Effect of propofol on human sphincter of Oddi. *Dig Dis Sci* 1995; 40: 2364–7.

47 Craig AG, Omari T, Lingenfelser T, Schloithe AC, Saccone GT, Dent J *et al.* Development of a sleeve sensor for measurement of sphincter of Oddi motility. *Endoscopy* 2001; 33: 651–7.

48 Blaut U, Sherman S, Fogel E, Lehman GA. Influence of cholangiography on biliary sphincter of Oddi manometric parameters. *Gastrointest Endosc* 2000; 52: 624–9.

49 Raddawi HM, Geenen JE, Hogan WJ, Dodds WJ, Venu RP, Johnson GK. Pressure measurements from biliary and pancreatic segments of sphincter of Oddi. Comparison between patients with functional abdominal pain, biliary, or pancreatic disease. *Dig Dis Sci* 1991; 36: 71–4.

50 Rolny P, Ärlebäck A, Funch-Jensen P, Kruse A, Jarnerot G. Clinical significance of manometric assessment of both pancreatic duct and bile duct sphincter in the same patient. *Scand J Gastroenterol* 1989; 24: 751–4.

51 Silverman WB, Ruffolo TA, Sherman S, Hawes RH, Lehman GA. Correlation of basal sphincter pressures measured from both the bile duct and pancreatic duct in patients with suspected sphincter of Oddi dysfunction. *Gastrointest Endosc* 1992; 38: 440–3.

52 Chan YK, Evans PR, Dowsett JF, Kellow JE, Badcock CA. Discordance of pressure recordings from biliary and pancreatic duct segments in patients with suspected sphincter of Oddi dysfunction. *Dig Dis Sci* 1997; 42: 1501–6.

53 Kalloo AN, Tietjen TG, Pasricha PJ. Does intrabiliary pressure predict basal sphincter of Oddi pressure? A study in patients with and without gallbladders. *Gastrointest Endosc* 1996; 44: 696–9.

54 Guelrud M, Mendoza S, Rossiter G, Villegas MI. Sphincter of Oddi manometry in healthy volunteers. *Dig Dis Sci* 1990; 35: 38–46.

55 Sherman S, Troiano FP, Hawes RH, Lehman GA. Sphincter of Oddi manometry: decreased risk of clinical pancreatitis with the use of a modified aspirating catheter. *Gastrointest Endosc* 1990; 36: 462–6.

56 Rolny P, Anderberg B, Ihse I, Lindstrom E, Olaison G, Arvill A. Pancreatitis after sphincter of Oddi manometry. *Gut* 1990; 31: 821–4.

57 Maldonado ME, Brady PG, Mamel JJ, Robinson B. Incidence of pancreatitis in patients undergoing sphincter of Oddi manometry (SOM). *Am J Gastroenterol* 1999; 94: 387–90.

58 Tarnasky PR, Palesch YY, Cunningham JT, Mauldin PD, Cotton PB, Hawes RH. Pancreatic stenting prevents pancreatitis after biliary sphincterotomy in patients with sphincter of Oddi dysfunction. *Gastroenterology* 1998; 115: 1518–24.

59 Sherman S, Ruffolo TA, Hawes RH, Lehman GA. Complications of endoscopic sphincterotomy. A prospective series with emphasis on the increased risk associated with sphincter of Oddi dysfunction and nondilated bile ducts. *Gastroenterology* 1991; 101: 1068–75.

60 Freeman ML, Nelson DB, Sherman S, Haber GB, Herman ME, Dorsher PJ *et al.* Complications of endoscopic biliary sphincterotomy: a prospective, multicenter study. *N Engl J Med* 1996; 335: 909–18.

61 Guelrud M, Mendoza S, Rossiter G, Ramirez L, Barkin J. Effect of nifedipine on sphincter of Oddi motor activity: studies in healthy volunteers and patients with biliary dyskinesia. *Gastroenterology* 1988; 95: 1050–5.

62 Khuroo MS, Zargar SA, Yattoo GN. Efficacy of nifedipine therapy in patients with sphincter of Oddi dysfunction: a prospective, double-blind, randomized, placebo-controlled, cross over trial. *Br J Clin Pharmacol* 1992; 33: 477–85.

63 Sand J, Nordback I, Koskinen M, Matikainen M, Lindholm TS. Nifedipine for suspected Type II sphincter of Oddi dyskinesia. *Am J Gastroenterol* 1993; 88: 530–5.

64 Guelrud M, Rossiter A, Souney P, Mendoza S, Mujica V. The effect of transcutaneous nerve stimulation on sphincter of Oddi pressure in patients with biliary dyskinesia. *Am J Gastroenterol* 1991; 86: 581–5.

65 Lee SK, Kim MH, Kim HJ, Seo DS, Yoo KS, Joo YH *et al*. Electroacupuncture may relax the sphincter of Oddi in humans. *Gastrointest Endosc* 2001; 53: 211–16.

66 Moody FG, Vecchio R, Calabuig R, Runkel N. Transduodenal sphincteroplasty with trans-ampullary septectomy for stenosing papillitis. *Am J Surg* 1991; 161: 213–18.

67 Sherman S, Hawes RH, Madura J, Lehman GA. Comparison of intraoperative and endoscopic manometry of the sphincter of Oddi. *Surg Gynecol Obstet* 1992; 175: 410–18.

68 Chen JW, Saccone GT, Toouli J. Sphincter of Oddi dysfunction and acute pancreatitis. *Gut* 1998; 43: 305–8.

69 Kozarek RA. Balloon dilation of the sphincter of Oddi. *Endoscopy* 1988; 20: 207–10.

70 Kozarek RA. Pancreatic stents can induce ductal changes consistent with chronic pancreatitis. *Gastrointest Endosc* 1990; 36: 93–5.

71 Fogel EL, Kwon E, Sherman S, Philips SD, Watkins JL, Paige-Ongay B *et al*. Pancreatic ductal alterations following small diameter, long length, unflanged pancreatic duct (PD) stent placement. *Gastrointest Endosc* 2001; 53: A86.

72 Goff JS. Common bile duct sphincter of Oddi stenting in patients with suspected sphincter of Oddi dysfunction. *Am J Gastroenterol* 1995; 90: 586–9.

73 Rolny P. Endoscopic bile duct stent placement as a predictor of outcome following endoscopic sphincterotomy in patients with suspected sphincter of Oddi dysfunction. *Eur J Gastroenterol Hepatol* 1997; 9: 467–71.

74 Rolny P, Geenen JE, Hogan WJ. Post-cholecystectomy patients with 'objective signs' of partial bile outflow obstruction: clinical characteristics, sphincter of Oddi manometry findings, and results of therapy. *Gastrointest Endosc* 1993; 39: 778–81.

75 Bozkurt T, Orth KH, Butsch B, Lux G. Long-term clinical outcome of post-cholecystectomy patients with biliary-type pain: results of manometry, non-invasive techniques and endoscopic sphincterotomy. *Eur J Gastroenterol Hepatol* 1996; 8: 245–9.

76 Wehrmann T, Wiemer K, Lembcke B, Caspary WF, Juno M. Do patients with sphincter of Oddi dysfunction benefit from endoscopic sphincterotomy? A 5-year prospective trial. *Eur J Gastroenterol Hepatol* 1996; 8: 251–6.

77 Geenen JE, Hogan WJ, Dodds WJ, Toouli J, Venu RP. The efficacy of endoscopic sphinctero-tomy after cholecystectomy in patients with sphincter of Oddi dysfunction. *N Engl J Med* 1989; 320: 82–7.

78 Toouli J, Roberts-Thomson I, Kellow J *et al*. Prospective randomized trial of endoscopic sphincterotomy for treatment of sphincter of Oddi dysfunction. *J Gastroenterol Hepatol* 1996; 11: A115.

79 Toouli J, Roberts-Thomson IC, Kellow J, Dowsett J, Saccone GTP, Evans P *et al*. Manometry based randomized trial of endoscopic sphincterotomy for sphincter of Oddi dysfunction. *Gut* 2000; 46: 98–102.

80 Sherman S, Lehman GA, Jamidar P, Hawes RH, Silverman W, Madura J *et al*. Efficacy of endoscopic sphincterotomy and surgical sphincteroplasty for patients with sphincter of Oddi dysfunction (SOD): randomized, controlled study. *Gastrointest Endosc* 1994; 40: A125.

81 Guelrud M, Plaz J, Mendoza S, Beker B, Rojas O, Rossiter G. Endoscopic treatment in Type II pancreatic sphincter dysfunction. *Gastrointest Endosc* 1995; 41: A398.

82 Soffer EE, Johlin FC. Intestinal dysmotility in patients with sphincter of Oddi dysfunction. A reason for failed response to sphincterotomy. *Dig Dis Sci* 1994; 39: 1942–6.

83 Eversman D, Fogel E, Philips S, Sherman S, Lehman G. Sphincter of Oddi dysfunction (SOD): long-term outcome of biliary sphincterotomy (BES) correlated with abnormal biliary and pan-creatic sphincters. *Gastrointest Endosc* 1999; 49: A78.

84 Elton E, Howell DA, Parsons WG, Qaseem T, Hanson BL. Endoscopic pancreatic sphinctero-tomy: indications, outcome, and a safe stentless technique. *Gastrointest Endosc* 1998; 47: 240–9.

85 Kaw M, Verma R, Brodmerkel GJ. Biliary and/or pancreatic sphincter of Oddi dysfunction (SOD). Response to endoscopic sphincterotomy (ES). *Gastrointest Endosc* 1996; 43: A384.

86 Freeman ML, DiSario JA, Nelson DB, Fennerty MB, Lee JG, Bjorkman DJ et al. Risk factors for post-ERCP pancreatitis: a prospective, multicenter study. *Gastrointest Endosc* 2001; 54: 425–34.

87 Gottlieb K, Sherman S. ERCP- and endoscopic sphincterotomy-induced pancreatitis. *Gastrointest Endosc Clin N Am* 1998; 8: 87–114.

88 Tarnasky P, Cunningham T, Cotton P, Hoffman B, Palesch Y, Freeman T et al. Pancreatic sphincter hypertension increases the risk of post-ERCP pancreatitis. *Endoscopy* 1997; 29: 252–7.

89 Sherman S, Lehman G, Freeman ML, Earle D, Watkins J, Barnett T et al. Risk factors for post-ERCP pancreatitis: a prospective multicenter study. *Am J Gastroenterol* 1997; 92: A1639.

90 Fogel EL, Devereaux BM, Rerknimitr R, Sherman S, Bucksot L, Lehman GA. Does placement of a small diameter, long length, unflanged pancreatic duct stent reduce the incidence of post-ERCP pancreatitis? *Gastrointest Endosc* 2000; 51: A182.

91 Pasricha PJ, Miskovsky EP, Kalloo AN. Intrasphincteric injection of botulinum toxin for suspected sphincter of Oddi dysfunction. *Gut* 1994; 35: 1319–21.

92 Wehrmann T, Seifert H, Seipp M, Lembcke B, Caspary WF. Endoscopic injection of botulinum toxin for biliary sphincter of Oddi dysfunction. *Endoscopy* 1998; 30: 702–7.

93 Kuo WH, Pasricha PJ, Kalloo AN. The role of sphincter of Oddi manometry in the diagnosis and therapy of pancreatic disease. *Gastrointest Endosc Clin N Am* 1998; 8: 79–85.

94 Ros E, Navarro S, Bru C, Garcia-Puges A, Valderrama R. Occult microlithiasis in 'idiopathic' acute pancreatitis: prevention of relapses by cholecystectomy or ursodeoxycholic acid therapy. *Gastroenterology* 1991; 101: 1701–9.

95 Kaw M, Brodmerkel GJ Jr. ERCP, biliary crystal analysis, and sphincter of Oddi manometry in idiopathic recurrent pancreatitis. *Gastrointest Endosc* 2002; 55: 157–62.

96 Toouli J, Di Francesco V, Saccone G, Kollias J, Schloithe A, Shanks N. Division of the sphincter of Oddi for treatment of dysfunction associated with recurrent pancreatitis. *Br J Surg* 1996; 83: 1205–10.

97 Okolo PI 3rd, Pasricha PJ, Kalloo AN. What are the long-term results of endoscopic pancreatic sphincterotomy? *Gastrointest Endosc* 2000; 52: 15–19.

98 Jacob L, Geenen JE, Catalano MF, Geenen DJ. Prevention of pancreatitis in patients with idiopathic recurrent pancreatitis: a prospective nonblinded randomized study using endoscopic stents. *Endoscopy* 2001; 33: 559–62.

99 Smith MT, Sherman S, Ikenberry SO, Hawes RH, Lehman GA. Alterations in pancreatic duct morphology following polyethylene pancreatic stent therapy. *Gastrointest Endosc* 1996; 44: 268–75.

100 Wehrmann T, Schmitt TH, Arndt A, Lembcke B, Caspary WF, Seifert H. Endoscopic injection of botulinum toxin in patients with recurrent acute pancreatitis due to pancreatic sphincter of Oddi dysfunction. *Aliment Pharmacol Ther* 2000; 14: 1469–77.

CHAPTER 9

ERCP in Acute Pancreatitis

MARTIN L. FREEMAN

Synopsis

ERCP plays an expanding role in both the diagnosis and therapy of acute and relapsing pancreatitis of various etiologies. Although initially used in the diagnosis and treatment of biliary disorders causing pancreatitis, endoscopic interventions are now increasingly directed towards the pancreatic sphincter and ducts as well. In certain settings, such as acute gallstone pancreatitis, the value of ERCP has been proven in randomized controlled trials. There are also data to support the role of ERCP in the treatment of acute relapsing pancreatitis due to various disorders, such as pancreas divisum and to a lesser degree sphincter of Oddi dysfunction. Other applications include the use of ERCP to treat smoldering pancreatitis and pancreatic ductal disruptions in the setting of acute and chronic pancreatitis, and most recently in the setting of evolving pancreatic necrosis. Many causes of otherwise unexplained acute recurrent pancreatitis can be found after an extensive evaluation and treated by advanced ERCP techniques. The role of ERCP in acute and especially recurrent pancreatitis should be primarily therapeutic, with diagnosis first established whenever possible by other techniques, including endoscopic ultrasound and MRCP. ERCP for the diagnosis and treatment of severe or acute relapsing pancreatitis is optimally performed in a multidisciplinary context involving primary or critical care, advanced hepato-biliary–pancreatic surgery, and interventional radiology when appropriate.

Introduction

ERCP appeared in the early 1970s and soon evolved as a diagnostic and therapeutic technique for biliary tract disorders. Biliary therapy including sphincterotomy was then applied to biliary causes of acute pancreatitis such as gallstone pancreatitis. Over the last decade, the application of pancreatic diagnostic and therapeutic techniques has expanded to incorporate a wider range of pancreatic methods including pancreatic sphincterotomy, stenting, stricture dilation, and stone extraction via the major and minor papillae. These techniques have allowed the endoscopist to approach the therapy of a wider range of causes of acute pancreatitis.

This chapter reviews the established and investigational applications of ERCP for the diagnosis and treatment of acute and recurrent acute pancreatitis.

Interdisciplinary management: complex ERCP

ERCP for the diagnosis and treatment of non-biliary acute or relapsing pancreatitis is optimally performed in a multidisciplinary context involving primary or critical care, advanced hepatobiliary–pancreatic surgery, and interventional radiology when appropriate (Fig. 9.1). The majority of endoscopists performing ERCP are capable of performing biliary therapy including sphincterotomy and stone extraction, affording them the ability to diagnose and treat biliary pancreatitis. However, performance of pancreatic endotherapy is considerably more technically challenging, requires more complex equipment and accessories, and generally carries higher risk, and is thus best performed primarily at tertiary centers with extensive expertise in these techniques (Table 9.1). The role of ERCP in acute pancreatitis should be primarily therapeutic, with diagnosis established whenever possible by other techniques, including endoscopic ultrasound and MRCP. It is also important to perform ERCP on the appropriate patients using optimal timing and techniques.

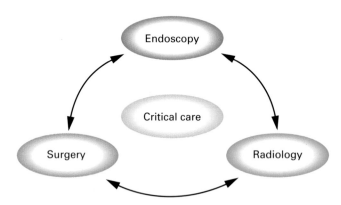

Fig. 9.1 Context for the management of complex pancreatic disease.

Table 9.1 Risks and settings for pancreatic endotherapy.

Substantially more difficult and risky than conventional biliary endotherapy
Should be performed in multidisciplinary context
Assess whether you and your center are appropriate before undertaking

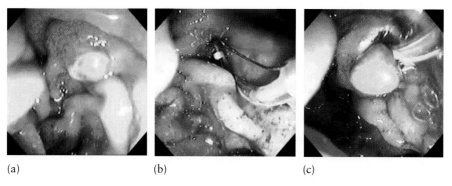

(a)   (b)   (c)

Fig. 9.2 Acute gallstone pancreatitis. This 48-year-old female presented with abdominal pain, tachycardia, hypoxemia, severe hyperamylasemia, mildly elevated transaminases, and normal bilirubin, and transabdominal ultrasound showed multiple gallstones with a shadowing stone in a mildly dilated common bile duct. Urgent ERCP showed a stone impacted in the ampulla (a), with a second floating stone in the bile duct (likely the one visualized by ultrasound). (b) ERCP with biliary sphincterotomy and (c) stone extraction was performed with gradual resolution of symptoms.

Acute gallstone pancreatitis

Gallstone disease accounts for approximately half of the cases of acute pancreatitis in the Western world [1–3]. Biliary pancreatitis may result in severe, necrotizing, life-threatening, or fatal pancreatitis as it often occurs in a previously healthy gland. As many as 25% of patients with biliary pancreatitis may develop severe pancreatitis and mortality may be as high as 10%. The role of ERCP in acute biliary pancreatitis has long been recognized and there is now substantial evidence from randomized controlled trials that early ERCP with biliary sphincterotomy and stone extraction (Fig. 9.2) can improve the outcome of properly selected patients with acute biliary pancreatitis.

Clinical diagnosis of acute gallstone pancreatitis

Biliary pancreatitis is usually suspected in the setting of acute abdominal pain with hyperamylasemia or hyperlipasemia, in the absence of another etiology such as alcohol, and in the presence of gallstones as documented by ultrasound, computed tomography (CT), or other imaging techniques [4,5]. There is usually elevation of liver chemistries although the pattern is not consistent, and may include elevated serum bilirubin, transaminase, or alkaline phosphatase. Jaundice and a dilated bile duct are further supporting evidence of biliary etiology in the context of biliary stone disease. The sensitivity and specificity of predictors of acute biliary pancreatitis are also variable but acute biliary pancreatitis is more likely in patients with markedly elevated serum amylase or elevated serum transaminase.

Predicting severity of acute pancreatitis

Assessment of the severity of acute pancreatitis is a complex topic beyond the scope of this chapter [6]. Various indices, including Ranson's criteria, Apache II score, presence of organ failure, and CT severity index [7,8], all have important prognostic value. Elevated serum hematocrit indicating hemoconcentration has recently been proposed as another predictor of poor outcome [9].

Acute treatment

In patients suspected to have severe pancreatitis, resuscitation is critical and intensive care unit management is advised. There is little role for early cholecystectomy in severe cases [10]. The relevant issue for the endoscopist is whether to perform ERCP in patients with acute suspected biliary pancreatitis.

The role of early ERCP

There are substantial data regarding the efficacy of ERCP in this setting, including four randomized controlled trials comparing early ERCP with biliary sphincterotomy to no intervention.

British study

A British group was the first to prospectively evaluate the role of ERCP in acute biliary pancreatitis [11]. In that study, 121 patients with acute pancreatitis and ultrasound evidence of gallstone disease were randomized to either conventional medical management or urgent ERCP within 72 h. Patients were stratified by severity of illness; one-half of the patients randomized to ERCP had severe pancreatitis. Common bile duck stones were found in 63% of patients with severe pancreatitis, but in only 25% of those with mild pancreatitis. Sphincterotomy was performed in those patients found to have bile duct stones. In the group randomized to intervention with ERCP and sphincterotomy, there was a significant reduction in complications in those with severe disease: 24% with 4% mortality vs. 61% with 18% mortality. However, there was no difference in the outcomes of patients with mild pancreatitis.

Hong Kong study

In a subsequent study from Hong Kong [12], 195 patients with acute pancreatitis were randomized to receive ERCP with sphincterotomy vs. conservative management within 24 h of admission. Stones were found in 65% of the patients. The major difference in outcome of the group undergoing ERCP was a reduction in biliary sepsis (0% after ERCP vs. 14% in the conservative group). There was a tendency towards fewer complications in the ERCP group vs. conservative management group, especially in those with severe pancreatitis, and a slight trend towards a reduction in mortality. The applicability of this study has been questioned as bile duct stones in Asians are more often primary bile duct stones rather than cholesterol stones originating from the gallbladder, thus reflecting different pathophysiology than in Western patients.

Polish study

A randomized controlled trial from Poland has been presented only in abstract form [13]; 280 patients with acute biliary pancreatitis all underwent ERCP within 24 h of admission. All patients with bile duct stones were treated with biliary sphincterotomy while the remaining patients without common bile duct stones were randomized to sphincterotomy or conventional treatment. There were significant reductions in complications in sphincterotomy-treated patients vs. conservatively treated patients (17% vs. 36%) and a significant reduction in mortality (2% vs. 13%). The benefits of intervention appeared to apply to patients with all severities of pancreatitis, including those with mild disease. Problems with this study include the fact that it has not been published in a peer-reviewed journal, a lack of true randomization, and the fact that some of the patients with empty ducts may have had more severe irreversible damage, or may have had pancreatitis due to etiologies other than stone disease.

German study

The most contentious study is the German multicenter study published in the *New England Journal of Medicine* [14], in which 238 patients with suspected biliary pancreatitis were randomized to early ERCP within 72 h of presentation or conservative management. Patients with jaundice were excluded. Fifty-eight of 121 patients randomized to the ERCP arm were found to have bile duct stones. In the control arm, 13 of 112 were crossed over to ERCP for apparent bile duct stones. In this study, there was no improvement in outcome from early sphincterotomy. Paradoxically, there appeared to be more severe complications, including respiratory failure, in the early ERCP group, and a numerically increased mortality. Major criticisms of this study have included the fact that patients most likely to benefit from ERCP, i.e. those with jaundice, were excluded from the study. Furthermore, many contributing centers enrolled fewer than two patients per year, raising questions about technical proficiency at ERCP.

Table 9.2 Meta-analysis of ERCP + biliary sphincterotomy (ES) versus conservative therapy for treatment of acute gallstone pancreatitis.

Reference	Complications (ERCP + ES)	Complications (control)	RRR	ARR	NNT
Neoptolemos et al. [11]	16.9%	33.9%	50.2	17.0	5.8
Fan et al. [12]	17.5%	28.6%	38.8	11.1	9
Folsch et al. [14]	46.0%	50.9%	19.6	4.9	20.4
Nowak et al. [13]	16.9%	36.3%	53.4	15.9	6.3
Pooled data	25%	38.2%	34.6	13.2	7.6

ARR, absolute risk reduction; NNT, number needed to treat; RRR, relative risk reduction.

Meta-analysis of studies of early ERCP, and current consensus

A meta-analysis of these randomized controlled trials has suggested that early intervention with ERCP in acute biliary pancreatitis results in a lower complication rate and a numerically lower mortality group rate [15] (Table 9.2). Meta-analysis found that complications occurred in 25% of treated patients vs. 38.2% of controls, $P < 0.001$, with a mortality of 5.2% in treated patients vs. 9.1% in control patients ($P = $ NS). The numbers needed to treat (NNT) for avoidance of complications and death were 7.6 and 25.6, respectively. Therefore, it is probably safe to say that early ERCP with sphincterotomy in patients with gallstone pancreatitis and persistent bile duct stones is effective in reducing complications, particularly in patients with severe pancreatitis.

ERCP is rarely indicated before cholecystectomy in patients with gallstone pancreatitis

Unless there is reasonably clear evidence of a persistent bile duct stone, such as a rising serum bilirubin or an imaging study clearly showing an intraductal stone, routine use of ERCP is unnecessary and adds avoidable risk in patients with mild to moderate biliary pancreatitis in whom cholecystectomy is planned. For the majority of patients with suspected biliary pancreatitis, bile duct stones have passed by the time cholangiography is performed. ERCP can be deferred and any remaining ductal stones can be identified at intraoperative cholangiography during laparoscopic cholecystectomy. These stones can then be removed by postoperative or even intraoperative ERCP, or, in those few centers with the appropriate expertise, by laparoscopic common bile duct exploration. If ERCP is unsuccessful, the patient can be referred to a tertiary endoscopy center where biliary access is virtually always possible.

Acute pancreatitis postcholecystectomy

ERCP is appropriate in postcholecystectomy patients with suspected biliary pancreatitis, but in many of these patients there is a non-biliary stone etiology, such as sphincter of Oddi dysfunction, a setting in which conventional diagnostic and therapeutic ERCP techniques can be highly risky [16,17], and protective measures, such as placement of a pancreatic stent, may be advisable [18,19].

Treatment by biliary sphincterotomy alone?

Empirical biliary sphincterotomy for suspected biliary pancreatitis may be appropriate in certain settings without cholecystectomy, especially in elderly patients who are not good candidates for surgery due to severe medical comorbidity [20–24]. Under these circumstances, biliary sphincterotomy is sometimes performed in the absence of demonstration of a definite bile duct stone or as a semidefinitive treatment in lieu of cholecystectomy. Several studies have suggested the effectiveness of endoscopic biliary sphincterotomy in preventing future episodes of acute biliary pancreatitis [25]. These uncontrolled case series mostly suggest a reduction in the frequency of pancreatitis attacks, although recurrent bile duct stones and cholecystitis may be problematic [26]. Caution must be applied to patients who might have other etiologies. Empirical biliary sphincterotomy in patients with recurrent pancreatitis and mildly abnormal enzymes may in fact be due to sphincter of Oddi dysfunction, especially in women, younger to middle-aged patients, and those who are postcholecystectomy or do not have clearly documented gallstone disease. Empirical biliary sphincterotomy and even diagnostic ERCP in this setting may be quite hazardous [16,17] and less likely to be of benefit.

Pancreatic duct disruptions

Acute disruptions of the main pancreatic duct or side branches may occur during acute pancreatitis of various etiologies, such as gallstones or alcohol, or may be the primary mechanism of pancreatitis in cases such as trauma. These disruptions may result in localized fluid collections, pseudocysts, ascites, or pancreatico-pleural or cutaneous fistulas.

Stenting for duct disruption

ERCP with transpapillary pancreatic duct stenting has been described as an effective technique to close pancreatic duct disruptions in a variety of settings in

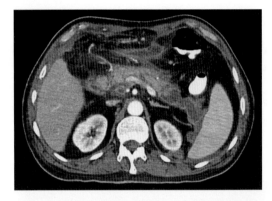

Fig. 9.3 CT scan showing a persistent leak from the pancreatic duct after surgical debridement of severe necrotizing medication-induced pancreatitis.

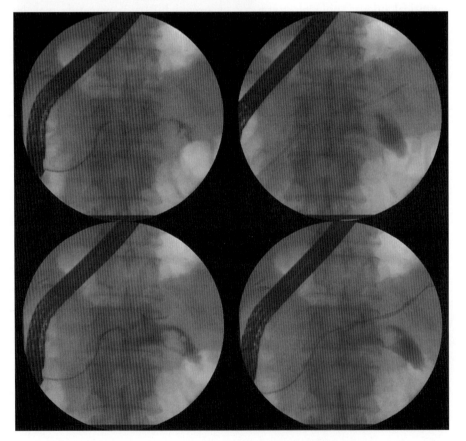

Fig. 9.4 ERCP showing bridging of the disrupted main pancreatic duct with a guidewire and stent, leading to ultimate closure of the leak.

acute and chronic pancreatitis [27–29] (Figs 9.3 and 9.4). Unlike for biliary strictures, it may often be necessary to bridge the main pancreatic duct beyond the point of disruption with a stent in order to obtain closure of a pancreatic duct leak, especially if there is a small-caliber, diseased, or strictured pancreatic duct.

The use of transpapillary pancreatic duct stenting in evolving acute necrosis or complicated pancreatitis has been recently reported [30]. This is based on the theory that main pancreatic ductal disruption is integral to the pathophysiology of acute pancreatic necrosis, and suggests that transpapillary pancreatic stenting might be beneficial in the course of this difficult group of patients by relieving downstream obstruction and thus reducing complications. In patients with pancreatic necrosis in various stages of evolution at the time of transfer to their institution, this group reported a management strategy including ERCP, with findings of main pancreatic duct disruptions in two-thirds of patients who were treated with transpapillary pancreatic stent plus/minus biliary sphincterotomy. In general, organized necrosis or fluid collections were drained separately by surgical, percutaneous, or endoscopic routes. They reported a very low mortality in this case series of over 100 patients. Although an intriguing concept, this approach deserves further study in a randomized controlled trial. Special concerns with performance of ERCP in the setting of acute necrosis include the risk of introducing infection into otherwise sterile pancreatic necrosis and/or fluid collections.

Smoldering pancreatitis

Rapid resolution of persistent smoldering pancreatitis without associated pancreatic duct disruption has been reported to occur with placement of a transpapillary stent. We and others have also found this to be quite effective in patients with a prolonged course of smoldering pancreatitis that persists for 2 to 3 weeks or more, with pain and hyperamylasemia despite fasting and total parenteral nutrition, and often without significant pancreatic injury evident by CT scan. Regardless of the etiology of pancreatitis, placement of a transpapillary stent can often interrupt and hasten resolution of the process [31,32]. There are limited data supporting this approach, with no randomized controlled trials.

Acute recurrent pancreatitis

Acute recurrent pancreatitis is most commonly the result of alcohol or gallstone disease. Other etiologies include medications such as azathioprine, tetracycline, or estrogens [33–35]. Metabolic causes such as severe hypertriglyceridemia [36] or hypercalcemia may be revealed by laboratory investigation.

'Idiopathic' pancreatitis

Some 10–30% of patients with acute recurrent pancreatitis may have no etiology apparent by history, laboratory, and non-invasive imaging studies such as CT or ultrasound. Such patients are often labeled as having 'idiopathic' pancreatitis. 'Unexplained acute pancreatitis' and 'unexplained acute recurrent pancreatitis' are more appropriate terms, reserving the label 'idiopathic' for pancreatitis whose etiology remains unidentified after a truly exhaustive and advanced evaluation. Advanced diagnostic investigation may reveal etiologies such as microlithiasis, sphincter of Oddi dysfunction, congenital anomalies such as pancreas divisum, annular pancreas, intraductal papillary mucinous neoplasia, occult malignancy, idiopathic chronic pancreatitis with ductal pathology such as stones or strictures, or anatomical causes such as choledochocele or anomalous pancreatico-biliary junction. An increasingly diagnosed cause of 'unexplained' pancreatitis is autoimmune, or lymphoplasmacytic sclerosing pancreatitis. Only the remainder with normal pancreatico-biliary ductal anatomy and no other etiology are appropriately labeled as 'idiopathic'.

Microlithiasis and occult gallstones

Microlithiasis, biliary sludge, and occult gallstones are part of a spectrum of biliary disorders that may cause acute recurrent pancreatitis. The perceived prevalence of these disorders as a cause for recurrent pancreatitis, and the appropriate strategy for diagnosis and therapy, are the matter of some debate [37–39]. Patients with microlithiasis as a cause of pancreatitis usually have an intact gallbladder, and may or may not have associated abnormalities in liver chemistries. The best known study linking biliary sludge to recurrent pancreatitis included many patients with fairly suggestive evidence of a biliary cause, such as visible sludge at ultrasonography or abnormal liver chemistries, and thus included patients whose pancreatitis would not be considered as 'unexplained' or 'idiopathic' in most centers [38].

Detecting microlithiasis

Imaging techniques such as transcutaneous ultrasound may reveal layering sludge in the gallbladder or be entirely normal. Alternative diagnostic strategies include endoscopic ultrasound, which may be more sensitive for subtle gallbladder stone disease than transcutaneous ultrasound [40–43], and analysis of bile for crystals.

Bile crystals Bile analysis may be performed directly on the bile duct aspirates via retrograde cannulation at ERCP [44], ideally after gallbladder contraction is induced with cholecystokinin, or on duodenal bile collected by tube or endoscopy after gallbladder contraction is induced [45]. Bile is analyzed by a polarizing microscope for the presence of crystals. Problems with bile analysis include: (1) interobserver variation in technique and interpretation of analysis; (2) sensitivity and specificity of microscopic analysis for detecting biliary stone disease

[46]; and (3) uncertain correlation between findings of bile abnormalities and response to therapeutic intervention such as cholecystectomy or biliary sphincterotomy [47]. In general, crystal analysis has been found to be of limited value with a very low prevalence after cholecystectomy [48,49]. Treatment of microlithiasis as a cause for acute pancreatitis can include cholecystectomy, endoscopic biliary sphincterotomy, or ursodeoxycholic acid [38,50].

Empiric cholecystectomy? In the patient with unexplained acute recurrent pancreatitis and intact gallbladder, and normal pancreatico-biliary ductal anatomy by EUS or MRCP, it may be more prudent to consider empiric laparoscopic cholecystectomy rather than subjecting the patient to a potentially risky ERCP just to perform bile analysis of unclear predictive value. In patients who are postcholecystectomy, the low probability of a positive finding and high risk of performing ERCP just to make this diagnosis make the practice of bile analysis questionable. Other less invasive diagnostic modalities such as endoscopic ultrasound (EUS) or MRCP may be indicated prior to considering cholecystectomy as the diagnosis of occult tumors may otherwise be delayed.

Sphincter of Oddi dysfunction

Sphincter of Oddi dysfunction is thought by many to be an important cause of acute recurrent pancreatitis, accounting for up to one-third of otherwise unexplained cases [51,52]. Approaches to suspected sphincter of Oddi dysfunction vary widely and are the subject of much controversy. This disorder is most often suspected as a cause of recurrent pancreatitis in women who are postcholecystectomy, often with relatively mild pancreatitis and intermittent or continuous abdominal pain between overt attacks of pancreatitis.

Diagnosis of sphincter of Oddi dysfunction

The diagnosis is generally based on findings of an abnormal sphincter of Oddi manometry with a basal pressure of greater than 40 mmHg [53–55]. A number of studies have demonstrated the discordance of manometric findings between the biliary and pancreatic sphincters, and thus stress the importance of assessing both sphincters [56–59] (Fig. 9.5).

Endoscopic therapy for sphincter of Oddi dysfunction

Although the traditional approach has been to perform biliary sphincterotomy or other biliary therapy to treat recurrent pancreatitis or other symptoms of sphincter of Oddi dysfunction [60–66], recent data suggest that combined

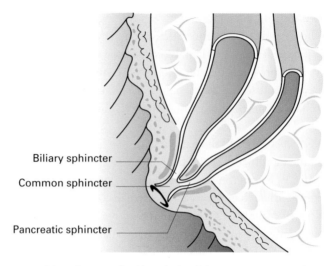

Biliary sphincter

Common sphincter

Pancreatic sphincter

Fig. 9.5 Anatomy of the sphincter of Oddi including biliary, pancreatic, and common sphincters.

pancreatic as well as biliary sphincterotomy, whether performed simultaneously (Fig. 9.6) or sequentially (Fig. 9.7), is optimal to treat patients who have concomitant pancreatic sphincter hypertension [67]. The desired result is a 'septotomy' in which a 'double-barrel' appearance of the biliary and pancreatic sphincters is achieved (Fig. 9.8). In one study, biliary sphincterotomy alone resulted in improvement in only 25% of patients; in contrast, either sequential biliary and pancreatic sphincterotomy (78% response) or simultaneous dual sphincterotomy (82% response) resulted in significantly better outcomes [67].

Sphincterotomy without sphincter manometry?

Some centers avoid sphincter of Oddi manometry or pancreatic endotherapy in these patients, advocating empiric biliary sphincterotomy [39,68] or alternative diagnostic tests such as quantitative scintigraphy [69], fatty-meal sonography, or secretin-stimulated assessment of pancreatic duct dilation [70].

Is sphincter manometry dangerous? This is based in part on the assumption that sphincter of Oddi manometry is the principal danger, and that merely avoiding this investigation will reduce risk [71]. The risk of any type of ERCP in these patients (women with recurrent abdominal pain and normal serum bilirubin) cannot be overemphasized; recent prospective multicenter multivariate studies [16,17] have shown clearly that diagnostic ERCP or empiric biliary sphincterotomy carries a substantial risk of pancreatitis (approximately

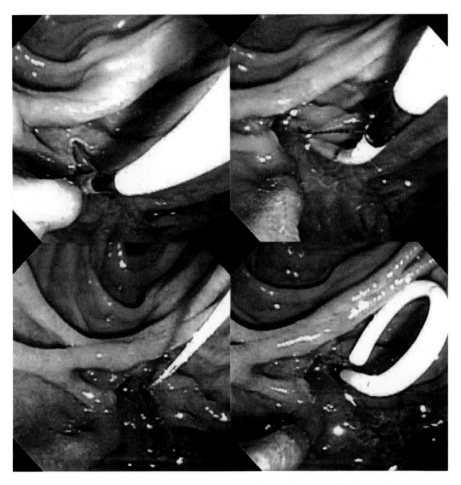

Fig. 9.6 Biliary and pancreatic sphincterotomies performed sequentially during the same procedure.

20% or higher), including the majority of severe and necrotizing cases. Newer techniques of aspirated sphincter manometry have been shown to add little or no independent risk to ERCP. Importantly, placement of a transpapillary pancreatic stent significantly reduces the risk of pancreatitis in patients with sphincter of Oddi dysfunction (from 27% to 7% in one randomized controlled trial) [72], and virtually eliminates the risk of severe post-ERCP pancreatitis (Fig. 9.9). Recent data suggest that, in patients with suspected sphincter of Oddi dysfunction, pancreatico-biliary manometry followed by combined pancreatico-biliary therapy that includes a pancreatic stent is actually safer than simple biliary sphincterotomy [73]. Prophylactic pancreatic stenting is now performed

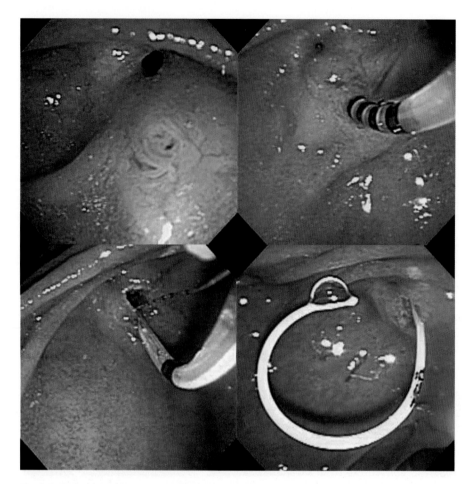

Fig. 9.7 Pancreatic manometry and sphincterotomy in a patient unresponsive to previous biliary sphincterotomy.

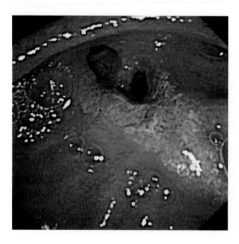

Fig. 9.8 Final appearance of pancreatic 'septotomy' after endoscopic biliary and pancreatic sphincterotomies for sphincter of Oddi dysfunction.

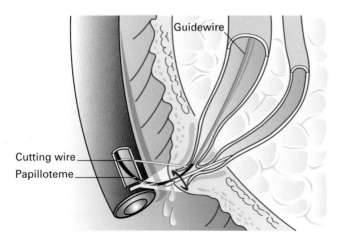

Fig. 9.9 Schematic diagram of pancreatic stent placement to reduce risk of post-ERCP pancreatitis.

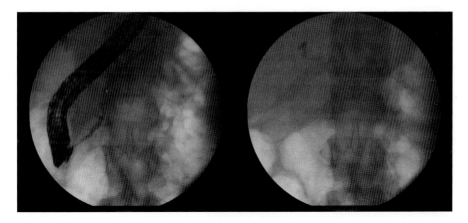

Fig. 9.10 Relatively easy pancreatic ductal anatomy for placement of pancreatic stent.

routinely in many centers after pancreatic investigation in these types of patients [18,74,75]. Placement of pancreatic stents can range from technically easy (Fig. 9.10) to very challenging (Fig. 9.11) depending on pancreatic ductal anatomy and endoscopic expertise. Pancreatic stents have potential to cause damage, especially to normal ducts [76–78] (Fig. 9.12), and should be removed within 10–14 days from normal ducts. The trend is now to use smaller stents (3 or 4 Fr) compared with traditional larger (5–7 Fr) stents, because they are thought to cause less ductal injury and lower post-ERCP pancreatitis rates [79].

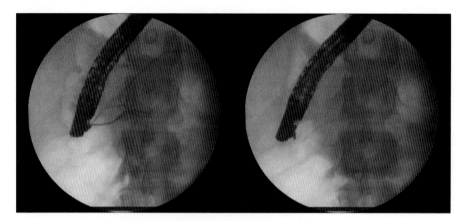

Fig. 9.11 Very difficult pancreatic ductal anatomy for placement of pancreatic stent.

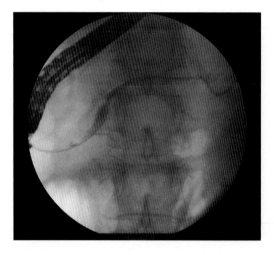

Fig. 9.12 Pancreatic stricture in a previously normal duct resulting from indwelling pancreatic stent for 4 weeks.

Many centers now use longer 3 Fr stents (8–12 cm long), without any internal flaps; most of these pass spontaneously in 1–3 weeks, and a simple abdominal radiograph is taken to confirm. This confers the same protection against pancreatitis, and removes the need for a second procedure in most cases. Short (2 cm) straight stents may still be necessary for the 15% of patients with very tortuous small-caliber ducts, in whom passage of a guidewire to the tail may be difficult or impossible [80]. Without any type of pancreatic stent, however, available data suggest that the risk of empiric biliary sphincterotomy for suspected sphincter of Oddi dysfunction (about 25% pancreatitis) is about equal to its efficacy (approximately 25%).

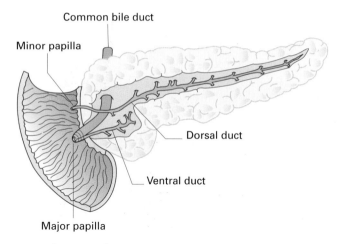

Fig. 9.13 Diagram of pancreas divisum.

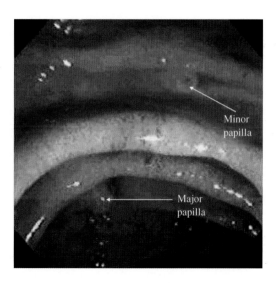

Fig. 9.14 Typical endoscopic appearance of major and minor papillae.

Sphincter of Oddi dysfunction in patients with intact gallbladders

Whether sphincter of Oddi dysfunction should be suspected in patients with an intact gallbladder is contentious. We generally recommend empiric cholecystectomy in most cases prior to investigation for sphincter of Oddi dysfunction as a cause for recurrent pancreatitis.

Pancreas divisum

Pancreas divisum is the most common congenital anomaly of the pancreas and may be present in up to 5% of the general population [81] (Figs 9.13 and 9.14).

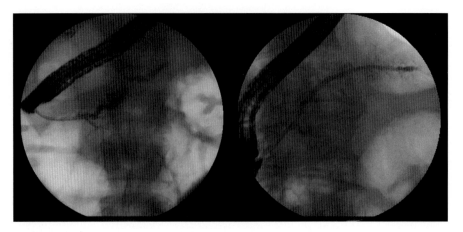

Fig. 9.15 Various appearances of the dorsal duct in patients with pancreas divisum and acute relapsing pancreatitis.

The diagnosis of pancreas divisum can be made by ERCP, MRCP [82–84], or EUS [85] demonstrating a small or absent ventral pancreatic duct draining into the major papilla that does not communicate with the dorsal duct draining entirely through the minor papilla. In patients with symptomatic pancreas divisum, the dorsal duct may be normal, dilated, or contain evidence of chronic pancreatitis including dorsal duct pancreatic stones (Fig. 9.15). Partial or vestigial communication between dorsal and ventral pancreatic ducts is called 'incomplete pancreas divisum' and behaves functionally similar to complete pancreas divisum [86]. Findings of apparent pancreas divisum at MRCP or ERCP can be mimicked by small tumors or strictures at the junction of the ducts of Wirsung and Santorini in patients with otherwise normal pancreatic ductal anatomy (see section on neoplastic disorders, p. 222).

Does pancreas divisum cause pancreatitis?

There has been some controversy about whether pancreas divisum is an innocent bystander or a cause of acute recurrent pancreatitis. The preponderance of evidence suggests that the dorsal duct outflow obstruction at the minor papilla can be the etiology of acute and chronic pancreatitis [4,87,88]. Evidence includes: an increased prevalence of pancreas divisum in patients with pancreatitis, the findings at autopsy of chronic pancreatitis isolated to the dorsal pancreas in patients with pancreas divisum, and data suggesting improved outcomes in patients undergoing minor papilla drainage procedures, either

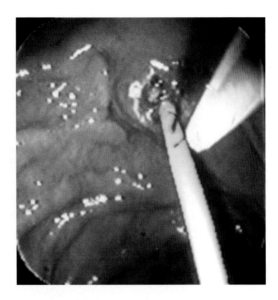

Fig. 9.16 Pancreatic sphincterotomy performed using a needle-knife over a pancreatic stent.

endoscopic or surgical [89–93]. Evidence for efficacy of endoscopic therapy includes a number of case series [94–99] and one randomized controlled trial [100] indicating improvement in frequency and severity of attacks after minor papillotomy and/or stenting.

Endoscopic treatment for pancreas divisum

Endoscopic therapy for symptomatic pancreas divisum consists of minor papilla sphincterotomy plus/minus dorsal duct pancreatic stenting or stone extraction [101] (Figs 9.16–9.18). Evidence suggests that results of minor papilla therapy for pancreas divisum are best in patients with acute recurrent pancreatitis, with improvement seen in up to 80% of patients (Table 9.3). In the sole randomized controlled trial of dorsal duct therapy for pancreas divisum, improvement was seen in 90% of treated patients vs. 11% of controls with reduction in hospitalizations for acute pancreatitis over a 12-month follow-up. Benefit is less evident in patients with chronic pancreatitis, with response rates of 40–50%. Whether or not there is any role for dorsal duct endotherapy in patients with pancreas divisum and pain only without evidence of pancreatic disease is controversial, but most series suggest responses of 20–30%, rates which may be no better than placebo. Furthermore, many patients do not fit neatly into one of the above three categories, but rather overlap features of all three patterns; they may have elevated amylase during pain attacks, but also have chronic pain, and/or EUS evidence of chronic pancreatitis. A new approach to select patients most likely to respond includes secretin-stimulated assessment of dorsal duct dilation. In

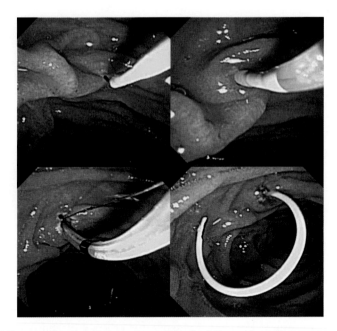

Fig. 9.17 Minor papilla cannulation using a glidewire followed by pull-type wire-guided sphincterotomy and stent placement in a patient with pancreas divisum and acute relapsing pancreatitis.

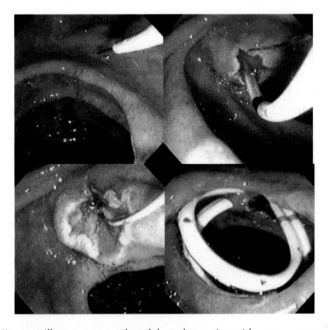

Fig. 9.18 Minor papillotomy to treat dorsal duct obstruction with acute recurrent pancreatitis in a patient with 'pseudodivisum' due to a small stone obstructing the pancreatic duct of Wirsung that could not be extracted.

Table 9.3 Results of minor papilla therapy for pancreas divisum.

Author	Year	Mean F/U (mo)	Acute recurrent pancreatitis		Pain only		Chronic pancreatitis	
			n	Improved (%)	n	Improved (%)	n	Improved (%)
Soehendra	1986	3	2	100	0	—	4	75
Ligoury	1986	24	8	63	0	—	0	—
McCarthy	1988	21	19	89	0	—	0	—
Lans	1992	30	10	90	0	—	0	—
Lehman	1993	22	17	76	23	26	11	27
Coleman	1994	23	9	78	5	0	20	60
Sherman	1994	28	0	—	16	44	0	—
Kozarek	1995	20	15	73	5	20	19	32
Ertan	2000	24	25	76	—	—	—	—
Total			95	79	49	29	54	44

one study, secretin-stimulated dilation of the dorsal pancreatic duct by EUS predicted favorable outcome to minor papilla therapy, a concept that deserves further scrutiny and corroboration [102].

Minor papilla therapy for pancreas divisum usually includes minor papilla sphincterotomy, which can be either performed after placement of a pancreatic stent using a needle-knife (Fig. 9.16), or using a conventional traction sphincterotome (Figs 9.17 and 9.18). Many endoscopists, including this author, now favor use of a wire-guided traction sphincterotome in most cases, as it assists with gauging the optimal extent and depth of the minor papilla sphincter incision. Eversion of the sphincter with a partially bowed papillotome may allow assessment of the length of the remaining sphincter segment.

Stenting for pancreas divisum A few centers advocate long-term pancreatic duct stenting; however, in the presence of a normal dorsal pancreatic duct, there is substantial risk of inducing pancreatic duct strictures or irregularities (up to 70% in one series) [75]. Most authorities recommend minor papillotomy with only short-term stenting, less than 2 weeks in most cases. Exceptions are the presence of a pancreatic duct stricture or a pancreatic duct stone in association with pancreas divisum (Fig. 9.15), in which case longer term stenting and/or adjunctive methods, such as extracorporeal shock-wave lithotripsy, may be necessary.

Problems with endoscopic therapy Major problems with dorsal duct therapy for pancreas divisum include technical difficulty, complications such as post-ERCP pancreatitis, and restenosis of the minor papillotomy. A recent large

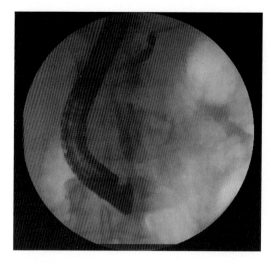

Fig. 9.19 Small main pancreatic duct stone in a young woman with acute recurrent pancreatitis due to idiopathic chronic pancreatitis.

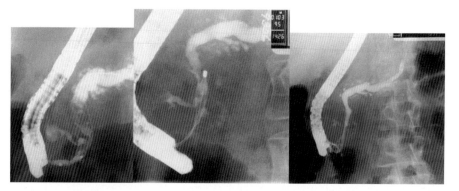

Fig. 9.20 Pancreatic duct stone extraction in a patient with acute recurrent pancreatitis due to hereditary pancreatitis.

series casts doubt on the long-term efficacy of minor papillotomy in relieving pain in any of the above groups, with eventual pain relapse in the majority. While initial response rates were consistent with previous studies, long-term pain relief was reported in only 43% of patients with relapsing pancreatitis, 21% of those with chronic pancreatitis, and 11% of those with pain only [103].

Chronic pancreatitis (idiopathic, alcohol, familial, other)

A relatively common finding in patients with acute recurrent pancreatitis is unsuspected chronic pancreatitis (Table 9.3 and Figs 9.19–9.22). Such patients may or may not have a history of alcohol abuse or family history of pancreatitis [104] and may have a normal or non-specific CT scan, but further investigation,

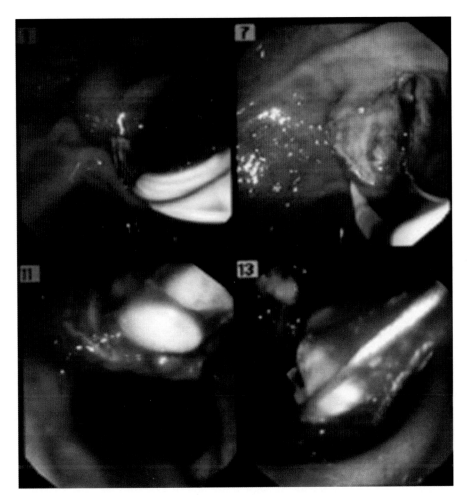

Fig. 9.21 Endoscopic view of pancreatic sphincterotomy and stone extraction for Fig. 9.20.

including EUS, may reveal moderate to severe chronic pancreatitis with normal-caliber or minimally dilated main pancreatic ducts, often with small intraductal stones and/or strictures [105–110]. The role of genetic abnormalities, such as CFTR mutations and cationic trypsinogen gene mutations, has been explored in the pathogenesis of idiopathic chronic and hereditary pancreatitis [15,111–116], but is of uncertain practical value in the management of patients with unexplained pancreatitis at present.

Endoscopic therapy for chronic pancreatitis

Pancreatic ductal abnormalities are often amenable to endoscopic therapy in the form of pancreatic sphincterotomy, pancreatic stone extraction with or without

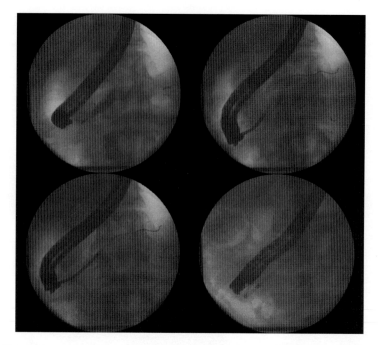

Fig. 9.22 Dilation and stenting of dorsal duct stricture via minor papilla in a patient with acute relapsing pancreatitis due to chronic alcoholic pancreatitis. A Soehendra 'screw' device is used to core through the stricture.

extracorporeal shock-wave lithotripsy, and/or stricture dilation with stenting [117–124]. Figures 9.19–9.22 show examples of endoscopic therapy in patients with acute relapsing pancreatitis due to chronic pancreatitis with intraductal stones or strictures of etiologies ranging from idiopathic (Fig. 9.19) to familial (Figs 9.20 and 9.21) to former alcohol abuse (Fig. 9.22).

Pancreatitis due to neoplastic obstruction

One of the most important and easily missed etiologies of unexplained acute pancreatitis is occult neoplastic disease. Ampullary tumors and larger solid and cystic pancreatic tumors are usually diagnosable by conventional techniques including ERCP [125–133]. However, CT scan, MRI, and diagnostic ERCP all are of limited value in the identification of small (less than 2 cm) solid tumors of the pancreas, such as pancreatic ductal adenocarcinoma, islet cell, or other neuroendocrine tumors, and for the diagnosis of early or side-branch variants of intraductal or papillary mucinous tumors of the pancreas [134,135]. Endosonography may be essential to diagnose these tumors [133,136–139] (Fig. 9.23). In our center's series of 102 patients with unexplained acute pancreatitis, none of whom had a mass on CT scan, 15 were diagnosed definitively to have occult neoplasms by linear-array EUS with fine-needle aspiration (FNA); nine could

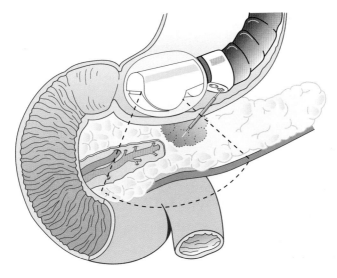

Fig. 9.23 Utility of linear-array EUS in the diagnosis of unexplained acute pancreatitis.

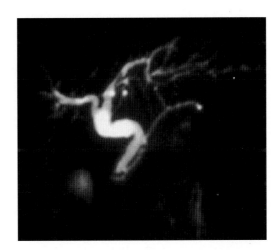

Fig. 9.24 MRCP in a patient with unexplained acute pancreatitis with normal CT scan. MRCP and ERCP suggested pancreas divisum (see Fig. 9.25).

not be diagnosed by any other technique including CT or ERCP [140] (Figs 9.24 and 9.25). The majority (eight of 10) were found to be resectable at the time of surgery.

Endoscopic management of neoplastic obstruction

There is a role for ERCP in the palliation of acute pancreatitis in certain patients with obstructing pancreatic neoplasms. In patients with recurrent pancreatitis due to obstructing ampullary adenomas, or in poor surgical candidates with ampullary carcinomas, endoscopic snare ampullectomy, often in combination

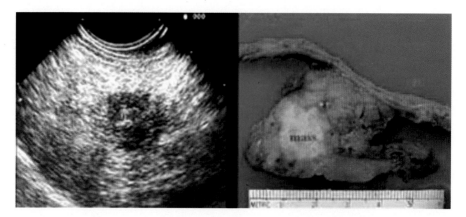

Fig. 9.25 Linear EUS of patient in Fig. 9.24 showing 15 mm mass with FNA positive for adenocarcinoma.

with ablative thermal therapy, such as argon plasma or bipolar coagulation, is a reasonable method to achieve palliation or cure of the underlying lesion [141–145]. The technique of ampullectomy increasingly includes pancreatic sphincterotomy and placement of a pancreatic stent to reduce the risk of both immediate and relapsing pancreatitis, which can otherwise be substantial [142]. There may also be a role for pancreatic sphincterotomy to palliate acute recurrent pancreatitis by preventing mucin impaction in patients with mucin-secreting tumors (intraductal papillary mucinous tumor, IPMT) who are not surgical candidates.

Stenting for smoldering pancreatitis due to malignancy

Some patients with pancreatic ductal adenocarcinoma or other solid tumors obstructing the pancreatic duct may present with acute or smoldering pancreatitis. ERCP in such cases often demonstrates a focal stricture with upstream dilation. In such patients, placement of a transpapillary stent through the pancreatic stricture may often interrupt or resolve the pancreatitis, either as a preoperative maneuver or as definitive palliation [146] (Fig. 9.26). In selected patients with unresectable pancreatic neoplasms and smoldering or acute pancreatitis, self-expanding metallic stents have been placed through pancreatic strictures for more long-term palliation (Fig. 9.27) [147].

Choledochocele

Cystic dilation of the intramural segment of the distal pancreatico-biliary segment is called a choledochocele (type III choledochal cyst). These may range in size from a few millimeters to several centimeters and may herniate in the duo-

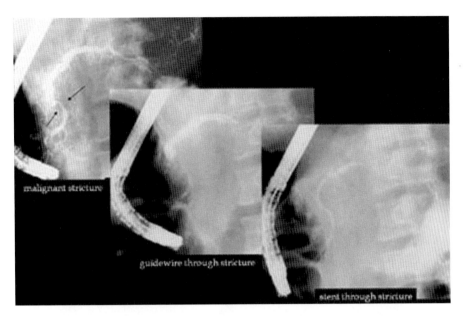

Fig. 9.26 ERCP in a young man with metastatic melanoma and intractable acute pancreatitis requiring TPN and continuous narcotics. Malignant stricture in the head of the pancreas with upstream dilation is traversed with a guidewire and stented, with resolution of pancreatitis and pain.

denum. These may be associated with both pancreatic and biliary obstruction and may cause acute recurrent pancreatitis [148–154]. Although biliary sphincterotomy is classically thought to be the definitive treatment, a substantial number of these patients eventually require pancreatic as well as biliary sphincterotomy for long-term palliation.

Other rare causes of pancreatitis

Other miscellaneous conditions such as annular pancreas [155–157], anomalous pancreatico-biliary junction [158], or pancreatic intraductal parasites have been reported to cause acute or recurrent pancreatitis. These may be diagnosed by EUS, MRCP, or ERCP and may sometimes be amenable to endoscopic intervention.

Overall approach to unexplained acute pancreatitis

The approach to unexplained acute or recurrent pancreatitis varies widely among centers and is the subject of substantial controversy [159]. Recommended approaches for endoscopy vary from treatment based on analysis of bile for

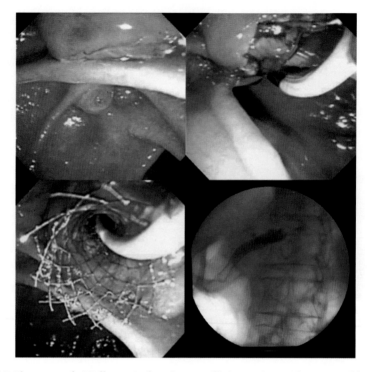

Fig. 9.27 Placement of a Wall stent in the minor papilla in a patient with unresectable pancreatic cancer obstructing the dorsal pancreatic duct who presented with pancreatitis and pancreatic duct disruption.

crystals, to empiric cholecystectomy, to ERCP with empiric biliary sphinctero-tomy [39], to ERCP with performance of sphincter of Oddi manometry focused on the biliary sphincter segment, to sphincter of Oddi manometry focused on the pancreatic sphincter segment. The use of alternative imaging techniques, such as MRCP [82,160–164] and EUS, in evaluating unexplained pancreatitis varies widely, often related more to local expertise and bias rather than data. Therapy at some centers is focused primarily at suspected biliary causes (either by cholecystectomy or endoscopic biliary sphincterotomy), while in most advanced centers the focus of diagnosis and treatment is usually to identify and correct pancreatic sphincter or ductal abnormalities. Many advanced centers have evolved to the opinion that, in most cases of recurrent pancreatitis, the problem lies in the pancreas itself and not in the biliary tract.

Concerns about ERCP and empiric sphincterotomy in recurrent acute pancreatitis

ERCP is often overused as a diagnostic and empiric biliary therapeutic modality in unexplained acute pancreatitis, potentially exposing the patient to unneces-sary risk for a limited therapeutic benefit. Systematic evaluation with multiple imaging techniques, especially EUS and secretin-enhanced MRCP, provides more useful anatomic information, particularly regarding occult tumors, chronic pancreatitis [106], occult biliary stone disease, and pancreas divisum, and in some cases eliminates the need for ERCP entirely [82,160]. In particular, the appropriateness of diagnostic ERCP and empiric biliary sphincterotomy for findings of normal ductal anatomy to treat presumed microlithiasis or sphincter of Oddi dysfunction, which is advocated even at some advanced centers, may be questioned.

Risks of ERCP

Available data suggest that the performance of empiric biliary sphincterotomy without pancreatic stenting incurs a risk of post-ERCP pancreatitis (20% in one multicenter study [16], including a 3–4% rate of severe pancreatitis) that may equal the chance of curing the underlying cause of pancreatitis (25% in the series of Guelrud). This risk may be even higher in patients with possible sphincter of Oddi dysfunction and small ducts [165]. Enduring but unsubstantiated beliefs are that diagnostic ERCP is safe—in fact the risk is as high as for therapeutic ERCP—and that sphincter of Oddi manometry is the primary culprit. In fact, two recent multivariate analyses have shown that sphincter of Oddi manometry utilizing the aspirating catheter in the pancreas adds no independent risk to ERCP [16,17]. Rather, it is the patient profile (female, recurrent abdominal pain, and absence of jaundice or advanced chronic pancreatitis) that places the patient at higher risk of any ERCP. Paradoxically, centers performing sphincter of Oddi manometry often have lower pancreatitis rates after ERCP in these patients than do referring community centers [16], probably because of the widespread use of pancreatic stents, which have been shown to significantly reduce the risk of post-ERCP pancreatitis in patients with sphincter of Oddi dysfunction (Fig. 9.9). Given the risk of diagnostic ERCP in these types of patients, ERCP merely for the purpose of collecting bile for crystal analysis in patients with intact gallbladders and recurrent pancreatitis seems questionable; performance of empiric cholecystectomy is probably safer and more definitive.

Investigations other than ERCP

Prior to considering ERCP for unexplained acute pancreatitis, we and others use a systematic approach, including advanced imaging techniques such as EUS, in most cases (Fig. 9.23). Initial evaluation of acute pancreatitis includes a detailed history regarding alcohol, medications, family history, and laboratory evaluation including liver chemistries and amylase, lipase, triglyceride, and calcium levels. Initial imaging studies should include transabdominal ultrasound, often repeated at least once if the initial study is negative, and abdominal CT scan.

MRCP

Magnetic resonance cholangiopancreatography [82,160] is quite useful as it can fairly reliably establish the anatomy of the bile and pancreatic ducts, identify pancreas divisum or pancreatic ductal strictures, diagnose bile duct stones, and image pancreatic or biliary duct dilation. Secretin administration not only improves imaging of the pancreatic duct, but may also provide functional information about the presence and severity of outflow obstruction at the level of the sphincter or stricture. The advantages of MRCP include its non-invasiveness and increasingly wide availability. MRCP is contraindicated in patients with pacemakers or cerebral aneurysm clips. The sensitivity and specificity of MRCP for the detection of small bile duct stones or microlithiasis, for small pancreatic tumors, and for pancreas divisum are limited, as MRCP cannot differentiate true divisum from 'pseudodivisum' due to a small obstructing pancreatic stone or tumor (Figs 9.24 and 9.25).

EUS

Endoscopic ultrasound is increasingly utilized, and in our opinion is the procedure of choice, for the initial evaluation of unexplained acute pancreatitis [40–43,87,106,108,166] (Fig. 9.23). Linear-array EUS can detect occult biliary tract disease, such as gallstones, biliary sludge, or occult common bile duct stones. It is the method of choice for diagnosing occult pancreatic tumors including neuroendocrine tumors and IPMT as well as small adenocarcinomas, with the advantage of tissue diagnosis via fine-needle aspirate. EUS is probably the most sensitive test for chronic pancreatitis and can identify intraductal pancreatic stones that may be missed by CT or even ERCP [105,106,108]. EUS is potentially accurate in the diagnosis of pancreas divisum and other congenital anomalies. Finally, EUS is useful for the identification of rare extrapancreatic disorders that may mimic acute pancreatitis with abdominal pain and mild hyperamylasemia, such as intravascular tumors. EUS carries minimal risk when compared to ERCP. A completely normal high-quality EUS essentially limits the diagnostic yield of ERCP to sphincter of Oddi dysfunction or microlithiasis. Limitations of EUS are primarily that there are relatively few endoscopists trained in its use.

Recommended approach to ERCP for acute recurrent pancreatitis

ERCP for acute recurrent pancreatitis at our center, and many others, is reserved for directed therapy if alternative advanced investigations reveal an anatomic cause, or for sphincter of Oddi manometry if the anatomy appears to be normal.

If the pancreatico-biliary anatomy is normal by EUS or MRCP, and the gallbladder is intact, we generally recommend empiric cholecystectomy in reasonable surgical candidates. In patients with apparently normal pancreatico-biliary anatomy who are postcholecystectomy or who are poor surgical candidates for cholecystectomy, we proceed with ERCP with sphincter of Oddi manometry with the primary goal of assessing for pancreatic sphincter hypertension, as increasing data and experience suggest that the response to dual sphincterotomy (pancreatic plus biliary) is substantially better than that for biliary sphincterotomy alone. Empiric biliary sphincterotomy may be a reasonable but unproven treatment in patients with normal sphincter of Oddi manometry who are suspected of microlithiasis. However, we recommend placement of a short-term pancreatic stent to reduce the risk of post-ERCP pancreatitis in this high-risk subgroup of patients with normal pancreatico-biliary ductal anatomy and recurrent pancreatitis (Figs 9.9–9.12).

Because of the risk of ERCP, most authors recommend performance of ERCP only after two attacks of unexplained pancreatitis, unless the first is severe [125,167]. This dilemma can be circumvented by performing EUS after any unexplained episode of pancreatitis. ERCP is either unnecessary or postponed until a second attack occurs in the majority of cases.

Final diagnosis in recurrent acute pancreatitis after extensive investigation

Final diagnoses in series of unexplained acute pancreatitis are highly variable, depending on the patient population, number of patients with intact gallbladders, methods used to evaluate the patients, and thoroughness of evaluation [19,52,168].

Our experience

In most series, less than 20% of patients remain 'idiopathic' after extensive investigation. Results of endoscopic and other therapies are also variable depending on those factors and types of therapy performed. In our series of 102 patients with unexplained acute pancreatitis over a 5-year period, only 8% of patients remained truly 'idiopathic' after extensive investigation. Diagnosis was made uniquely by ERCP in 66%, uniquely by EUS in 21%, uniquely by MRCP in 0%, and uniquely at surgery in 6% [140]. Diagnoses were sphincter of Oddi dysfunction in 28% (mostly treated with combined pancreatic and biliary sphincterotomy), anatomic causes in 23% (including primarily idiopathic chronic pancreatitis with endoscopically treatable findings such as main pancreatic duct stone or stricture in the majority), and pancreas divisum in 16%. Occult biliary stone disease was found in only 6%, usually gallbladder disease diagnosed by EUS and thus amenable to cholecystectomy.

Occult neoplasms Of great importance was that occult neoplasms were found in 15% of our patients and included six adenocarcinomas, six IPMT of the pancreas, one islet cell tumor, and two ampullary tumors. All had CT scans that were normal or showed non-specific pancreatic duct dilation, and nine out of 15 of these tumors were diagnosable (i.e. with positive cytology) only by linear-array EUS and not by ERCP. Eight of 10 of these patients who were surgically explored were successfully resected.

Endoscopic treatment and results Endoscopic therapy was performed in 76% of all patients, but consisted of biliary sphincterotomy alone in only 18, with the remaining 59 patients requiring advanced pancreatic endotherapeutic techniques including pancreatic sphincterotomy, pancreatic stenting, pancreateutic stone extraction with or without extracorporeal shock-wave lithotripsy, endoscopic ampullectomy including a pancreatic sphincterotomy and stent, transpapillary and/or transmural pseudocyst drainage [169–171], etc. Overall long-term outcomes were good with 88% long-term improvement after endoscopic therapy, similar in all major diagnostic groups. The impression from our data was that EUS is the most appropriate first test for unexplained pancreatitis, and that endoscopic diagnosis and therapy must be focused primarily on the pancreas itself, with a limited role for purely biliary diagnosis and treatment. The ultimate inference is that unexplained acute pancreatitis is best evaluated and treated at advanced centers with the capability to perform advanced EUS and pancreatic ERCP techniques, as well as complex pancreatico-biliary surgery. Standard diagnostic and therapeutic ERCP for acute recurrent pancreatitis using conventional biliary techniques has limited benefit and significant risk, and should probably be avoided.

Outstanding issues and future trends

There are many issues that demand further clinical investigation, and further techniques that need to be developed with respect to ERCP in acute pancreatitis. A substantial body of prospective data exists only for ERCP in acute biliary pancreatitis. There is much controversy and a paucity of data regarding endoscopic therapy in other settings, such as pancreas divisum, and especially the role of pancreatic sphincterotomy in the treatment of sphincter of Oddi dysfunction. Future studies will hopefully clarify these murky areas. The importance of pancreatic duct disruption and the need for endoscopic therapy in pancreatic necrosis require further evaluation. The evolution of strategies to evaluate and treat acute and relapsing pancreatitis will increasingly emphasize diagnosis and the prediction of need for endoscopic therapy using less invasive imaging techniques such as EUS and MRCP. Secretin-stimulated EUS and MRCP will play an increasingly important role in diagnosing the cause of pancreatitis, and in assessing the functional significance of duct obstruction. ERCP will hopefully then be relegated to a purely therapeutic modality in patients who are highly likely to benefit from directed endoscopic therapy. Further development of pancreatic stent technology should allow increased safety. Collaboration with laparoscopic surgery and other disciplines will open up new areas for minimally invasive treatment of pancreatic disease. Finally, new techniques to achieve sphincter ablation and stricture dilation may borrow from existing technology in minimally invasive surgery and vascular interventional radiology and cardiology.

References

1 Gorelick F. Acute pancreatitis. In: Yamada T, ed. *Textbook of Gastroenterology*, 2nd edn. Philadelphia: Lippincott 1995, 2064–5.
2 Sakorafas GH, Tsiotou AG. Etiology and pathogenesis of acute pancreatitis: current concepts. *J Clin Gastroenterol* 2000; 30: 343–56.
3 Steinberg W, Tenner S. Acute pancreatitis. *N Engl J Med* 1994; 330: 1198–2100.
4 Bank S, Indaram A. Causes of acute and recurrent pancreatitis. Clinical considerations and clues to diagnosis. *Gastroenterol Clin North Am* 1999; 28: 571–89.
5 Frakes JT. Biliary pancreatitis: a review emphasizing appropriate endoscopic intervention. *J Clin Gastroenterol* 1999; 28 (2): 97–109.
6 Banks PA. Practice guidelines in acute pancreatitis. *Am J Gastroenterol* 1997; 92: 377–86.
7 Balthazar E, Robinson D, Megibow A *et al.* Acute pancreatitis: value of CT in establishing a prognosis. *Radiology* 1990; 174: 331–6.
8 Bradley EL III. A clinically based classification system for acute pancreatitis. *Arch Surg* 1993; 128: 586–90.
9 Baillargeon JD, Orav J, Ramagopal V, Tenner SM, Banks PA. Hemoconcentration as an early risk factor for necrotizing pancreatitis. *Am J Gastroenterol* 1998; 93: 2130–4.
10 Kelly TR, Wagner DS. Gallstone pancreatitis: a prospective randomized trial of the timing of surgery. *Surgery* 1988; 104: 600–4.
11 Neoptolemos JP, Carr-Locke DL, London NJ, Bailey IA, James D, Fossard DP. Controlled trial of urgent endoscopic retrograde cholangiopancreatography and endoscopic sphincterotomy versus conservative treatment for acute pancreatitis due to gallstones. *Lancet* 1988; II: 979–83.
12 Fan S-T, Lai ECS, Mok FPT, Lo C-M, Zheng S-S, Wong T. Early treatment of acute biliary pancreatitis by endoscopic papillotomy. *N Engl J Med* 1993; 328: 228–32.
13 Nowak A, Sowakowska-Dulawa E, Marek T, Rybicka J. Final results of the prospective, randomized, controlled study on endoscopic sphincterotomy versus conventional management in acute biliary pancreatitis [Abstract]. *Gastroenterology* 1995; 108 (Suppl.): A380.
14 Folsch UR, Nitsche R, Ludtke R, Hilgers RA, Creutzfeldt W. Early ERCP and papillotomy compared with conservative treatment for acute biliary pancreatitis. *N Engl J Med* 1997; 336: 237–42.
15 Choudari CP, Lehman GA, Sherman S. Pancreatitis and cystic fibrosis gene mutations. *Gastroenterol Clin North Am* 1999; 28: 543–9.
16 Freeman MF, Nelson DB, Sherman S *et al.* Complications of endoscopic biliary sphincterotomy. *N Engl J Med* 1996; 335: 909–18.
17 Freeman ML, DiSario JA, Nelson DB *et al.* Risk factors for post-ERCP pancreatitis: a prospective, multicenter study. *Gastrointest Endosc* 2001; 54: 425–34.

18 Sherman S, Lehman GA. Endoscopic therapy of pancreatic disease. *Gastroenterologist* 1997; 5: 262–77.

19 Tarnasky PR, Hawes RH. Endoscopic diagnosis and therapy of unexplained (idiopathic) acute pancreatitis. *Gastrointest Endosc Clin North Am* 1998; 8: 13–37.

20 Escourrou J, Cordova JA, Lazorthes F *et al*. Early and late complications after endoscopic sphincterotomy for biliary lithiasis with and without the gallbladder 'in situ'. *Gut* 1984; 25: 598–602.

21 May GR, Shaffer EH. Should elective endoscopic sphincterotomy replace cholecystectomy for the treatment of high-risk patients with gallstone pancreatitis? *J Clin Gastroenterol* 1991; 13: 125–8.

22 Siegel JH, Veerappan A, Cohen SA, Kasmin FE. Endoscopic sphincterotomy for biliary pancreatitis: an alternative to cholecystectomy in high-risk patients. *Gastrointest Endosc* 1994; 40: 573–5.

23 Uomo G, Manes G, Laccetti M, Cavallera A, Rabitti PG. Endoscopic sphincterotomy and recurrence of acute pancreatitis in gallstone patients considered unfit for surgery. *Pancreas* 1997; 14 (1): 28–31.

24 Welbourn CR, Beckly DE, Eyre-Brook IA. Endoscopic sphincterotomy without cholecystectomy for gallstone pancreatitis. *Gut* 1995; 37: 119–20.

25 Hammarstrom LE, Stridbeck H, Ihse I. Effect of endoscopic sphincterotomy and interval cholecystectomy on late outcome after gallstone pancreatitis. *Br J Surg* 1988; 85: 333–6.

26 Hill J, Martin DF, Tweedle DE. Risks of leaving the gallbladder in situ after endoscopic sphincterotomy for bile duct stones. *Br J Surg* 1991; 78: 554–7.

27 Kozarek RA. Endoscopic therapy of complete and partial pancreatic duct disruptions. *Gastrointest Endosc Clin N Am* 1998; 8: 39–53.

28 Kozarek RA, Ball TJ, Patterson DJ *et al*. Endoscopic transpapillary therapy for disrupted pancreatic duct and peripancreatic fluid collections. *Gastroenterology* 1991; 100: 1362–70.

29 Traverso LW, Newman RM, Kozarek RA. Pancreatic ductal disruptions leading to pancreatic fistula, pancreatic ascites or pleural effusions. In: Cameron JL, ed. *Current Surgical Therapy*, 6th edn. St. Louis: Mosby 1988, 510–4.

30 Kozarek RA, Attia FM, Traverso LW *et al*. Pancreatic duct leak in necrotizing pancreatitis: role of diagnostic and therapeutic ERCP as part of a multidisciplinary approach (Abstract). *Gastrointest Endosc* 2000, 51: AB138.

31 Jacob L, Geenen JE, Catalano MF, Geenen DJ. Prevention of pancreatitis in patients with idiopathic recurrent pancreatitis: a prospective nonblinded randomized study using endoscopic stents. *Endoscopy* 2001; 33: 559–62.

32 KaiKaus RM, Jacob L, Geenen JE *et al*. 'Smoldering pancreatitis': rapid resolution with pancreatic duct stent therapy [Abstract]. *Gastrointest Endosc* 1995; 41 (4): 425.

33 Tenner SM, Steinberg WM. Drug-induced acute pancreatitis. In: Berger HG, Warshaw AL, Russell RCG, Buchler M, Carr-Locke DL, Neoptolemos JP, Sarr MG, eds. *The Pancreas*. Oxford: Blackwell Science 1998, 331–42.

34 Runzi M, Layer P. Drug-associated pancreatitis. *Pancreas* 1996; 13: 100–9.

35 Underwood TW, Frye CB. Drug-induced pancreatitis. *Clin Pharm* 1993; 12: 440–8.

36 Toskes PP. Hyperlipidemic pancreatitis. *Gastroenterol Clin North Am* 1990; 19: 783–91.

37 Hernandez CA, Lerch MM. Sphincter stenosis and gallstone migration through the biliary tract. *Lancet* 1993; 341: 1371–3.

38 Lee SP, Nichols JF, Park HZ. Biliary sludge as a cause of acute pancreatitis. *N Engl J Med* 1992; 326: 589–93.

39 Somogyi L, Martin SP, Venkatesan T, Ulrich CD. Recurrent acute pancreatitis: an algorithmic approach to identification and elimination of inciting factors. *Gastroenterology* 2001; 120: 708–17.

40 Dahan P, Andant C, Levy P *et al*. Prospective evaluation of endoscopic ultrasonography and microscopic examination of duodenal bile in the diagnosis of cholecystolithiasis in 45 patients with normal conventional ultrasonography. *Gut* 1996; 38: 277–81.

41 Dill JE, Hill S, Callis J et al. Combined endoscopic ultrasound and stimulated biliary drainage in cholecystitis and microlithiasis—diagnosis and outcomes. *Endoscopy* 1995; 27: 424–7.

42 Liu CL, Lo CM, Chan JKF et al. EUS for detection of occult cholelithiasis in patients with idiopathic pancreatitis. *Gastrointest Endosc* 2000; 51: 28–32.

43 Tandon M, Topazian M. Endoscopic ultrasound in idiopathic acute pancreatitis. *Am J Gastroenterol* 2001; 96: 705–9.

44 Geenen JE, Nash JA. The role of sphincter of Oddi manometry and biliary microscopy in evaluating idiopathic recurrent pancreatitis. *Endoscopy* 1998; 30 (Suppl. 1): 237–41.

45 Neoptolemos JP, Davidson BR, Winder AF, Vallance D. Role of duodenal bile crystal analysis in the investigation of 'idiopathic' pancreatitis. *Br J Surg* 1988; 75: 450–3.

46 Marks JW, Bonorris G. Intermittency of cholesterol crystals in duodenal bile from gallstone patients. *Gastroenterology* 1984; 87: 622–7.

47 Rubin M, Pakula R, Konikoff FM. Microstructural analysis of bile: relevance to cholesterol gallstone pathogenesis. *Histol Histopathol* 2000; 15: 761–70.

48 Kaw M, Brodmerkel GJ. ERCP, biliary crystal analysis, and sphincter of Oddi manometry in idiopathic recurrent pancreatitis. *Gastrointest Endosc* 2002; 55: 157–62.

49 Quallich LG, Stern MA, Rich M, Chey WD, Barnett JL, Elta GH. Bile duct crystals do not contribute to sphincter of Oddi dysfunction. *Gastrointest Endosc* 2002; 55: 163–6.

50 Ros E, Navarro S, Bru C, Garcia-Puges A, Valderrama R. Occult microlithiasis in 'idiopathic' acute pancreatitis: prevention of relapses by cholecystectomy or ursodeoxycholic acid therapy. *Gastroenterology* 1991; 101: 1701–9.

51 Lehman GA, Sherman S. Sphincter of Oddi dysfunction. *Int J Pancreatol* 1996; 20: 11–25.

52 Levy MJ, Geenen JE. Idiopathic acute recurrent pancreatitis. *Am J Gastroenterol* 2001; 96 (9): 2540–55.

53 Geenen JE, Hogan WJ, Dodds WJ et al. The efficacy of endoscopic sphincterotomy after cholecystectomy in patients with suspected sphincter of Oddi dysfunction. *N Engl J Med* 1989; 320: 82–7.

54 Hogan WJ, Sherman S, Pasricha P, Carr-Locke D. Sphincter of Oddi manometry. *Gastrointest Endosc* 1997; 45: 342–8.

55 Kuo W-H, Pasricha P, Kalloo A. The role of sphincter of Oddi manometry in the diagnosis and therapy of pancreatic disease. *Gastrointest Endosc Clin North Am* 1998; 8: 79–85.

56 Eversman D, Fogel EL, Rusche M, Sherman S, Lehman G. Frequency of abnormal pancreatic and biliary sphincter manometry compared with clinical suspicion of sphincter of Oddi dysfunction. *Gastrointest Endosc* 1999; 50: 637–41.

57 Funch-Jensen P, Kruse A. Manometric activity of the pancreatic duct sphincter in patients with total bile duct sphincterotomy for sphincter of Oddi dyskinesia. *Scand J Gastroenterol* 1987; 22: 1067–70.

58 Sherman S, Troiano FP, Hawes RH, O'Connor KW, Lehman GA. Frequency of abnormal sphincter of Oddi manometry compared with the clinical suspicion of sphincter of Oddi dysfunction. *Am J Gastroenterol* 1991; 86: 586–9.

59 Silverman WB, Ruffolo TA, Sherman S et al. Correlation of basal sphincter pressures measured from both the bile duct and pancreatic duct in patients with suspected sphincter of Oddi dysfunction. *Gastrointest Endosc* 1992; 38: 440–3.

60 Catalano MF, Sivak MV, Falk GW et al. Idiopathic pancreatitis (IP): diagnostic role of sphincter of Oddi manometry (SOM) and response to endoscopic sphincterotomy (ES). *Gastrointest Endosc* 1993; 39: 310A.

61 Goff JS. Common bile duct sphincter of Oddi stenting in patients with suspected sphincter dysfunction. *Am J Gastroenterol* 1995; 90: 586–9.

62 Neoptolemos JP, Bailey IS, Carr-Locke DL. Sphincter of Oddi dysfunction: results of treatment by endoscopic sphincterotomy. *Br J Surg* 1988; 75: 454–9.

63 Rolny P. Endoscopic bile duct stent placement as a predictor of outcome following endoscopic sphincterotomy in patients with suspected sphincter of Oddi dysfunction. *Eur J Gastroenterol Hepatol* 1997; 9: 467–71.

64 Toouli J, Di Francesco V, Saccone G et al. Division of the sphincter of Oddi for treatment of dysfunction associated with recurrent pancreatitis. *Br J Surg* 1996; 83: 1205–10.

65 Toouli J, Roberts-Thomson IC, Dent J, Lee J. Sphincter of Oddi motility disorders in patients with idiopathic recurrent pancreatitis. *Br J Surg* 1985; 72: 859–63.

66 Wehrmann T, Seifert H, Seipp M *et al.* Endoscopic injection of botulinum toxin for biliary sphincter of Oddi dysfunction. *Endoscopy* 1998; 30: 702–7.

67 Guelrud M, Plaz J, Mendoza S, Beker B, Rojas O, Rossiter G. Endoscopic treatment in Type II pancreatic sphincter dysfunction (Abstract). *Gastrointest Endosc* 1995; 52: 398A.

68 Testoni PA, Caporuscio S, Bagnolo F, Lella F. Idiopathic recurrent pancreatitis: long-term results after ERCP, endoscopic sphincterotomy, or ursodeoxycholic acid treatment. *Am J Gastroenterol* 2000; 95: 1702–7.

69 Kalloo AN, Pasricha PJ. Therapy of sphincter of Oddi dysfunction. *Gastrointest Endosc Clin North Am* 1996; 6: 117–25.

70 Di Francesco V, Brunori MP, Rigo L *et al.* Comparison of ultrasound-secretin test and sphincter of Oddi manometry in patients with recurrent acute pancreatitis. *Dig Dis Sci* 1999; 44: 336–40.

71 Cotton PB, Lehman G, Vennes J *et al.* Endoscopic sphincterotomy, complications and their management: an attempt at consensus. *Gastrointest Endosc* 1991; 37: 383–93.

72 Tarnasky PR, Palesch YY, Cunningham JT, Mauldin P, Cotton P, Hawes R. Pancreatic stenting prevents pancreatitis after biliary sphincterotomy in patients with sphincter of Oddi dysfunction. *Gastroenterology* 1998; 115: 1518–24.

73 Sherman S, Eversman D, Fogel E, Gottlieb K, Earle D. Sphincter of Oddi dysfunction (SOD): needle-knife pancreaticobiliary sphincterotomy over pancreatic stent (NKOPS) has a lower post-procedure pancreatitis rate than pull-type biliary sphincterotomy (BES). *Gastrointest Endosc* 1997; 45: 148A.

74 Shakoor T, Hogan WJ, Geenen JE. Efficacy of nasopancreatic catheter in the prevention of post-ERCP pancreatitis: a prospective randomized controlled trial. *Gastrointest Endosc* 1992; 38: 251A.

75 Freeman ML. Role of pancreatic stents in prevention of post-ERCP pancreatitis. *JOP* 2004; 5: 322–7.

76 Kozarek RA. Pancreatic stents can induce ductal changes consistent with chronic pancreatitis. *Gastrointest Endosc* 1990; 36: 93–5.

77 Siegel JH, Veerappan A. Endoscopic management of pancreatic disorders: potential risks of pancreatic prosthesis. *Endoscopy* 1991; 23: 177–80.

78 Smith MT, Sherman S, Ikenberry SO, Hawes RH, Lehman GA. Alternations in pancreatic ductal morphology following polyethylene pancreatic stent therapy. *Gastrointest Endosc* 1996; 44: 268–75.

79 Rashdan A, Fogel EL, McHenry L Jr, Sherman S, Temkit M, Lehman GA. Improved stent characteristics for prophylaxis of post-ERCP pancreatitis. *Clin Gastroenterol Hepatol* 2004; 2: 322–9.

80 Freeman ML, Overby C, Qi D. Pancreatic stent insertion: consequences of failure and results of a modified technique to maximize success. *Gastrointest Endosc* 2004; 59: 8–14.

81 Hill ID, Lebenthal E. Congenital abnormalities of the exocrine pancreas. In: Go VLW, ed. *The Pancreas: Biology, Pathobiology and Disease*. New York: Raven 1993, 1029–40.

82 Barish MA, Yucel EK, Ferrucci J. Magnetic resonance cholangiopancreatography. *N Engl J Med* 1999; 341: 258–64.

83 Bret PM, Reinhold C, Taourel P *et al.* Pancreas divisum: evaluation with MR cholangiopancreatography. *Radiology* 1996; 199: 99–103.

84 Lai R, Freeman ML, Cass OW, Mallery S. Accurate diagnosis of pancreas divisum by linear-array endoscopic ultrasonography. *Endoscopy* 2004; 36: 705–9.

85 Bhutani MS, Hoffman BJ, Hawes RH. Diagnosis of pancreas divisum by endoscopic ultrasonography. *Endoscopy* 1999; 31: 167–9.

86 Jacob L, Geenen JE, Catalano MF *et al.* Clinical presentation and short-term outcome of endoscopic therapy of patients with symptomatic and incomplete pancreas divisum. *Gastrointest Endosc* 1999; 49: 53–7.

87 Bernard JP, Sahel J, Giovannini M, Sarles H. Pancreas divisum is a probable cause of acute pancreatitis: a report of 137 cases. *Pancreas* 1990; 5: 248–54.

88 Warshaw AL. Pancreas divisum and pancreatitis. In: Beger HG, Warshaw AL, Russel RCG, Buchler M, Carr-Locke DL, Neoptolemos JP, Sarr MG, eds. *The Pancreas*. Oxford: Blackwell Science 1998, 364–374.

89 Bradley EL III, Stephan RN. Accessory duct sphincteroplasty is preferred for long-term prevention of recurrent acute pancreatitis in patients with pancreas divisum. *J Am Coll Surg* 1996; 183: 65–70.

90 Brenner P, Duncombe V, Ham JM. Pancreatitis and pancreas divisum: etiological and surgical considerations. *Aust N Z J Surg* 1990; 60: 899–903.

91 Keith RG, Shapero TF, Saibil FG. Dorsal duct sphincterotomy is effective long-term treatment of acute pancreatitis associated with pancreas divisum. *Surgery* 1989; 106: 660–7.

92 Lehman GA, Sherman S. Diagnosis and therapy of pancreas divisum. *Gastrointest Endosc Clin North Am* 1998; 8: 55–77.

93 Richter JM, Schapiro RH, Mulley AG, Warshaw AL. Association of pancreas divisum and pancreatitis, and its treatment by sphincteroplasty of the accessory ampulla. *Gastroenterology* 1981; 81: 1104–10.

94 Coleman SD, Eisen GM, Troughton AB *et al*. Endoscopic treatment in pancreas divisum. *Am J Gastroenterol* 1994; 89: 1152–5.

95 Cotton PB. Congenital anomaly of pancreas divisum as a cause of obstructive pain and pancreatitis. *Gut* 1980; 21: 105–14.

96 Ertan A. Long-term results after endoscopic pancreatic stent placement without pancreatic papillotomy in acute recurrent pancreatitis due to pancreas divisum. *Gastrointest Endosc* 2000; 52: 9–14.

97 Lehman GA, Sherman S, Nisi R, Hawes RH. Pancreas divisum: results of minor papilla sphincterotomy. *Gastrointest Endosc* 1993; 39: 1–8.

98 Ligoury C, Lefebvre JF, Canard JM *et al*. Pancreas divisum: therapeutic results in 12 patients. *Gastrointest Endosc* 1986; 10: 530S.

99 Soehendra N, Kempeneers I, Nam VC *et al*. Endoscopic dilation and papillotomy of the accessory papilla and internal drainage in pancreas divisum. *Endoscopy* 1986; 18: 129–32.

100 Lans JI, Geenen JE, Johanson JF, Hogan WJ. Endoscopic therapy in patients with pancreas divisum and acute pancreatitis: a prospective, randomized, controlled clinical trial. *Gastrointest Endosc* 1992; 38: 430–4.

101 Kozarek RA, Ball TJ, Patterson DJ *et al*. Endoscopic approaches to pancreas divisum. *Dig Dis Sci* 1995; 40: 1974–81.

102 Catalano MF, Rosenblatt ML, Geenen JE, Hogan WJ. Pancreatic endotherapy of pancreas divisum; response based on clinical presentation and results of secretin-stimulated endoscopic ultrasound (Abstract). *Gastrointest Endosc* 2001, 53: AB133.

103 Gerke H, Byrne MF, Stiffler HL *et al*. Outcome of endoscopic minor papillotomy in patients with symptomatic pancreas divisum. *JOP* 2004; 5: 122–31.

104 Perrault J. Hereditary pancreatitis: historical perspectives. *Med Clin North Am* 2000; 84: 519–29.

105 Buscail L, Escourrou J, Moreau J *et al*. Endoscopic ultrasonography in chronic pancreatitis: a comparative prospective study with conventional ultrasonography, computed tomography and ERCP. *Pancreas* 1995; 10: 251–7.

106 Catalano MF, Lahoti S, Geenen JE, Hogan WJ. Prospective evaluation of endoscopic ultrasonography, endoscopic retrograde pancreatography, and secretin test in the diagnosis of chronic pancreatitis. *Gastrointest Endosc* 1998; 48: 11–7.

107 Forsmark CE. The diagnosis of chronic pancreatitis. *Gastrointest Endosc* 2000; 52: 293–8.

108 Sahai AV, Zimmerman M, Aabakken L *et al*. Prospective assessment of the ability of endoscopic ultrasound to diagnose, exclude or establish the severity of chronic pancreatitis found by endoscopic retrograde pancreatography. *Gastrointest Endosc* 1998; 48: 18–25.

109 Steer ML, Waxman I, Freedman S. Chronic pancreatitis. *N Engl J Med* 1995; 332: 1482–90.

110 Wiersema MJ, Hawes RH, Lehman GA, Kochman ML, Sherman S, Kipecky KK. Prospective evaluation of endoscopic ultrasonography and endoscopic retrograde cholangiopancreatography in patients with chronic abdominal pain of suspected pancreatic origin. *Endoscopy* 1993; 25: 555–64.

111 Cohn JA, Bornstein JD, Jowell PS. Cystic fibrosis mutations and genetic predisposition to idio-pathic chronic pancreatitis. *Med Clin North Am* 2000; 84: 621–31.

112 Cohn JA, Friedman KJ, Noone PG, Knowles MR, Silverman LM, Jowell PS. Relation between mutations of the cystic fibrosis gene and idiopathic pancreatitis. *N Engl J Med* 1998; 339: 653–8.

113 Gorry MC, Gabbaizedeh D, Furey W *et al*. Mutations in the cationic trypsinogen gene are associated with recurrent acute and chronic pancreatitis. *Gastroenterology* 1997; 113: 1063–8.

114 Sharer N, Schwarz M, Malone G *et al*. Mutations of the cystic fibrosis gene in patients with chronic pancreatitis. *N Engl J Med* 1989; 339: 645–52.

115 Whitcomb DC, Gorry MC, Preston RA *et al*. Hereditary pancreatitis is caused by a mutation in the cationic trypsinogen gene. *Nat Genet* 1996; 14: 141–5.

116 Whitcomb DC, Preston RA, Aston CE *et al*. A gene for hereditary pancreatitis maps to chro-mosome 7q35. *Gastroenterology* 1996; 110: 1975–80.

117 Binmoeller KF, Jue P, Seifert H *et al*. Endoscopic pancreatic stent drainage in chronic pan-creatitis and a dominant stricture: long-term results. *Endoscopy* 1995; 27: 638–44.

118 Cremer M, Deviere J, Delhaye M, Baize M, Vandermeeren A. Stenting in severe chronic pan-creatitis: results of medium-term follow-up in 76 patients. *Endoscopy* 1991; 23: 171–6.

119 Dumonceau JM, Deviere J, Le Moine O *et al*. Endoscopic pancreatic drainage in chronic pan-creatitis associated with ductal stones: long-term results. *Gastrointest Endosc* 1996; 43: 547–55.

120 Kozarek RA, Ball TJ, Patterson DJ *et al*. Endoscopic approach to pancreatic duct calculi and obstructive pancreatitis. *Am J Gastroenterol* 1992; 87: 600–3.

121 Kozarek RA, Traverso LW. Endotherapy of chronic pancreatitis. *Int J Pancreatol* 1996; 19: 93–102.

122 Ponchon T, Bory R, Hedelius F *et al*. Endoscopic stenting for pain relief in chronic pancreatitis: results of a standardized protocol. *Gastrointest Endosc* 1995; 42: 452–6.

123 Smits ME, Badiga SM, Rauws EAJ, Tytgat GNJ, Huibregtse K. Long-term results of pancreatic stents in chronic pancreatitis. *Gastrointest Endosc* 1995; 42: 461–7.

124 Smits ME, Rauws EA, Tytgat GNJ *et al*. Endoscopic treatment of pancreatic stones in patients with chronic pancreatitis. *Gastrointest Endosc* 1996; 43: 556–60.

125 Ballinger AB, Barnes E, Alstead EM, Fairclough PD. Is intervention necessary after a first episode of acute idiopathic pancreatitis? *Gut* 1996; 38: 293–5.

126 Procacci C, Biasiutti C, Carbognin G *et al*. Characterization of cystic tumors of the pancreas: CT accuracy. *J Comput Assist Tomogr* 1999; 23: 906–12.

127 Sand JA, Hyoty MK, Mattila J *et al*. Clinical assessment compared with cyst fluid analysis in the differential diagnosis of cystic lesions in the pancreas. *Surgery* 1996; 119: 275–80.

128 Sarr MG, Carpenter HA, Prabhakar LP *et al*. Clinical and pathologic correlation of 84 mucin-ous cystic neoplasms of the pancreas: can one reliably differentiate benign from malignant (or premalignant) neoplasms? *Ann Surg* 2000; 231: 205–12.

129 Sawada T, Muto T. Familial adenomatous polyposis: should patients undergo surveillance of the upper gastrointestinal tract? *Endoscopy* 1995; 27: 6–11.

130 Siech M, Tripp K, Schmidt-Rohlfing B *et al*. Cystic tumors of the pancreas: diagnostic accuracy, pathologic observations and surgical consequences. *Langenbecks Arch Surg* 1998; 383: 56–61.

131 Simpson WF, Adams DB, Metcalf JF, Anderson MC. Nonfunctioning pancreatic neuro-endocrine tumors presenting as pancreatitis: report of four cases. *Pancreas* 1988; 3: 223–31.

132 Vandervoort J, Soetikno RM, Mones H *et al*. Accuracy and complication rate of brush cyto-logy from bile duct versus pancreatic duct. *Gastrointest Endosc* 1999; 49: 322–7.

133 Wiersema MJ, Vilmann P, Giovannini M *et al*. Endosonography-guided fine-needle aspiration biopsy: diagnostic accuracy and complication assessment. *Gastroenterology* 1997; 112: 1087–95.

134 Adamek HE, Albert J, Breer H, Weitz M, Schilling D, Riemann JF. Pancreatic cancer detection with magnetic resonance cholangiopancreatography and endoscopic retrograde cholangio-pancreatography: a prospective controlled study. *Lancet* 2000; 356: 190–3.

135 Legmann P, Vignaux O, Dousset B *et al.* Pancreatic tumors: comparison of dual-phase helical CT and endoscopic sonography. *Am J Roentgenol* 1998; 170: 1315–22.

136 Palazzo L, Roseau G, Gayet B *et al.* Endosonographic ultrasonography in the diagnosis and staging of pancreatic adenocarcinoma. *Endoscopy* 1993; 25: 143–50.

137 Rosch T. Staging of pancreatic cancer: analysis of literature results. *Gastrointest Endosc Clin North Am* 1995; 5: 735–9.

138 Rosch T, Braig C, Gain J *et al.* Staging of pancreatic and ampullary carcinoma by endoscopic ultrasonography. Comparison with conventional sonography, computed tomography and angiography. *Gastroenterology* 1992; 102: 188–99.

139 Rosch T, Lightdale CJ, Botet JF *et al.* Localization of pancreatic endocrine tumors by endoscopic ultrasonography. *N Engl J Med* 1992; 326: 1721–6.

140 Sandozi IK, Freeman ML, Cass OW, Mallery JS. Long term outcome of unexplained acute pancreatitis (UAP) utilizing advanced endoscopic diagnosis and treatment (Abstract). *Gastrointest Endosc* 2001.

141 Binmoeller KF, Boaventura S, Ramsperger K, Soehendra N. Endoscopic snare excision of benign adenomas of the papilla of Vater. *Gastrointest Endosc* 1993; 39: 127–31.

142 Howell DA, Desilets DJ, Dy RM *et al.* Endoscopic management of tumors of the major duodenal papilla: refined techniques to improve outcome and avoid complications. *Gastrointest Endosc* 2001; 54: 202–8.

143 Lambert R, Ponchon T, Chavaillon A, Berger F. Laser treatment of tumors of the papilla of Vater. *Endoscopy* 1988; 20 (Suppl. 1): 227–31.

144 Ponchon T, Berger F, Chavaillon A *et al.* Contribution of endoscopy to diagnosis and treatment of tumors of the ampulla of Vater. *Cancer* 1989; 64: 161–7.

145 Robertson JF, Imrie CW. Acute pancreatitis associated with carcinoma of the ampulla of Vater. *Br J Surg* 1987; 74: 395–7.

146 Tham TC, Lichtenstein DR, Vandervoort J *et al.* Pancreatic duct stents for 'obstructive type' pain in pancreatic malignancy. *Am J Gastroenterol* 2000; 95: 956–60.

147 Keeley SP, Freeman ML. Placement of self-expanding metallic stents in the pancreatic duct for treatment of obstructive complications of pancreatic cancer. *Gastrointest Endosc* 2003; 57: 756–9.

148 Goldberg PB, Long WB, Oleaga JA, Mackie JA. Choledochocele as a cause of recurrent pancreatitis. *Gastroenterology* 1980; 78: 1041–5.

149 Greene FL, Brown JJ, Rubinstein P, Anderson MC. Choledochocele and recurrent pancreatitis. *Am J Surg* 1985; 149: 306–9.

150 Heikkinen ES, Salminen PM. Congenital choledochal cyst opening into the intraduodenal part of the common bile duct and complicated by cystolithiasis and acute pancreatitis. *Acta Chir Scand* 1984; 150: 183–5.

151 Lopez RR, Pinson CW, Campbell JR *et al.* Variation in management based on type of choledochal cyst. *Am J Surg* 1991; 161: 612–5.

152 Okada A, Higaki J, Nakamura T *et al.* Pancreatitis associated with choledochal cyst and other anomalies in childhood. *Br J Surg* 1995; 82: 829–32.

153 Taylor RG, Auldish AW. Choledochal cyst presenting as acute pancreatitis. *Aust N Z J Surg* 1985; 55: 611–2.

154 Venu RP, Geenen JE, Hogan W *et al.* Role of endoscopic retrograde cholangiopancreatography in the diagnosis and treatment of choledochocele. *Gastroenterology* 1984; 87: 1144–9.

155 Dowsett JF, Rode J, Russell RC. Annular pancreas: a clinical, endoscopic and immunohistochemical study. *Gut* 1989; 30: 130–5.

156 Gress F, Yiengpruksawan A, Sherman S *et al.* Diagnosis of annular pancreas by endoscopic ultrasound. *Gastrointest Endosc* 1996; 44: 485–9.

157 Lloyd-Jones W, Mountain JC, Warren KW. Annular pancreas in the adult. *Ann Surg* 1972; 176: 163–70.

158 Kochhar R, Nagi B, Chawla S *et al.* The clinical spectrum of anomalous pancreatobiliary junction. *Surg Endosc* 1989; 3: 83–6.

159 Toskes PP. Approach to the patient with acute relapsing pancreatitis. *Gastrointest Dis Today* 1994; 3: 8–15.

160 Barish MA, Soto JA, Yucel EK. Magnetic resonance cholangiopancreatography of the biliary ducts. Techniques, clinical applications and limitations. *Top Magn Reson Imaging* 1996; 8: 302–11.

161 Bret PM, Reinhold C. Magnetic resonance cholangiopancreatography. *Endoscopy* 1997; 29: 472–86.

162 Sica GT, Braver J, Cooney MJ, Miller FH, Chai JL, Adams DF. Comparison of endoscopic retrograde cholangiopancreatography with MR cholangiopancreatography in patients with pancreatitis. *Radiology* 1999; 210: 605–10.

163 Soto JA, Barish MA, Yucel EK *et al.* Magnetic resonance cholangiography: comparison with endoscopic retrograde cholangiopancreatography. *Gastroenterology* 1996; 110: 589–97.

164 Varghese JC, Liddell RP, Farrell MA, Murray FE, Osborne H, Lee MJ. The diagnostic accuracy of magnetic resonance cholangiopancreatography and ultrasound compared with direct cholangiography in the detection of choledocholithiasis. *Clin Radiol* 1999; 54: 604–14.

165 Sherman S, Ruffolo TA, Hawes RH *et al.* Complications of endoscopic sphincterotomy: a prospective series with emphasis on the increased risk associated with sphincter of Oddi dysfunction and nondilated bile ducts. *Gastroenterology* 1991; 101: 1068–75.

166 Froussard JL, Sosa-Valencia L, Amouyal G *et al.* Usefulness of endoscopic ultrasonography in patients with 'idiopathic' acute pancreatitis. *Am J Med* 2000; 109: 196–200.

167 Gregor JC, Ponich TP, Detsky AS. Should ERCP be routine after an episode of 'idiopathic' pancreatitis? A cost-utility analysis. *Gastrointest Endosc* 1996; 44: 118–23.

168 Venu RP, Geenen JE, Hogan W, Stone J, Johnson GK, Soergel K. Idiopathic recurrent pancreatitis: an approach to diagnosis and treatment. *Dig Dis Sci* 1989; 34: 56–60.

169 Binmoeller KF, Seifert H, Walter A *et al.* Transpapillary and transmural drainage of pancreatic pseudocysts. *Gastrointest Endosc* 1995; 42: 219–24.

170 Catalano MF, Geenen JE, Schmalz MJ *et al.* Treatment of pancreatic pseudocysts with ductal communication by transpapillary pancreatic duct endoprosthesis. *Gastrointest Endosc* 1995; 42: 214–8.

171 Cremer M, Deviere J, Engelholm L. Endoscopic management of cysts and pseudocysts in chronic pancreatitis: long-term follow-up after 7 years of experience. *Gastrointest Endosc* 1989; 35: 1–9.

CHAPTER 10

Endoscopy in Chronic Pancreatitis

LEE MCHENRY, STUART SHERMAN, AND GLEN LEHMAN

Synopsis

Chronic pancreatitis is an inflammatory process of the pancreas characterized pathologically by irreversible destruction of parenchymal and ductal architecture. Clinically, pain is the predominant symptom. Pain may be due to elevated pancreatic ductal or parenchymal pressure, and therapeutic efforts are directed at reducing pancreatic secretion or reducing pancreatic ductal or parenchymal pressure. A variety of interventions are utilized, including pharmacological therapy (pancreatic enzymes, octreotide), surgical procedures (resective, decompressive, and denervative), and endoscopic techniques.

Endoscopic therapy for chronic pancreatitis has evolved over the past 15 years, with the incorporation of endoscopic techniques previously reserved for the treatment of biliary tract disorders such as bile duct stones, strictures, and leaks. Endoscopic therapy for chronic pancreatitis is highlighted in this chapter and an extensive literature review accompanies the discussion of a variety of techniques. The endoscopic techniques, safety, and clinical efficacy of the endoscopic management of pancreatic duct strictures are reviewed. Particular attention is paid to the duration of stenting, complications associated with stents, and the long-term follow-up of patients undergoing endoscopic therapy. Management of pancreatic duct stones utilizing various stone extraction techniques and the usefulness of incorporating extracorporeal shock-wave lithotripsy into the armamentarium are also discussed. The role of sphincter of Oddi dysfunction in pancreatic disease and the technique of pancreatic sphincterotomy are highlighted. The management of biliary obstruction as a complication of chronic pancreatitis is also discussed. The results of endoscopic management of pancreatic pseudocysts are briefly reviewed; however, more exhaustive discussion of the technique appears in a subsequent chapter. Endoscopic therapy of chronic pancreatitis is an expanding area for the interventional endoscopist. The appropriate selection of candidates for various pancreatic interventions is important to achieve the best results.

Table 10.1 Abdominal pain in chronic pancreatitis.

Pancreatic causes	Extrapancreatic causes
Acute inflammation	Common bile duct obstruction
Increased intrapancreatic pressure	Descending duodenal obstruction
Ducts	Colonic obstruction
Pseudocysts	Duodenal/gastric ulcer
Parenchyma	
Perineural inflammation	
Pancreatic ischemia	

Chronic pancreatitis

Chronic pancreatitis is an inflammatory process of the pancreas that may result in chronic, disabling abdominal pain, fat and protein maldigestion, and diabetes mellitus. The histological hallmarks of chronic pancreatitis are irreversible destruction of the pancreatic parenchyma and ductal architecture associated with fibrosis, protein plugs, and ductal calculi [1]. Pain is the predominant symptom of chronic pancreatitis and its pathogenesis is multifactorial. Pain may be caused by pancreatic or extrapancreatic processes (Table 10.1) [2,3]. Pancreatic duct and parenchymal pressures are generally increased in chronic pancreatitis, whether the main pancreatic duct is dilated or normal in diameter [4]. Such elevated parenchymal and duct pressures contribute to pancreatic ischemia, which appears to play a significant role in the pain of chronic pancreatitis [5,6]. Therapeutic efforts are directed at reducing pancreatic parenchymal and ductal hypertension. Pharmacological agents, endoscopic techniques, and surgical procedures (resective, drainage, and denervative) have been employed to reduce pain, with variable results. The complexity and multiplicity of the causes of pain in chronic pancreatitis may well explain the mixed results achieved by current methods of therapy.

Treatments for chronic pancreatitis

Most therapeutic efforts in the treatment of chronic pancreatitis are directed toward the correction of the etiological factors, including relief of obstructions and control of symptoms.

Medical therapy

Medical therapy consisting of analgesics, dietary alterations, nerve blocks, enzyme supplements, intervals of pancreatic rest, and suppression of pancreatic secretion (octreotide) is variably effective in relieving pain. Further options or alternatives to medical therapy are sought by patients with uncontrolled, persistent pain.

Surgical therapy

Surgical therapy has been the main therapeutic recourse for patients with disabling symptoms that fail to improve with standard medical therapy. A surgical drainage procedure is usually performed in the setting of a dilated main pancreatic duct, whereas pancreatic resection and/or denervation are reserved for those patients with normal or small diameter ducts. Immediate pain relief is seen in 70–90% of patients following surgical drainage procedures. However, pain recurs in 20–50% of patients during long-term follow-up. Surgical drainage procedures are associated with a morbidity of 20–40%, and a mortality averaging 4% [7].

Endoscopic treatment for chronic pancreatitis

Since its inception and initial application in the early 1970s, endoscopic therapy has revolutionized the approach to a variety of biliary tract disorders. Within the past 10 years, similar endoscopic techniques have been applied and adapted to diseases of the pancreas [8].

Safety issues

These techniques, however, have not been widely utilized because of concern about prohibitive morbidity and the difficulty in achieving technical success. It was not until the relative safety of endoscopic retrograde cholangiopancreatography (ERCP) and endoscopic sphincterotomy in acute gallstone pancreatitis was recognized that the indications for endoscopic therapy in disorders of the pancreas were expanded [8–10]. Pharmacological agents such as gabexate and interleukin-10 have shown promise in reducing the incidence and severity of pancreatitis in patients undergoing therapeutic ERCP and may add further safety to endoscopic interventions of the pancreas [11,12].

Indications for endoscopic treatment

Endoscopic therapy is now being applied in the setting of chronic pancreatitis for patients presenting with pain and/or clinical episodes of acute pancreatitis [13,14]. One of the aims of endoscopic therapy is to alleviate the obstruction to exocrine juice flow. Certain pathological alterations of the pancreatic duct, the bile duct, and/or the sphincter lend themselves to endoscopic therapy. Outflow obstruction may be caused by ductal strictures (biliary or pancreatic), pancreatic stones, pseudocysts, and minor or major papilla stenosis. Although the endoscopic approach has never been directly compared with surgery, endoscopic drainage is appealing in that it may offer an alternative to surgical drainage procedures, with generally less morbidity and mortality. Furthermore, endoscopic procedures do not preclude subsequent surgery, should that be necessary. Moreover, the outcome from reducing the intraductal pressure by endoscopic methods may be a predictor for the success of surgical drainage [15].

Results of endoscopic treatment

Outcome data following endoscopic therapy in chronic pancreatitis are rapidly accumulating. The data in this area, however, are often difficult to interpret because of the heterogeneous populations with one or more pathological processes being treated (e.g. pancreatic duct stones, strictures, pseudocysts) and because of the multiple therapies performed in a given patient (e.g. stricture dilation, stone extraction, biliary and/or pancreatic sphincterotomy).

Table 10.2 lists the currently available endoscopic techniques for the treatment of acute and chronic pancreatitis, and their complications. This table is (intentionally) all-inclusive, because differentiating acute recurrent pancreatitis

Table 10.2 Endoscopic interventions for pancreatic diseases.

Clinical condition	Endoscopic therapy
Acute pancreatitis	Endoscopic sphincterotomy (bile duct and/or pancreatic duct), sphincter dilation, bile duct or pancreatic duct stent or nasobiliary/nasopancreatic drain, gallstone removal, *Ascaris* parasite removal
Chronic pancreatitis	Endoscopic sphincterotomy (bile duct and/or pancreatic duct), stricture dilation, bile duct or pancreatic duct stents, pancreatic stone extraction ± ESWL, endoscopic ultrasound-guided celiac plexus block
Pancreatic pseudocysts, duct disruption, pancreatic ascites	Endoscopic cystgastrostomy or cystduodenostomy, transpapillary stents, or nasopancreatic drainage
Pancreas divisum	Minor papilla sphincterotomy, stent, sphincter dilation
Ampullary tumors	Endoscopic ampullectomy, stenting, thermal ablation
Pancreatic cancer	Bile duct plastic or metallic stent, pancreatic duct plastic stent, endoscopic ultrasound-guided celiac plexus block

from exacerbations of chronic pancreatitis may be clinically difficult [16]. In this chapter, we analyse the current state of the art of some of these exciting new applications of endoscopy in the treatment of chronic pancreatitis.

Pancreatic ductal strictures

Benign strictures of the main pancreatic duct may be a consequence of generalized or focal inflammation, or necrosis around the main pancreatic duct. Given the putative role of ductal hypertension in the genesis of symptoms (at least in a subpopulation of patients), the utility of pancreatic duct stents for treatment of dominant pancreatic duct strictures is being evaluated [17–26]. In experimental models, pancreatic duct stents have been shown to reduce elevated ductal pressures significantly, although not as effectively as surgical measures [27]. The best candidates for stenting are those patients with a distal stricture (in the pancreatic head) and upstream dilation (type IV lesion) [17]. The majority of patients with a stricture have associated calcified pancreatic duct stones. For optimal results, the therapy must address both the stones and stricture. Underlying malignancy as the cause of the pancreatic stricture must be excluded by non-invasive and tissue sampling means [28–30].

Pancreatic stent placement techniques

Most pancreatic stents are simply standard polyethylene biliary stents with extra side-holes at approximately 1-cm intervals to permit better side-branch juice flow (Fig. 10.1). Stents made of other materials have received limited evaluation.

The technique for placing a stent in the pancreatic duct is similar to that used for inserting a biliary stent. In most patients, a pancreatic sphincterotomy (with or without a biliary sphincterotomy) via the major or minor papilla is performed to facilitate placement of accessories and stents. A guidewire must be maneuvered upstream to the narrowing. Hydrophilic flexible tip wires are especially helpful for bypassing strictures. Torqueable wires are occasionally necessary to achieve this goal. High-grade strictures require dilation prior to insertion of the endoprosthesis. This may be performed with hydrostatic balloon dilating catheters or graduated dilating catheters (Figs 10.2 and 10.3).

Extremely tight strictures may permit passage of only a small-caliber guidewire. Such wires may be left *in situ* overnight and usually permit dilator passage the next day. Alternatively, 3 Fr angioplasty balloons or the Soehendra stent retriever may be helpful [31]. The Soehendra stent retriever is rarely used due to concern about excessive duct damage from the device [32,33]. Although one preliminary report [34] suggested that luminal patency of the duct persisted

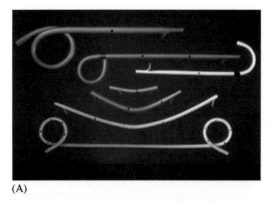

(A)

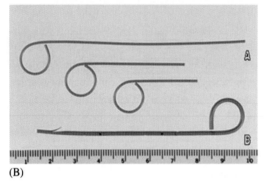

(B)

Fig. 10.1 (A) Pancreatic stents of various sizes. From top to bottom: 10 Fr, 8.5 Fr, and 5 Fr diameter stents. Note the external ^{3}/$_4$ pigtail to prevent proximal migration of the stent into the pancreatic duct and the single flange for anchoring the stent in the pancreatic duct. (B) Comparison of (*top three*) protective pancreatic stents with ^{3}/$_4$ external pigtail and without internal flange (3 Fr) to allow for spontaneous dislodgement and (*bottom*) 5 Fr flanged pancreatic stent with ^{3}/$_4$ external pigtail used for longer term stenting.

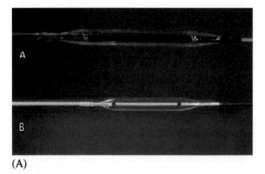

(A)

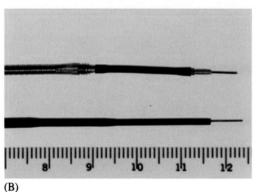

(B)

Fig. 10.2 (A) Hydrostatic dilation balloons for pancreatic stricture dilation. *Top*: 5 Fr catheter with 3 cm long balloon of 6 mm outer diameter. Accepts a 0.035 inch diameter guidewire. *Bottom*: 3 Fr angioplasty catheter with balloon of 2 cm length and 4 mm outer diameter. Accepts a 0.018 inch diameter guidewire and is used for tight strictures that will not accommodate a 5 Fr catheter. (B) Catheter dilation devices for pancreatic strictures. *Top*: Soehendra stent extraction device utilized for stricture dilation with 7 Fr screw at tip and 10 Fr screw located 2.5 cm proximal. This device is rarely used due to concern about excessive pancreatic ductal trauma. *Bottom*: Graduated dilation catheter pictured with 5-7-8 Fr outer diameter that accommodates a 0.035 inch diameter guidewire.

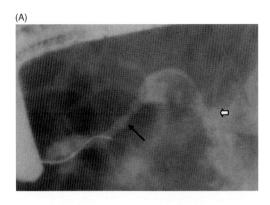

(A)

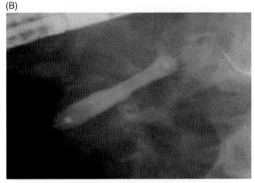

(B)

Fig. 10.3 A 45-year-old male with chronic calcific pancreatitis from pancreatic trauma 20 years earlier. Distal pancreatectomy and pancreatico-jejunostomy were performed. Now presents with recurrent pancreatitis and continuous abdominal pain. (A) Pancreatogram obtained through the minor papilla reveals segmental narrowing of the pancreatic duct, upstream stone, and patent pancreatico-jejunostomy. (B) Dilation of pancreatic duct stricture performed with 6 mm diameter hydrostatic balloon. Note the persistent waistline of the balloon. (C) A 5 Fr by 6 cm intraductal, flanged, duodenal pigtail pancreatic stent placed into dorsal duct with proximal tip traversing pancreatico-jejunostomy. (D) Follow-up pancreatogram 2 months later revealed improvement of the pancreatic stricture and widely patent pancreatico-jejunostomy (*arrow*). No further stents were placed. The patient had marked reduction in pain and no further pancreatitis over the ensuing 1 year.

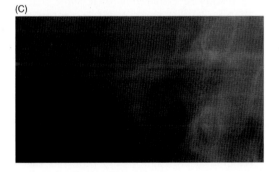

(C)

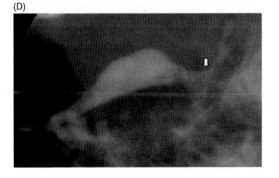

(D)

at a mean time of 5 months following balloon dilation alone, most authorities have observed recurrence of strictures after one-time dilation and therefore advocate stenting [15].

As a rule, the diameter of the stent should not exceed the size of the downstream duct. Therefore, 5, 7, or 8.5 Fr stents are commonly used in smaller ducts, whereas 10–11.5 Fr stents or dual side-by-side 5–7 Fr stents may be inserted in patients with severe chronic pancreatitis and a dilated main pancreatic duct. The tip of the stent in the pancreas must extend upstream to the narrowed segment and into a straight portion of the pancreatic duct to avoid stent tip erosion through the duct wall.

For diagnostic trials of pancreatic stenting in patients with nearly daily pain, most stents are left in place for 3–4 weeks. When long-term pancreatic stents are placed for therapy, stents have remained in place for 3–116 months [17,24].

Stents are known to occlude within the first several weeks [35]; however, clinical improvement may persist for much longer, possibly due to siphoning of the pancreatic juice along the stent. At this time, self-expanding metallic stents play no role in the management of refractory pancreatic strictures due to the high occlusion rate from mucosal hyperplasia [36].

Efficacy of pancreatic duct stenting

The results of pancreatic duct stent placement (usually with ancillary procedures) are detailed in Table 10.3 [17–26]. Successful stent placement was achieved in 82–100% of patients. Sixty-six per cent of patients with successful stent placement were reported to benefit from therapy during a mean follow-up to 8–39 months (N.B., many patients still had their stent in place during the follow-up period).

Cremer and colleagues

Cremer and colleagues [17] reported their experience with pancreatic duct stenting in 76 patients with severe chronic pancreatitis (primarily alcohol related) complicated by a distal pancreatic duct stricture and upstream dilation. A 10 Fr stent was successfully placed in 75 patients (98.7%) through the major ($n = 54$) or minor ($n = 21$) papilla. All patients had undergone biliary and pancreatic sphincterotomy, stricture dilation, and extracorporeal shock-wave lithotripsy (ESWL) (most patients) to fragment pancreatic duct stones.

A dramatic decrease or complete relief of pain was initially observed in 94% of patients and was associated with a decrease in the main pancreatic duct diameter. Clinically, stents were thought to remain patent for a mean time of 12 months (range: 2–38 months). Disappearance of the stricture was observed in only seven of 64 non-operated patients after 13 months (range: 2–30 months).

Table 10.3 Selected series reporting the results of pancreatic duct stenting for dominant strictures.

Reference	No. of patients	Technical success[a]	Mean follow-up (months)	No. of patients symptomatically improved	Major complications	Deaths
McCarthy et al. 1988 [21]	5	5	14	4	2[b]	0
Grimm et al. 1989 [18]	63	55	19	31[b]	20[b]	1
Cremer et al. 1991 [17]	76	75	37	41	12	1
Kozarek et al. 1989 [20]	N/A	17	8	13	3	0
Binmoeller et al. 1995 [23]	93	84	39	61	6	0
Ponchon et al. 1995 [25]	28	23	26	12	10	0
Smits et al. 1995 [24]	51	49	34	40	8	0
Total	311[c]	308	34[b]	202[d] (66%)	61[b] (19%)	2 (1%)

[a]Technical success refers to the number of patients successfully stented.
[b]Estimate.
[c]Does not include the studies from which the number of patients attempted is not available.
[d]Percentage improved refers to the number of patients who benefited (during the follow-up period) of the total number of patients successfully stented.
N/A, not available.

Eleven patients underwent pancreatico-jejunostomy after confirmation of pain reduction with main pancreatic duct decompression. The remainder required repeated stent changes. Fifty-five per cent of non-operated patients remained symptom-free at a mean follow-up of 3 years [19].

Early complications were related to pancreatic and/or biliary sphincterotomy (cholangitis in three patients and hemobilia in 10). Intraductal infection due to stent clogging developed in eight patients, and three had their stent migrate inwardly. Stent therapy was believed by the authors to be an acceptable medium-term treatment of pain associated with main pancreatic duct stricture. Unfortunately, because the stricture persists in the majority of patients, compliance with long-term use of plastic stents (i.e. multiple stent changes are required) would be difficult. As a result, expandable stents (18 Fr diameter, 23 mm long) have been tried in 29 patients [19].

Early follow-up to 6 months was encouraging, because stent clogging did not occur during this short follow-up interval. However, during longer term follow-up, mucosal hyperplasia (i.e. tissue ingrowth) resulted in stent occlusion in the majority of patients [36]. Because these stents are not removable by endoscopic techniques, their use should be limited, perhaps, to patients in whom resective therapy (during which the stent and head of the pancreas would both be removed) is the next step. Evaluation of covered metal stents is in progress.

Ponchon and colleagues

Ponchon and colleagues [25] successfully placed 10 Fr multi-side-hole stents after biliary and pancreatic sphincterotomy and balloon dilation of strictures in 28 of 33 patients (85%) with a distal pancreatic duct stricture and upstream dilation. This was a highly selected subgroup, because patients with multiple sites of strictures, pancreatic duct stones, pancreas divisum, common bile duct narrowing with cholestasis, any duodenal impingement, or the presence of a pseudocyst larger than 1 cm were excluded. The stents were exchanged at 2-month intervals for a total stenting duration of 6 months.

Twenty-three patients were observed for at least 1 year after removal of the stent and comprised the basis of the report. During the stenting period, 21 of 23 patients (91%) had resolution or reduction in pain, usually within days of stent insertion, and 17 patients (74%) discontinued analgesic medications. Initial relief of symptoms correlated with a decreased diameter (2 mm; $P < 0.01$) of the main pancreatic duct. Twelve patients (52%) had a persistent beneficial outcome for at least 1 year after stent removal. Disappearance of the stenosis on pancreatography at stent removal ($P < 0.05$) and 1 year later ($P < 0.005$) and reduction in the pancreatic duct diameter (2 mm) were significantly associated with pain relief. Complications of therapy occurred in 10 patients (30%), and included mild pancreatitis (resolved within 48 h) in nine and development of a communicating pseudocyst in one.

Smits and colleagues

Smits and colleagues [24] evaluated the long-term efficacy of pancreatic duct stenting (5 or 7 Fr in nine patients and 10 Fr in 40) in a heterogeneous group of 51 patients with pancreatic duct strictures (44 dominant, seven multiple) located in the head ($n = 38$), body ($n = 14$), or tail ($n = 6$), and upstream dilation. Associated pancreatic pathology treated at the time of stenting included pancreatic duct stones ($n = 17$), pseudocysts ($n = 10$), common bile duct strictures with concomitant cholestasis ($n = 12$), and pancreas divisum ($n = 3$). Stents were successfully placed in 49 patients (96%) after pancreatic sphincterotomy ($n = 31$) and stricture dilation ($n = 9$).

Patients were re-evaluated within 3 months of stent placement and were followed for a median duration of 34 months. Responders underwent stent exchanges (approximately every 3 months) until such time as the stricture patency had improved. Clinical benefit was noted in 40 of 49 patients (82%) during the stenting period. In 16 of these 40 patients, the stents were still *in situ* at the time of the report and offered continued clinical improvement over periods ranging from 6 to 116 months. In 22 of the 40 patients, the stents were electively removed. All 22 patients experienced persistent clinical improvement during periods ranging between 6 and 41 months (median: 28.5 months) after stent removal. There were no demographic factors (age, sex, duration of pancreatitis, alcohol abuse), ERCP findings (single or multiple strictures, presence of pancreatic duct stones, pseudocyst, or biliary stricture), or additional interventions (stricture dilation, removal of stones, drainage of pseudocyst, stenting of bile duct stricture) that predicted the clinical outcome.

Ashby and Lo

Ashby and Lo [40], from the United States, reported results of pancreatic stenting for strictures that differed from the European experience. Although relief of symptoms was common (86% had significant improvement in their symptom score), this was usually not evident until day 7. More disappointing was the lack of long-term benefit, with recurrence of symptoms within 1 month of stenting. This study was relatively small (21 successfully stented patients) and included five patients with pancreatic cancer. Possible explanations for the less favorable results were that sphincterotomy was not performed and strictures were not dilated routinely before stent placement (to improve pancreatic duct drainage).

Hereditary and early onset pancreatitis

Pancreatic endotherapy was evaluated in patients with hereditary pancreatitis and idiopathic early onset chronic pancreatitis. In a report by Choudari *et al.*, 27 consecutive patients with hereditary chronic pancreatitis underwent endoscopic or surgical therapy of the pancreatic duct. Nineteen (70%) underwent endoscopic therapy and eight (30%) underwent surgery as their primary treatment. After a mean follow-up of 32 months, 50% of patients undergoing endoscopic therapy were symptom free, 38% were improved, and 12% were unchanged with respect to pain. After surgery, 38% were symptom free, 25% were improved, and 37% were unchanged [38]. In a cohort of patients with painful, early onset idiopathic chronic pancreatitis (aged 16–34 years) and a dilated pancreatic duct, 11 patients underwent endoscopic therapy and were followed for over 6 years. The median interval between onset of symptoms and endoscopic therapy was 5 years (3–10 years). Pancreatic sphincterotomy and stent insertion provided short-term relief in 11 patients (100%).

Complications included fever in three patients and cholecystitis in one patient. Four patients (37%) developed recurrent pain felt to be due to recurrent pancreatic strictures or stones, and underwent further endoscopic therapy [39]. These two patient populations of hereditary and early onset idiopathic chronic pancreatitis illustrate the value of endoscopic therapy in affording short-term and medium-term pain relief. Repeat endoscopic therapy is not uncommon.

Predicting the outcome of pancreatic stenting

There are few studies that have been designed to identify subgroups of patients with chronic pancreatitis who are most likely to benefit from stenting. In a preliminary report, 65 chronic pancreatitis patients with duct dilation (> or = to 6 mm), obstruction (usually a stricture with a diameter of 1 mm or less), obstruction and dilation, or no obstruction or dilation underwent pancreatic duct stenting for 3–6 months [37]. The presence of both obstruction and dilation was a significant predictor of improvement.

Duration of stenting

The appropriate duration of pancreatic stent placement and the interval from placement to change of the pancreatic stent are not known. Two options are available [15]: (1) the stent can be left in place until symptoms or complications occur; (2) the stent can be left in place for a predetermined interval (e.g. 3 months). If the patient fails to improve, the stent should be removed because ductal hypertension is unlikely to be the cause of pain. If the patient has benefited from stenting, one can remove the stent and follow the patient clinically, continue stenting for a more prolonged period, or perform a surgical drainage procedure. (This latter option assumes that the results of endoscopic stenting will predict the surgical outcome.) There are limited data to support any of these options.

In a recent preliminary report, Borel *et al.* [42] evaluated the effect of definitive pancreatic duct stent placement only exchanged on demand when symptoms recurred. In 42 patients, a single 10 Fr stent was inserted into the main pancreatic duct following pancreatic sphincterotomy. The patients were followed for a median of 33 months with respect to pain reduction, weight gain or loss, and recurrence of symptoms. With recurrence of symptoms, the stent was exchanged. Of the 42 patients, 72% had pain relief with pancreatic stenting (pain score reduced > 50%) and 69% gained weight. Two-thirds of the patients ($n = 28$) required only the single pancreatic stent placement and 12 patients required a stent exchange after a median of 15 months. Two patients required repeated stent exchanges for recurrence of pain. Persistence or recurrence of pain was significantly associated with the development of cholestasis and continued alcohol abuse. These authors concluded that long-term pancreatic stenting appears to be an effective, and possibly a superior, option compared to temporary stenting [42].

Does response to stenting predict the outcome of surgery?

The question may be posed: in patients with chronic pancreatitis and a dilated pancreatic duct, will the response to pancreatic stent placement predict the response to surgical duct decompression? In a preliminary report of a randomized controlled trial ($n = 8$), McHenry and associates evaluated the utility of short-term (12 weeks) pancreatic duct stenting to relieve pain and to predict the response to surgical decompression in patients with chronic pancreatitis and a dilated main pancreatic duct [43]. Four of eight patients benefited from stenting, while no control patient improved. Among five patients who underwent a Puestow procedure following stent therapy, four had pain relief. Improvement with the pancreatic stent was seen in two of four patients responding to surgery; one patient benefited from the stent but did not improve with surgery. In another preliminary series, reported by DuVall and colleagues [44], endoscopic therapy predicted the outcome from surgical decompression in nine of 11 patients (82%; positive and negative predictive values were 80% and 83%, respectively) during a 2-year postoperative follow-up interval.

Several institutions have recently reported that symptomatic improvement may persist after pancreatic stent removal despite stricture persistence [17,23–25]. When summarizing the results of two studies ($n = 54$) that evaluated the efficacy of pancreatic duct stenting for dominant strictures, 65% of patients had persistent symptom improvement after stent removal, although the stricture resolved in only 33% (Table 10.4). Although these data indicate that complete stricture resolution is not a prerequisite for symptom improvement, several other factors may account for this outcome. First, other therapies performed at the time of stenting (e.g. pancreatic stone removal, pancreatic sphincterotomy)

Table 10.4 Pancreatic duct stenting for dominant strictures: clinical outcome and stricture resolution after stent removal.

Reference	Persistent improvement after stent removal	Median follow-up after stent removal (months)	Stricture resolution
Smits *et al*. 1995 [24]	23/33 (70%)	29	10/33 (20%)
Ponchon *et al*. 1995 [25]	12/21 (57%)	14	8/21 (38%)
Total	35/54 (65%)	23	18/54 (33%)

may contribute to patient benefit. Second, many of the unresolved strictures had improved luminal patency (but without return of lumen diameter to normal). Third, the pain of chronic pancreatitis tends to decrease with time and may resolve when marked deterioration of pancreatic function occurs [40].

Long-term follow-up

In the largest multicenter trial, Rosch *et al.* [26] reported on the long-term follow-up of over 1000 patients with chronic pancreatitis undergoing initial endoscopic therapy during the period 1989–95. Some of these patients were previously reported with shorter follow-up as noted in Table 10.3.

A total of 1211 patients from eight centers in Europe with pain and obstructive chronic pancreatitis underwent endoscopic therapy including endoscopic pancreatic sphincterotomy, pancreatic stricture dilation, pancreatic stone removal, pancreatic stent placement, or a combination of these methods. Over a mean period of 4.9 years (range: 2–12 years), 1118 patients (84%) were followed for symptomatic improvement and need for pancreatic surgery. Success of endoscopic therapy was defined as a significant reduction or elimination of pain and reduction in pain medication. Partial success was defined as reduction in pain although further interventions were necessary for pain relief. Failure of endoscopic therapy was defined as the need for pancreatic decompressive surgery or patients that were lost to follow-up.

Over long-term follow-up, 69% of patients were successfully treated with endoscopic therapy and 15% experienced a partial success. Twenty per cent of patients required surgery with a 55% significant reduction in pain. Five per cent of patients were lost to follow-up. The patients with the highest frequency of completed treatment were those with stones alone (76%) as compared to those with strictures alone (57%) and those with strictures and stones (57%) ($P < 0.001$). Interestingly, the percentage of patients with no or minimal residual pain at follow-up was similar in all groups (strictures alone 84%, stones alone 84%, and strictures plus stones 87%) ($P = 0.677$). The authors of this report concluded that endoscopic therapy of chronic pancreatitis in experienced centers is effective in the majority of patients, and the beneficial response to successful endoscopic therapy in chronic pancreatitis is durable and long-term [26].

Only randomized controlled studies comparing surgical, medical, and endoscopic techniques will allow us to determine the true long-term efficacy of pancreatic duct stenting for stricture therapy. There remain many unanswered questions. Which patients are the best candidates? Is proximal pancreatic ductal dilation a prerequisite? Does the response to stenting depend on the etiology of the chronic pancreatitis? Finally, as noted, how does endoscopic therapy compare with medical and surgical management?

Table 10.5 Complications directly related to pancreatic duct stents.

Occlusion, which may result in pain and/or pancreatitis
Migration into or out of duct
Duodenal erosions
Pancreatic infection
Ductal perforation
Ductal and parenchymal changes
Stone formation

Complications associated with pancreatic stents

True complication rates are difficult to decipher due to: (1) the simultaneous performance of other procedures (e.g. pancreatic sphincterotomy, stricture dilation); (2) the heterogeneous patient populations treated (i.e. patients with acute or chronic pancreatitis); and (3) the lack of uniform definitions of complications and a grading system of their severity [47]. Complications related directly to stent therapy are listed in Table 10.5 [47,49].

Occlusion

The pathogenesis of pancreatic stent occlusion on scanning electron microscopy mirrors biliary stent blockage with typical biofilm and microcolonies of bacteria mixed with crystals, similar to biliary sludge. The rate of pancreatic stent occlusion appears to be similar to that for biliary stents [35]. We found that 50% of pancreatic stents (primarily 5–7 Fr) were occluded within 6 weeks of placement and 100% of stents were occluded at more than 9 weeks when carefully evaluated by water flow methods. More than 80% of these early occlusions were not associated with adverse clinical events. In such circumstances, the stent is perhaps serving as a dilator or a wick. Similarly, stents reported to be patent for as long as 38 months [17] are clinically patent but would presumably be occluded by water flow testing.

Migration

Stent migration may be upstream (i.e. into the duct) or downstream (i.e. into the duodenum). Migration in either direction may be heralded by the return of pain or pancreatitis. Johanson and associates [50] reported inward migration in 5.2% of patients and duodenal migration in 7.5%. These events occurred with single intraductal and single duodenal stent flanges. Rarely, surgery is needed to remove a proximally migrated stent. Modifications in pancreatic stent design have greatly reduced the frequency of such occurrences. Dean and associates [51] reported no inward migration in 112 patients stented with a four-barbed (two internal and two external) stent. We have had no inward migration in greater than 3000 stents with a duodenal pigtail.

Stent-induced duct changes

Although therapeutic benefit has been reported for pancreatic stenting, it is evident that morphological changes of the pancreatic duct directly related to this therapy occur in the majority of patients. In summarizing the results of seven published series [52–55,57–59], new ductal changes were seen in 54% (range: 33–83%) of 297 patients. Limited observations to date indicate a tendency of these ductal changes to improve with time following stent change and/or removal [44,45,47,50,52,53,55,57–59].

The long-term consequences of these stent-induced ductal changes remain uncertain. Moreover, the long-term parenchymal effects have not been studied in humans. In a pilot study, six mongrel dogs underwent pancreatic duct stenting for 2–4 months [49]. Radiographic, gross, and histological abnormalities developed in all dogs. The radiographic findings (stenosis in the stented region with upstream dilation) were associated with gross evidence of fibrosis, which increased proportionally with the length of the stenting period. Histological changes of obstructive pancreatitis were present in most experimental dogs.

Although follow-up after stent removal was short, the atrophy and fibrosis seen were not likely to be reversible. In a recently reported study [59], parenchymal changes (hypoechoic area around the stent, heterogeneity, and cystic changes) were seen on endoscopic ultrasound in 17 of 25 patients undergoing short-term pancreatic duct stenting. Four patients who had parenchymal changes at stent removal had a follow-up study at a mean time of 16 months. Two patients had (new) changes suggestive of chronic pancreatitis (heterogeneous echotexture, echogenic foci in the parenchyma, and a thickened hyperechoic irregular pancreatic duct) in the stented region. While such damage in a normal pancreas may have significant long-term consequences, the outcome in patients with advanced chronic pancreatitis may be inconsequential.

Brief mini-stents

If brief interval stenting is needed, such as for pancreatic sphincterotomy, we now commonly use small-diameter stents (3 or 4 Fr) with no intraductal barb [83] (Fig. 10.1). Depending on their length, 80–90% of these stents migrate out of the duct spontaneously. Further studies addressing issues of stent diameter as well as composition and duration of therapy as they relate to safety and efficacy are needed. Additionally, further evaluation of expandable stents, particularly the coated models, is awaited.

Pancreatic ductal stones

Causes of pancreatic ductal stones

Worldwide, alcohol consumption appears to be the most important factor associated with chronic calcifying pancreatitis. Although the exact mechanism of intraductal stone formation has not been clearly elucidated, considerable progress in this area has been made [60]. Alcohol appears to be directly toxic to the pancreas and produces a dysregulation of secretion of pancreatic enzymes (including zymogens), citrate (a potent calcium chelator), lithostathine (pancreatic stone protein), and calcium. These changes favor the formation of a nidus (a protein plug), followed by precipitation of calcium carbonate to form a stone [60,61].

Stones cause obstruction

The rationale for intervention is based on the premise that pancreatic stones increase the intraductal pressure (and probably the parenchymal pressure, with resultant pancreatic ischemia) proximal to the obstructed focus. Reports indicating that endoscopic (with or without ESWL) or surgical removal of pancreatic calculi results in improvement of symptoms support this notion [15]. Moreover, stone impaction may cause further trauma to the pancreatic duct, with epithelial destruction and stricture formation [53,55]. Thus, identification of pancreatic ductal stones in a symptomatic patient warrants consideration of removal. One or more large stones in the head with upstream asymptomatic parenchymal atrophy probably warrant therapy also.

Endoscopic techniques for stone extraction

Pancreatic sphincterotomy

A major papilla pancreatic sphincterotomy (in patients with normal anatomy, i.e. no pancreas divisum) is usually performed to facilitate access to the duct prior to attempts at stone removal. There are two methods available to cut the major pancreatic sphincter [63,64]. A standard pull-type sphincterotome (with or without a wire guide) is inserted into the pancreatic duct and orientated along the axis of the pancreatic duct (usually in the 12–1 o'clock position). Although the landmarks to determine the length of incision are imprecise, authorities recommend cutting 5–10 mm [63] (Fig. 10.4). The cutting wire should not extend more than 6–7 mm up the duct when applying electrocautery so as to prevent deep ductal injury. Alternatively, a needle-knife can be used to perform the sphincterotomy over a previously placed pancreatic stent [63,64].

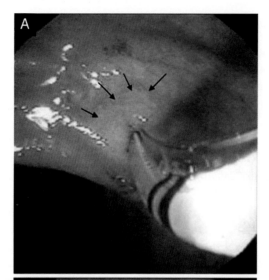

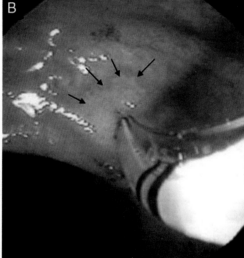

Fig. 10.4 (A) Technique of major papilla pancreatic sphincterotomy using a pull-type sphincterotome. *Left top*: Biliary sphincterotomy is performed using a standard pull-type sphincterotome. *Right top*: Pancreatic sphincterotomy is performed with a pull-type sphincterotome cutting in the 1 o'clock direction. *Left bottom*: Completed biliary and pancreatic sphincterotomy. A guidewire is in the pancreatic duct. *Right bottom*: A 6 Fr pancreatic stent is placed following performance of the pancreatic sphincterotomy. (B) Technique of minor papilla pancreatic sphincterotomy. 1. Traction sphincterotome positioned in minor papilla. Note the extent of the minor papilla mound (*arrows*). Duodenal juice at the minor papilla orifice is aspirated away before cutting to prevent heat dissipation to juice and boiling the adjacent tissues during the sphincterotomy. 2. Wire is bowed taut and cut is performed rapidly with minimal coagulation utilizing the ERBE generator. The optimal cut length in this setting is unknown. The 5 mm length minor papilla sphincterotomy is complete without white tissue coagulum. 3. White pancreatic stone removed through patent sphincterotomy orifice with balloon catheter. 4. Excessive white coagulum at the cut edge of the sphincterotomy in a patient who underwent minor papilla sphincterotomy. This may potentially lead to restenosis of the sphincterotomy orifice.

Biliary sphincterotomy also? Some authorities favor performing a biliary sphincterotomy prior to the pancreatic sphincterotomy because of the high incidence of cholangitis if this is not done [64]. Patients with alkaline phosphatase elevation from chronic pancreatitis-induced biliary strictures are especially at risk for cholangitis (if no biliary sphincterotomy is performed) [65]. Such complications were not found by others [23,24,64,65]. Performing a biliary sphincterotomy first, however, can expose the pancreatico-biliary septum and allow the length of the cut to be gauged more accurately.

Pancreas divisum In patients with pancreas divisum, a minor papilla sphincterotomy is usually necessary. The technique is similar to that of major papilla sphincterotomy, except that the direction of the incision is usually in the 10–12 o'clock position and the length of the sphincterotomy is limited to 4–8 mm.

Stone removal The ability to remove a stone by endoscopic methods alone is dependent on the stone size and number, duct location, presence of downstream stricture, and the degree of impaction [67,68]. Downstream strictures usually require dilation with either catheters or hydrostatic balloons. Standard stone-retrieval balloons and baskets are the most common accessories used to remove stones. Passage of these instruments around a tortuous duct can be difficult, but use of over-the-wire accessories is usually helpful. Stone removal is then performed in a fashion similar to bile duct stone extraction (Fig. 10.5). Occasionally, mechanical lithotripsy is necessary, particularly when the stone is larger in diameter than the downstream duct or the stone is proximal to a stricture. A rat tooth forceps may be helpful when a stone is located in the head of the pancreas close to the pancreatic orifice.

Results of endoscopic treatment for stones

Sherman and colleagues Sherman and colleagues attempted to identify those patients with predominantly main pancreatic duct stones most amenable to endoscopic removal and to determine the effects of such removal on the patients' clinical course [67].

Thirty-two patients with ductographic evidence of chronic pancreatitis and pancreatic duct stones underwent attempted endoscopic removal using various techniques, including bile duct and/or pancreatic duct sphincterotomy, stricture dilation, pancreatic duct stenting, stone basketing, balloon extraction, and/or flushing. Of these patients, 72% had complete or partial stone removal, and 68% had significant symptomatic improvement after endoscopic therapy. Symptomatic improvement was most evident in the group of patients with chronic relapsing pancreatitis (vs. those presenting with chronic continuous pain alone; 83% vs. 46%).

Factors favoring complete stone removal included: (1) three or fewer stones; (2) stones confined to the head or body of the pancreas; (3) absence of a downstream stricture; (4) stone diameter less than or equal to 10 mm; and (5) absence of impacted stones.

(a)

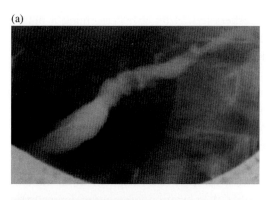

(b)

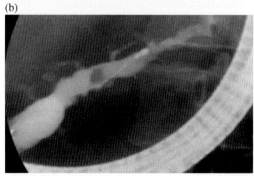

(c)

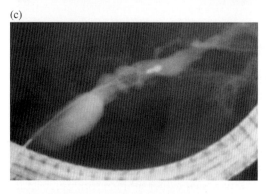

(d)

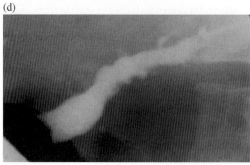

Fig. 10.5 A 40-year-old female with alcohol-induced chronic pancreatitis complicated by pancreatic main duct stones. (a) Pancreatogram revealing dilated pancreatic duct with 5 mm diameter filling defect consistent with a pancreatic stone. (b) After pancreatic sphincterotomy, a non-wire-guided stone extraction basket was utilized. The basket is opened fully in the dilated pancreatic duct and the stone is engaged. (c) Basket is slowly closed on the stone. (d) Stone is extracted and follow-up pancreatogram with a balloon catheter reveals no residual filling defects. No further stenting was performed.

After successful stone removal, 25% of patients had regression of the ducto-graphic changes of chronic pancreatitis, and 42% had a decrease in the main pancreatic duct diameter. The only complication from therapy was mild pancreatitis, occurring in 8%.

Smits and colleagues Smits and colleagues [68] reported the results of 53 patients with pancreatic duct stones treated primarily by endoscopic methods alone (eight had ESWL). Stone removal was successful in 42 patients (79%; complete in 39 and partial in three), with initial relief of symptoms in 38 (90%). Similar to the results reported by Sherman *et al.* [67], in this series, three of 11 patients (27%) with failed stone removal had improvement in symptoms, suggesting that some of the clinical response may be related to other therapies performed at the time of attempted stone removal (e.g. pancreatic sphincterotomy).

During a median follow-up of 33 months, 13 patients had recurrent symptoms due to stone recurrence. The stones were successfully removed in 10 (77%). No factor evaluated (etiology of pancreatitis, presentation with pain or pancreatitis, presence of single or multiple stones, location of stones, presence or absence of a stricture) was shown to predict successful stone treatment (defined as complete or partial removal of stones, resulting in relief of symptoms).

Cremer and colleagues Cremer and colleagues [37] reported the results of 40 patients with pancreatic duct stones who were treated by endoscopic methods alone. Complete stone clearance was achieved in only 18 (45%). However, immediate resolution of pain occurred in 77%. During a 3-year follow-up, 63% remained symptom free. Clinical steatorrhea improved in 11 of 15 patients (73%).

Summary results Table 10.6 summarizes six selected series [37,67–71] reporting the results of pancreatic stone removal by endoscopic methods alone. Complete stone clearance was achieved in 93 of 147 patients (63%). The major complication rate was 9% (primarily pancreatitis), and the mortality rate was 0%. Cremer *et al.* [37] reported bleeding in 3% and retroperitoneal perforation in 1.4%. Sepsis was an infrequent complication. During a 2.5-year (approximate) follow-up, 74% of patients had improvement in their symptoms.

Endoscopic therapy with ESWL

As noted, endoscopic methods alone will likely fail in the presence of large or impacted stones and stones proximal to a stricture. ESWL can be used to fragment stones and facilitate their removal (Fig. 10.6). Thus, this procedure is complementary to endoscopic techniques and improves the success of non-surgical ductal decompression.

Table 10.6 Selected series reporting the results of endoscopic therapy of pancreatic ductal stones (using ERCP techniques alone).

Reference	No. of patients	Complete stone clearance (%)	Major complications (%)	Mortality (%)	Mean follow-up (months)	Symptom improvement (%)
Schneider and Lux 1985 [69]	3	100	0	0	N/A	N/A
Fuji *et al*. 1989 [70]	11	55	0	0	N/A	N/A
Sherman *et al*. 1991 [67]	32	59	8	0	26	68
Kozarek *et al*. 1992 [71]	8	88	13	0	17	88
Cremer *et al*. 1993 [37]	40	45	10	0	36	63
Smits *et al*. 1996 [68]	53[b]	74	9	0	33	81
Total	147	63	9	0	31[a]	74

[a]Estimate.
[b]Eight also had ESWL.
N/A, not available.

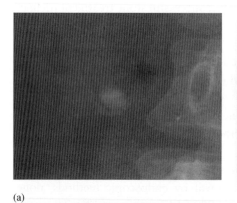

(a)

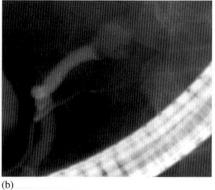

(b)

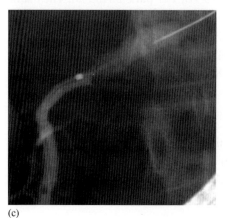

(c)

Fig. 10.6 A 41-year-old female with a history of abdominal pain, pancreatitis, and pancreatic calcification on CT scan. (a) Abdominal radiograph reveals solitary radiopaque stone in head/body region. (b) Pancreatogram reveals an 8 mm obstructing stone in body of pancreas pancreatic duct. (c) A 0.018 inch diameter guidewire was advanced beyond the stone. Further contrast filling of duct demonstrating upstream dilation. Following pancreatic sphincterotomy, stone extraction with basket was unsuccessful.

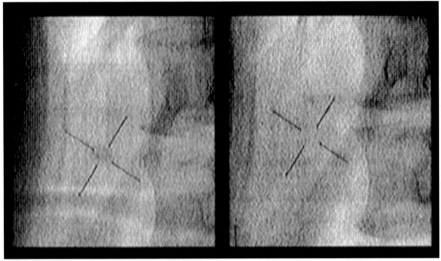

(d)

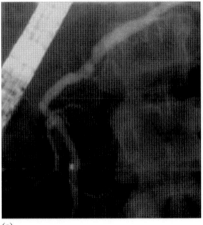

(e)

Fig. 10.6 (*cont'd*) (d) ESWL performed with Healthronics Lithotron spark-gap lithotriptor at a setting of 26 kV for a total of 2500 shocks. Fragmentation of the stone demonstrated post-ESWL. (e) Endoscopic view of small stone fragments removed from the pancreatic duct post-ESWL.

Sauerbruch and colleagues Sauerbruch and colleagues [76] were the first (in 1987) to report the successful use of ESWL in the treatment of pancreatic duct stones. Since that time, more than 400 patients have been reported in the literature [66,74–81]. Patients with obstructing prepapillary concrement and upstream ductal dilation appear to be the best candidates for ESWL. In the largest

Table 10.7 Selected series reporting the results of endoscopic therapy of pancreatic ductal stones using adjunctive ESWL.

Reference	No. of patients	Mean no. ESWL sessions	Complete stone clearance (%)	Major complications (%)	Mortality (%)	Mean follow-up (months)	Symptom improvement (%)
Neuhaus 1989 [74]	12	1.6	67	0	0	8	91
Soehendra et al. 1989 [73]	8	N/A	100	0	0	6	75
Delhaye et al. 1992 [66]	123	1.8	59	36	0	14	63
Sauerbruch et al. 1992 [76]	24	1.5	42	0	0	24	83
Schneider et al. 1994 [77]	50	2.4	60	0	0	20	90
van der Hul et al. 1994 [78]	17	1.9	41	6	0	30	65
Sherman et al. 1991 [67]	26	1.2	61	12	0	26	81
Kozarek et al. 2002 [80]	40	1.1	100	20	0	29	80
Farnbacher et al. 2002 [81]	125	2.5	51	0	0	29	93
Total	425	2.0	60	9	0	21[a]	80

[a]Estimate.
N/A, not available.

reported series, 123 patients with main pancreatic duct stones and proximal dilation were treated with an electromagnetic lithotriptor, usually before pancreatic duct sphincterotomy [66]. Stones were successfully fragmented in 99%, resulting in a decrease in duct dilation in 90%. The main pancreatic duct was completely cleared of all stones in 59%. Eighty-five per cent of patients noted pain improvement during a mean follow-up of 14 months. However, 41% of patients had a clinical relapse due to stone migration into the main pancreatic duct, progressive stricture, or stent occlusion.

This same center compared their results of pancreatic stone removal prior to the availability of ESWL and after the introduction of adjunctive ESWL therapy [37]. Stones were successfully cleared in 18 of 40 patients (45%) by endoscopic methods alone, compared with 22 of 28 (78.6%) with ESWL. Table 10.7 summarizes the results of nine selected series reporting the efficacy and safety of adjunctive ESWL [66,67,73,74,76–78,80,81]. Complications in these series were related primarily to the endoscopic procedure.

Although ultrasound-focused ESWL has been reported to achieve stone fragmentation, such focusing is clearly more difficult. In the series reported by Schneider and associates [77], stone localization was achieved in 17 of 119 sessions (14%) when only ultrasonography was used to monitor the position of the stone.

The Brussels group The Brussels group [79] studied 70 pancreatic stone patients who underwent attempts at endoscopic removal, with adjunctive ESWL used in 41 (59%). This was a fairly homogeneous group of patients in that those with strictures, previous pancreatic surgery, and failed pancreatic sphincterotomy were excluded. The authors evaluated the immediate technical and clinical results and reviewed the long-term outcome in patients followed for more than 2 years.

Complete ($n = 35$) or partial ($n = 20$) stone removal was achieved in 79%, and was more frequently observed when ESWL was performed ($P < 0.005$) and in the absence of a non-papillary ductal substenosis or complete main duct obstruction ($P < 0.05$). Complete stone clearance was most frequently observed with single stones or stones confined to the head ($P < 0.05$). In the multivariate analysis, ESWL was the only independent factor influencing the technical results of endoscopic management. In this series, the number of ERCPs performed per patient was reduced from 3.4 to 2.7 after the introduction of ESWL ($P < 0.01$). Of the 56 patients with pain on admission, 53 (95%) were pain free ($n = 41$) or had a reduction in pain ($n = 12$).

In both the univariate and multivariate analyses, a significant association was found between immediate disappearance of pain and complete or partial main pancreatic duct clearance. During the first 2 years of follow-up after therapy, 25 of 46 (54%) patients were totally pain free, whereas the frequency of pain attacks in the remaining 21 was halved. This frequency of recurrent symptoms (46%) is comparable to that of surgical series [82].

Long-term pain relief was associated with: (1) earlier treatment after disease onset ($P < 0.005$); (2) a low frequency of pain attacks before therapy ($P < 0.05$); and (3) absence of non-papillary substenosis of the main pancreatic duct ($P < 0.05$).

Interestingly, outcome was not associated with prior or continued alcohol intake. In the multivariate analysis, pain recurrence was independently associated with the frequency of pain attacks before therapy, the duration of disease, and the presence of non-papillary substenosis of the main pancreatic duct. It was suggested that such substenosis can induce ductal hypertension by blocking migration of fragmented stones or by progressing to higher grade stenosis. Twenty per cent underwent subsequent pancreatic surgical procedures. Of the remaining 28 patients, there was statistically significant improvement in mean pain scores, narcotic use, and hospitalizations when comparing intervals before and after stone therapy [83].

Kozarek and colleagues Kozarek and colleagues performed a retrospective review of the efficacy of ESWL as an adjunct to endoscopic therapy in 40 patients who underwent a total of 46 ESWL sessions (an average of 1.15 sessions/patient). Eighty per cent of patients did not require surgery and had significant pain relief, reduced number of hospitalizations, and reduced narcotic use as compared to the pre-ESWL period over a mean 2.4-year follow-up [80].

Farnbacher and colleagues Farnbacher and colleagues retrospectively reviewed the efficacy of pancreatic stone clearance with endoscopic and ESWL therapy. Technical success was achieved in 85% of the 125 patients. The majority of the patients (111 of 125) required piezoelectric ESWL for stone fragmentation. ESWL was safe, without any serious complications. Middle-aged patients in the early stages of chronic pancreatitis with stones in a prepapillary location were the best candidates for successful treatment and required the least number of ESWL treatment sessions [81].

These aforementioned studies reaffirm that ESWL as an adjunct to endoscopic pancreatic therapy is effective, and the results of the combined modality may obviate the need for surgery. The results of endoscopic therapy in conjunction with ESWL for pancreatic stone disease compare favorably to the outcomes in surgically treated patients.

Intraductal lithotripsy

Intraductal lithotripsy via mother–baby scope systems has largely failed due to inability to maneuver within the relatively narrow ductal system. Results with fluoroscopy-guided laser lithotripsy were similarly poor [71]. Pancreatoscopy (via a 'mother–baby' scope system) can be used to directly visualize laser fiber contact with the stone and fragmentation. Experience is limited to date [70,83].

Medical treatment for stones

Stone dissolution via ductal irrigation (contact dissolution) or oral agent is an attractive endoscopic adjunct for stone removal.

Citrate Sahel and Sarles found that intraduodenal infusion of citrate in dogs significantly increased the citrate concentration in pancreatic juice [85]. This led to a non-randomized study of oral citrate in 18 patients with chronic pancreatitis, 17 of whom had pancreatic duct stones. Seven patients responded during a mean duration of therapy of 9.5 months, with a mean stone size reduction of 21% and an improvement in symptoms [61].

Berger *et al.* [86] performed nasopancreatic drainage in six patients with main pancreatic duct stones. The pancreatic duct was perfused with a mixture of isotonic citrate and saline at 3 ml/min for 4 days. A stone-free state was achieved in all cases.

Pancreatic pain disappeared during the perfusion, and four patients remained free of pain during the follow-up period (1–12 months). The remaining two patients had repeat therapy, which resulted in pain resolution. Pancreatic exocrine function was evaluated by the Lundh test in five patients before and after therapy. An increase of 50–360% was observed in enzyme output in three patients, while no improvement was noted in the remaining two patients.

Trimethadione Trimethadione, an epileptic agent and a weak organic acid, has been shown *in vitro* to induce a concentration-dependent increase in calcium solubility [61]. Noda *et al.* [87] showed promising results for trimethadione in a dog model of pancreatic stones. Unfortunately, the doses used in the dogs, if extrapolated to humans, could potentially be toxic. At the present time, no rapidly effective solvent for human use is available to treat pancreatic stones. Further trials in humans are needed to establish a role for medical therapy (either alone or as an aid to endoscopic measures) in treating patients with symptomatic pancreatic duct stones.

Overall results for stone treatment

These data suggest that removal of pancreatic duct stones may result in symptomatic benefit. Longer follow-up is necessary to determine the stone recurrence rate and whether endoscopic success results in long-standing clinical improvement or permanent regression of the morphological changes. Overall, endoscopists are encouraged to remove pancreatic duct stones in symptomatic patients when the stones are located in the main duct (in the head, body, or both) and are thus readily accessible.

The currently available data suggest that the clinical outcome after successful endoscopic removal is similar to the surgical outcome, with lower morbidity and mortality [88]. Moreover, recurrence of symptoms due to migrated stone fragments can be treated again by endoscopy with or without ESWL.

On the other hand, re-operation rates for recurrent pain after surgery are as high as 20%, with a striking increase in morbidity and mortality after repeated surgery [82]. Controlled trials comparing endoscopic, surgical, and medical therapies are awaited.

Pancreatic pseudocysts

Pancreatic pseudocysts may complicate the course of chronic pancreatitis in 20–40% of cases [89,90]. Traditionally, surgery has been the treatment of choice for such patients. The introduction of ultrasound- and CT-guided needle and catheter drainage techniques provided a non-operative alternative for managing patients with pseudocysts.

Endoscopic treatment for pseudocysts

More recently, an endoscopic approach has been applied for this indication. The aim of endoscopic therapy is to create a communication between the pseudocyst cavity and the bowel lumen. This can be done by a transpapillary and/or a transmural approach. The route taken depends on the location of the pseudocyst and whether it communicates with the pancreatic duct or compresses the gut lumen. More than 400 cases of endoscopically managed pseudocysts have been reported (Table 10.8) [91–100]. The results indicate that endoscopic therapy is associated with a high technical success rate (80–95%), acceptably low complication rates (equal to or less than surgical rates), and a pseudocyst recurrence rate of 10–20% [95].

In the largest series reported [97], 100 of 108 patients (93%) had their pseudocysts successfully drained. Pseudocysts recurred in 13 (13%). The presence of chronic pancreatitis, obstructed pancreatic duct, ductal stricture, necrosis on CT scan, and a pseudocyst greater than 10 cm in size was not predictive of recurrent pseudocyst disease. Endoscopic therapy has also been shown to be effective in the management of partial [100] and complete pancreatic ductal disruptions [101], pancreatico-cutaneous fistulas, infected fluid collections [102], pancreatic ascites, pancreatic pleural effusions [9,103], and traumatic duct dis-

Table 10.8 Selected series reporting the results of endoscopic therapy of pseudocysts.

Reference	Technical success	Method of pseudocyst decompression			Complications	Deaths
		No. transpapillary	No. ECG	No. ECD		
Grimm et al. 1989 [18]	14/16	5	1	8	5	1
Cremer et al. 1989 [99]	32/33	0	11	21	3	0
Kozarek et al. 1991 [100]	12/14	12	0	0	5	0
Sahel 1991 [98]	58/67[a]	26	1	31	9	1
Catalano et al. 1995 [93]	17/21	17	0	0	1	0
Smits et al. 1995 [91]	31/37[a]	16	8	7	6	0
Binmoeller et al. 1995 [94]	47/53	31	6	10	6	0
Barthet et al. 1995 [92]	30/30[a]	30	10	0	13	0
Howell et al. 1996 [97]	100/108	37	38	25	25	0
Total	341/379 (90%)	174	75	102	79 (20%)	2 (1%)

[a]Estimate.

ruptions [103,104]. These studies and others [105] confirm the relative safety of endoscopic intervention in peripancreatic fluid collections (Table 10.8).

This topic is reviewed in detail by Howell in Chapter 11.

Biliary obstruction in chronic pancreatitis

Intrapancreatic common bile duct strictures have been reported to occur in 2.7–45.6% of patients with chronic pancreatitis (Fig. 10.7). Such strictures are a result of a fibrotic inflammatory restriction or compression by a pseudocyst [107]. In one ERCP series, a common bile duct stricture was seen in 30% of patients, and was associated with persistent cholestasis, jaundice, or cholangitis in 9% [108]. Because long-standing biliary obstruction can lead to secondary biliary cirrhosis and/or recurrent cholangitis, biliary decompression has been recommended. Surgical therapy has been the traditional approach. Based on the excellent outcome (with low morbidity) from endoscopic biliary stenting in postoperative stricture [109], however, evaluation of similar techniques for bile duct strictures complicating chronic pancreatitis was undertaken.

Standard biliary stents

Deviere and colleagues

Deviere and colleagues [108] evaluated the use of biliary stenting (one or two plastic 10 Fr C-shaped stents) in 25 chronic pancreatitis patients with bile duct obstruction and significant cholestasis (alkaline phosphatase > two times the

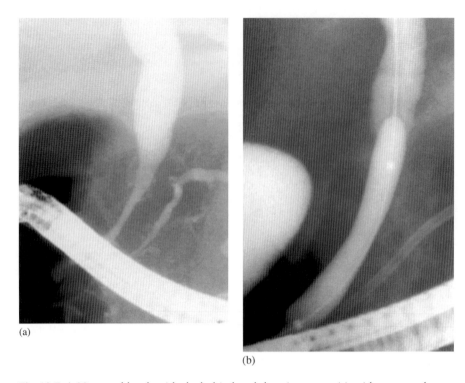

(a)

(b)

Fig. 10.7 A 38-year-old male with alcohol-induced chronic pancreatitis with recurrent bouts of pain, cholestatic serum liver chemistries, and elevated serum amylase. CT scan revealed enlarged head of pancreas, calcifications, and new biliary dilation. (a) Cholangiogram revealed smooth, 3 cm long narrowing of the distal common bile duct within the head of the pancreas, with upstream dilation typical of benign biliary stricture complicating chronic pancreatitis. Biliary intraductal brush cytology was negative. Pancreatogram revealed narrowing of the head of pancreas pancreatic duct, dilated secondary branches, and calcifications. (b) A 7 Fr multiple side-hole pancreatic stent in place. Balloon dilation of the bile duct stricture was performed with a 10 mm hydrostatic balloon.

upper limits of normal). Nineteen patients had jaundice and seven presented with cholangitis.

Following stent placement, cholestasis, hyperbilirubinemia, and cholangitis resolved in all patients. Late follow-up (mean: 14 months; range: 4–72 months) of 22 patients was much less satisfactory. One patient died of acute cholecystitis and postsurgical complications, whereas a second died of sepsis 10 months after stenting, which was believed to be due to stent blockage or dislodgement. Stent migration occurred in 10 patients and stent occlusion in eight, resulting in cholestasis with or without jaundice ($n = 12$), cholangitis ($n = 4$), or no symptoms ($n = 2$).

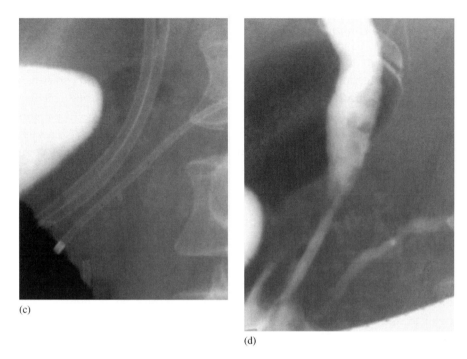

(c)

(d)

Fig. 10.7 (*cont'd*) (c) Placement of two 10 Fr polyethylene stents into bile duct and a 7 Fr multiple side-hole pancreatic stent into pancreatic duct. Serum liver chemistries normalized and abdominal pain improved. (d) Six months later, the patient's daily pain was moderately improved and ERCP was performed for possible bile duct and pancreatic stent removal. Cholangiogram revealed persistent bile duct narrowing requiring further bile duct stenting. Pancreatic ductal stricture in the head was improved and did not require further pancreatic stenting.

These patients were treated with stent replacement, surgery, or both ($n = 7$). Ten patients continued to have a stent in place (mean follow-up: 8 months) and remained asymptomatic. Because of resolution of their biliary stricture, only three patients required no further stents. The initial observation of this study is that biliary drainage is an effective therapy for resolving cholangitis or jaundice in patients with chronic pancreatitis and a biliary stricture. The long-term efficacy of this treatment, however, is much less satisfactory, because stricture resolution rarely occurs.

The Amsterdam group

The Amsterdam group reported their results of placing 10 Fr biliary stents in 52 chronic pancreatitis patients with cholestasis [15]. Jaundice and cholestasis disappeared within 2 weeks after stent insertion in all patients. During a median follow-up duration of 32 months (range: 3 months to 10 years), 17 patients (33%) had their stent removed without return of cholestasis. Complete resolution of the stricture was seen in 10 of the 17 patients. This suggested that complete resolution of the stricture was not necessary for long-term relief of symptoms and cholestasis.

Barthet and colleagues

Barthet and colleagues [110] also found that biliary stenting is not a definitive therapy for chronic pancreatitis patients with a distal common bile duct stricture. In their series of 19 patients (mean duration of stenting: 10 months), only two had complete clinical (resolution of symptoms), biological (normalization of cholestatic liver tests), and radiological (resolution of biliary stricture and upstream dilation) recovery. Six of 10 (60%) possible clinical successes, eight of 19 (42%) possible biological successes, and three of 19 (16%) possible radiological successes were obtained.

Metal stents for biliary obstruction?

Because of the disappointing results with plastic stents and the concern about the high morbidity associated with surgically performed biliary drainage procedures in alcoholic (frequently debilitated) patients, the group from Brussels evaluated the use of uncoated expandable metal stents for this indication [112].

Twenty patients were treated with a 34 mm long metal stent, which becomes 10 mm in diameter when fully expanded. The short length of the stent was chosen so that surgical bypass (e.g. choledochoduodenostomy) would still be possible if necessary. Cholestasis ($n = 20$), jaundice ($n = 7$), and cholangitis ($n = 3$) resolved in all patients. Eighteen patients had no further biliary problems during a follow-up period of 33 months (range: 24–42 months). Two patients (10%) developed epithelial hyperplasia within the stent, resulting in recurrent cholestasis in one and jaundice in the other. These patients were treated endoscopically with standard plastic stents, with one ultimately requiring surgical drainage. The authors concluded that this therapy could be an effective alternative to surgical biliary diversion, but longer follow-up and controlled trials are necessary to confirm these results.

In a recent abstract report, the Amsterdam group reported the long-term follow-up (mean: 50 months) of a cohort of 13 patients with chronic pancreatitis-induced biliary strictures who had undergone uncovered biliary Wallstent placement. Endoscopic Wallstent was successfully placed in all patients between 1994 and 1999. Nine patients (69%) were successfully treated and four patients failed Wallstent therapy. Of the nine patients treated successfully, four (44%) patients required repeated endoscopic intervention (three with a second Wallstent and one requiring cleaning with a balloon). One patient eventually required surgical biliary diversion and three patients are continuing to need endoscopic plastic stents through the Wallstent to maintain biliary patency [136].

Biodegradable stents

A recent exciting development in stent technology, utilizing bioabsorbable poly-L-lactide (PLLA) polymer strands woven into the tubular mesh design similar to the metallic stent, was reported by Haber *et al.* [111]. The PLLA stent is unique in that it undergoes slow hydrolytic degradation and disintegration after 6–18 months. In the feasibility study in patients with malignant obstructive jaundice, the endoscopic technique for placement of the bioabsorbable biliary stent was similar to present expandable stents and was technically successful in 48 of 50 patients. The unique feature of this stent is that it may obviate the need for follow-up endoscopy to remove/replace the stent and may potentially be an effective long-term option in benign, chronic pancreatitis-induced biliary strictures.

Stenting for biliary strictures and chronic pancreatitis: conclusion

The aforementioned studies indicate that plastic biliary stents are a useful alternative to surgery for short-term treatment of chronic pancreatitis-induced common bile duct strictures complicated by cholestasis, jaundice, and cholangitis. This therapy also should be considered for high-risk surgical patients. Because the long-term efficacy of this treatment is much less satisfactory, however, operative intervention appears to be a better long-term solution for this problem in average-risk patients. More data on the long-term outcome, preferably in controlled trials, are necessary before expandable metal stents can be advocated for this indication. Trials of membrane-coated metal stents, bioabsorbable stents, and removable coil spring stents are awaited.

Sphincter of Oddi dysfunction in chronic pancreatitis

Although sphincter of Oddi dysfunction (SOD) is a known cause of acute recurrent pancreatitis, its role in the pathogenesis of chronic pancreatitis is much less certain [113].

Pathogenesis of SOD in chronic pancreatitis

A direct effect of alcohol on the sphincter of Oddi has been postulated [114]. In studies performed in humans with T-tubes, it was demonstrated that intragastric or intravenous [115] administration of alcohol increased the sphincter tone.

Moreover, Guelrud and colleagues [116] showed that local instillation of alcohol on the papilla of Vater produced a significant increase in the basal pancreatic sphincter pressure at sphincter of Oddi manometry in both cholecystectomy patients and patients with chronic pancreatitis. The authors postulated that the increased motor activity of the sphincter of Oddi may raise the intraductular pancreatic pressure and result in disruption of small pancreatic ductules, and back flow of pancreatic juice into the parenchyma, with subsequent injury.

Other investigators have refuted these findings by showing that intravenous or intragastric administration of alcohol in humans results in a decrease in sphincter of Oddi basal pressures at manometry [117].

In a preliminary study, Morita *et al.* showed that chronic alcohol administration in the Japanese monkey resulted in an increase in sphincter of Oddi mean basal pressure from 9 to 20 mmHg ($P < 0.01$), while the phasic amplitude decreased by 75% and the pancreatic ductal secretory rate nearly doubled [118].

Frequency of SOD in chronic pancreatitis

More recent studies using modern manometric techniques have shown a high frequency of basal sphincter pressure abnormalities, especially the pancreatic sphincter, in patients with established chronic pancreatitis [119]. Results of other studies using sphincter of Oddi manometry refute these findings and have shown no difference in the dynamics of the pancreatic sphincter in patients with chronic pancreatitis and controls [120]. Such data suggest that the sphincter, at times, becomes dysfunctional as part of the overall general scarring process or has a role in the pathogenesis of chronic pancreatitis.

Surgical sphincter ablation

The surgical literature, although limited, suggests that sphincter ablation therapy (both the biliary and pancreatic sphincters) alone for patients with chronic pancreatitis and manometrically documented or suspected SOD benefits 30–60% of patients [121,122]. Bagley and associates [123] reported a surgical series of 67 patients with mild to moderate chronic pancreatitis undergoing empirical biliary and pancreatic sphincterotomy ($n = 33$) or sphincteroplasty ($n = 34$). During a 5-year follow-up, 44% of patients had pain relief. The outcome for patients with idiopathic chronic pancreatitis was similar to that for patients with alcohol-induced chronic pancreatitis. However, 92% (11/12) of patients who stopped alcohol consumption were clinically improved, compared with 12.5% (2/16) of those who continued to drink.

Endoscopic pancreatic sphincterotomy

Because endoscopic pancreatic sphincterotomy has been performed infrequently in most institutions, its role in the management of pancreatic sphincter stenosis has not been defined. Kozarek *et al.* reported resolution of pain and clinical episodes of pancreatitis after pancreatic sphincterotomy in six of 10 patients (1-year follow-up) with chronic pancreatitis and suspected or manometrically documented pancreatic SOD [63]. Okolo *et al.* retrospectively evaluated 55 patients who had undergone endoscopic pancreatic sphincterotomy over a 4-year period. After a median follow-up of 16 months, 62% of patients reported improvement of pain scores. Patients with pancreatic sphincter dysfunction (*n* = 15) had significant improvement in pain (73%) compared to patients with pancreato-graphic evidence of chronic pancreatitis (58%) [137]. The utility of endoscopic sphincter ablation as the only therapy in patients with chronic pancreatitis awaits further study, preferably in controlled randomized trials.

Pancreas divisum

Pancreas divisum is the most common congenital variant of pancreatic ductal anatomy, occurring in 7% of autopsy series [124]. Most commonly, in the setting of chronic pancreatitis, minor papilla sphincterotomy is performed to provide access to the duct to effect stone retrieval or facilitate endoprosthesis placement [9].

Pancreas divisum: a cause of pancreatitis?

It has been postulated that, in a subpopulation of pancreas divisum patients, the minor papilla orifice appears to be critically small, such that excessively high intrapancreatic dorsal duct pressures occur during active secretion [124]. This may result in pancreatic pain or pancreatitis [125]. Although most authorities agree that pancreas divisum is a definite cause of acute recurrent pancreatitis, its role in the pathogenesis of chronic pancreatitis is much more controversial. Several lines of evidence favor the association of pancreas divisum and pancreatitis, including: (1) the presence of pancreatographic and histological changes of chronic pancreatitis isolated to the dorsal pancreas; (2) an increased incidence of pancreas divisum in patients with idiopathic pancreatitis; and (3) symptomatic benefit following dorsal duct drainage, endoscopically or surgically [124].

Table 10.9 Selected series reporting the results of minor papilla therapy for pancreas divisum.

Reference	Mean follow-up (months)	Acute recurrent pancreatitis		Pain alone		Chronic pancreatitis	
		No.	Improved (%)	No.	Improved (%)	No.	Improved (%)
Soehendra et al. 1986 [126]	3	2	100	0	—	4	75
Ligoury et al. 1986 [127]	24	8	63	0	—	0	—
McCarthy et al. 1988 [21]	21	19	89	0	—	0	—
Lans et al. 1992 [128]	30	10	90	0	—	0	—
Lehman et al. 1993 [56]	22	17	76	23	26	11	27
Coleman et al. 1994 [129]	23	9	78	5	0	20	60
Sherman et al. 1994 [130]	28	0	—	16	44	0	—
Kozarek et al. 1995 [131]	20	15	73	5	20	19	32
Total		80	80	49	29	54	44

Minor papilla ablation

Although minor papilla sphincter therapy by endoscopic or surgical techniques has been shown to be effective for patients with pancreas divisum and acute recurrent pancreatitis, the outcome for patients with chronic pancreatitis has usually been much less satisfactory [21,56,126–132] (Table 10.9). In summarizing 54 patients undergoing dorsal duct decompressive therapy by minor papilla sphincterotomy and/or dorsal duct stenting, only 44% improved during a mean follow-up of 22 months.

A recent 4-year follow-up summary from our institution showed a similar 62–70% symptom improvement rate for pancreas divisum patients with and without dorsal duct chronic pancreatitis changes. These data suggest that methods used to select patients with pancreas divisum and chronic pancreatitis who are likely to benefit from endoscopic therapy need further investigation. The role of botulinum toxin use in predicting pain relief warrants further study [133].

Until such methods are identified, minor papilla sphincterotomy (as the only therapy) for patients with chronic pancreatitis should preferably be performed in a research setting and restricted to patients who are disabled by pain.

Outstanding issues and future trends

Endoscopic therapy of chronic pancreatitis is an expanding area for the interventional endoscopist. The techniques employed are very similar to the endoscopic interventions utilized in the biliary tree but tend to be more tedious. The appropriate selection of candidates for the various pancreatic interventions appears to be important to obtain optimal results of therapy. The continued improvement in resolution of magnetic resonance cholangiopancreatography may allow for suitable patient selection for endoscopic therapy without the need to perform an initial diagnostic ERCP [134,135].

Over the past decade, multiple series totaling a few thousand patients have demonstrated the medium-term effectiveness of endoscopic interventions in chronic pancreatitis, rivaling the medium-term outcomes from surgery in this disease. ESWL has proven to be indispensable in the management of patients with pancreatic stones. However, well-designed, long-term controlled studies comparing endoscopy to surgery in the management of patients with chronic pancreatitis are lacking. Further outcome and cost efficacy studies are awaited. The inexperienced endoscopist should exercise caution in the application of newer pancreatic techniques as they are technically demanding and associated with a small but significant complication rate.

Acknowledgment

We greatly appreciate the assistance of Joyce Eggleston in the preparation of this chapter.

References

1 Sarles H, Bernard JP, Johnson C. Pathogenesis and epidemiology of chronic pancreatitis. *Annu Rev Med* 1989; 40: 453–68.
2 Banks PA. Management of pancreatic pain. *Pancreas* 1991; 6 (Suppl. 1): S52–S59.
3 Steer ML, Waxman I, Freedman S. Chronic pancreatitis. *N Engl J Med* 1995; 332: 1482–90.
4 Widdison AL, Alvarez C, Karanjia ND, Reber HA. Experimental evidence of beneficial effects of ductal decompression in chronic pancreatitis. *Endoscopy* 1991; 23: 151–4.
5 Karanjia ND, Reber HA. The cause and management of the pain of chronic pancreatitis. *Gastrointest Clin North Am* 1990; 19: 895–904.
6 Lo SK, Lewis MPN, Reber PU *et al.* In-vivo endoscopic trans-sphincteric measurement of pancreatic blood flow (PBF) in humans. *Gastrointest Endosc* 1996; 43: 409A.
7 Malfertheiner P, Buchler M. Indications for endoscopic or surgical therapy in chronic pancreatitis. *Endoscopy* 1991; 23: 185–90.
8 Bedford RA, Howerton DH, Geenen JE. The current role of ERCP in the treatment of benign pancreatic disease. *Endoscopy* 1994; 26: 113–19.
9 Kozarek RA, Traverso LW. Endotherapy of chronic pancreatitis. *Int J Pancreatol* 1996; 19: 93–102.
10 Kaikaus RM, Geenen JE. Current role of ERCP in the management of benign pancreatic disease. *Endoscopy* 1996; 28: 131–7.
11 Cavallini G, Tittobello A, Frulloni L *et al.* Gabexate for the prevention of pancreatic damage related to ERCP. *N Engl J Med* 1996; 335: 919–23.
12 Deviere J, Le Moine O, Van Laethem JL *et al.* Interleukin-10 reduces the incidence of pancreatitis after therapeutic endoscopic retrograde cholangiopancreatography. *Gastroenterology* 2001; 120 (2): 498–505.

13 Sherman S, Lehman GA. Endoscopic therapy of pancreatic disease. *Gastroenterologist* 1993; 1: 5–17.

14 Kozarek RA. Chronic pancreatitis in 1994: is there a role for endoscopic treatment? *Endoscopy* 1994; 26: 625–8.

15 Huibregtse K, Smits ME. Endoscopic management of diseases of the pancreas. *Am J Gastroenterol* 1994; 89 (Suppl.): S66–S77.

16 Jacob L, Geenen JE, Catalano MF, Geenen DJ. Prevention of pancreatitis in patients with idiopathic recurrent pancreatitis: a prospective nonblinded randomized study using endoscopic stents. *Endoscopy* 2001; 33: 559–62.

17 Cremer M, Deviere J, Delhaye M *et al.* Stenting in severe chronic pancreatitis: results of medium-term follow-up in 76 patients. *Endoscopy* 1991; 23: 171–6.

18 Grimm H, Meyer WH, Nam VC, Soehendra N. New modalities for treating chronic pancreatitis. *Endoscopy* 1989; 21: 70–4.

19 Cremer M, Deviere J, Delhaye M *et al.* Nonsurgical management of severe chronic pancreatitis. *Scand J Gastroenterol* 1990; 25 (Suppl. 175): 77–84.

20 Kozarek RA, Patterson DJ, Ball TJ, Traverso LW. Endoscopic placement of pancreatic stents and drains in the management of pancreatitis. *Ann Surg* 1989; 209: 261–6.

21 McCarthy J, Geenen JE, Hogan WJ. Preliminary experience with stent placement in benign pancreatic diseases. *Gastrointest Endosc* 1988; 34: 16–18.

22 Geenen JE, Rolny P. Endoscopic therapy of acute and chronic pancreatitis. *Gastrointest Endosc* 1991; 37: 377–82.

23 Binmoeller KF, Jue P, Seifert H *et al.* Endoscopic pancreatic stent drainage in chronic pancreatitis and a dominant stricture: longterm results. *Endoscopy* 1995; 27: 638–44.

24 Smits ME, Badiga SM, Rauws EAJ *et al.* Longterm results of pancreatic stents in chronic pancreatitis. *Gastrointest Endosc* 1995; 42: 461–7.

25 Ponchon T, Bory R, Hedelius F *et al.* Endoscopic stenting for pain relief in chronic pancreatitis: results of a standardized protocol. *Gastrointest Endosc* 1995; 42: 452–6.

26 Rosch T, Daniel S, Scholz M *et al.* Endoscopic treatment of chronic pancreatitis: a multicenter study of 1000 patients with long-term follow-up. *Endoscopy* 2002; 34 (10): 765–71.

27 Reber PU, Patel AG, Kusske AM *et al.* Stenting does not decompress the pancreatic duct as effectively as surgery in experimental chronic pancreatitis. *Gastroenterology* 1995; 128: 386A.

28 Nakaizumi A, Uehara H, Takensaka A *et al.* Diagnosis of pancreatic cancer by cytology and measurement of oncogene and tumor markers in pure pancreatic juice aspirated by endoscopy. *Hepatogastroenterology* 1999; 46: 31–7.

29 Brandwein SL, Farrell JJ, Centeno BA, Brugge WR. Detection and tumor staging of malignancy in cystic intraductal, and solid tumors of the pancreas by EUS. *Gastrointest Endosc* 2001; 53: 722–7.

30 Lohr M, Muller P, Mora J *et al.* p53 and K-ras mutations in pancreatic juice samples from patients with chronic pancreatitis. *Gastrointest Endosc* 2001; 53: 734–43.

31 Freeman M, Cass OW, Dailey J. Dilation of high-grade pancreatic and biliary ductal strictures with small-caliber angioplasty balloons. *Gastrointest Endosc* 2001; 54: 89–92.

32 Van Someren R, Benson M, Glynn M, Ashraf W, Swain P. A novel technique for dilating difficult malignant biliary strictures during therapeutic ERCP. *Gastrointest Endosc* 1996; 43: 495–8.

33 Baron T, Morgan D. Dilation of a difficult benign pancreatic duct stricture using the Soehendra stent extractor. *Gastrointest Endosc* 1997; 46: 178–80.

34 Pasricha PJ, Kalloo AN. Successful endoscopic management of complete obstruction of the main pancreatic duct (MPD) in patients with chronic pancreatitis. *Gastrointest Endosc* 1993; 39: 320A.

35 Ikenberry SO, Sherman S, Hawes RH *et al.* The occlusion rate of pancreatic stents. *Gastrointest Endosc* 1994; 40: 611–13.

36 Cremer M, Suge B, Delhaye M *et al.* Expandable pancreatic metal stents (Wallstent) for chronic pancreatitis: first world series. *Gastroenterology* 1990; 98: 215A.

37 Cremer M, Deviere J, Delhaye M *et al.* Endoscopic management of chronic pancreatitis. *Acta Gastroenterol Belg* 1993; 56: 192–200.

38 Choudari C, Nickl N, Fogel E *et al.* Hereditary pancreatitis: clinical presentation, ERCP findings and outcome of endoscopic therapy. *Gastrointest Endosc* 2002; 56: 66–71.

39 Gabbrielli A, Mutignani M, Pandolfi M *et al.* Endotherapy of early onset idiopathic chronic pancreatitis: results with long-term follow-up. *Gastrointest Endosc* 2002; 55: 488–93.

40 Ashby K, Lo SK. The role of pancreatic stenting in obstructive ductal disorders other than pancreas divisum. *Gastrointest Endosc* 1996; 42: 306–11.

41 Burdick JS, Geenen JE, Hogan W *et al.* Pancreatic stent therapy in chronic pancreatitis: which patients benefit? *Gastrointest Endosc* 1993; 39: 309A.

42 Borel I, Saurin J-C, Napoleon B *et al.* Treatment of chronic pancreatitis using definitive stenting of the main pancreatic duct. *Gastrointest Endosc* 2001; 53 (5): 139A.

43 McHenry L, Gore DC, DeMaria EJ, Zfass AM. Endoscopic treatment of dilated duct chronic pancreatitis with pancreatic stents: preliminary results of a sham controlled, blinded, crossover trial to predict surgical outcome. *Am J Gastroenterol* 1993; 88: 1536A.

44 DuVall GA, Scheider DM, Kortan P, Haber GB. Is the outcome of endoscopic therapy of chronic pancreatitis predictive of surgical success? *Gastrointest Endosc* 1996; 43: 405A.

45 Ammann RW, Akovbiantz A, Larglader F, Schueler G. Course and outcome of chronic pancreatitis: longitudinal study of a mixed medical-surgical series of 245 patients. *Gastroenterology* 1984; 86: 820–8.

46 Cotton PB, Lehman G, Vennes J *et al.* Endoscopic sphincterotomy complications and their management: an attempt at consensus. *Gastrointest Endosc* 1991; 37: 383–93.

47 Siegel J, Veerappan A. Endoscopic management of pancreatic disorders: potential risks of pancreatic prostheses. *Endoscopy* 1991; 23: 177–80.

48 Leung J, Liu Y, Herrera J *et al.* Bacteriological and scanning electron microscopy (SEM) analyses of pancreatic stents. *Gastrointest Endosc* 2001; 53 (5): 138A.

49 Sherman S, Alvarez C, Robert M *et al.* Polyethylene pancreatic stent-induced changes in the normal dog pancreas. *Gastrointest Endosc* 1993; 39: 658–64.

50 Johanson JF, Schmalz MJ, Geenen JE. Incidence and risk factors for biliary and pancreatic stent migration. *Gastrointest Endosc* 1992; 38: 341–6.

51 Dean RS, Geenen JE, Hogan WJ *et al.* Pancreatic stent modification to prevent stent migration in patients with benign pancreatic disease. *Gastrointest Endosc* 1994; 40: 19A.

52 Kozarek RA. Pancreatic stents can induce ductal changes consistent with chronic pancreatitis. *Gastrointest Endosc* 1990; 36: 93–5.

53 Derfus GA, Geenen JE, Hogan WJ. Effect of endoscopic pancreatic duct stent placement on pancreatic ductal morphology. *Gastrointest Endosc* 1990; 36: 206A.

54 Rossos PG, Kortan P, Haber GB. Complications associated with pancreatic duct stenting. *Gastrointest Endosc* 1992; 38: 252A.

55 Burdick JS, Geenen JE, Venu RP *et al.* Ductal morphological changes due to pancreatic stent therapy: a randomized controlled study. *Am J Gastroenterol* 1992; 87: 155A.

56 Lehman GA, Sherman S, Nisi R, Hawes RH. Pancreas divisum: results of minor papilla sphincterotomy. *Gastrointest Endosc* 1993; 39: 1–8.

57 Smith MT, Sherman S, Ikenberry SO *et al.* Alterations in pancreatic ductal morphology following polyethylene pancreatic duct stenting. *Gastrointest Endosc* 1996; 44: 268–75.

58 Eisen G, Coleman S, Troughton A, Cotton PB. Morphological changes in the pancreatic duct after stent placement for benign pancreatic disease. *Gastrointest Endosc* 1994; 40: 107A.

59 Sherman S, Hawes RH, Savides TJ *et al.* Stent-induced pancreatic ductal and parenchymal changes: correlation of endoscopic ultrasound with ERCP. *Gastrointest Endosc* 1996; 4: 276–82.

60 Deviere J, Delhaye M, Cremer M. Pancreatic duct stones management. *Gastrointest Endosc Clin N Am* 1998; 8: 163–79.

61 Sarles A, Bernard JP. Lithostathine and pancreatic lithogenesis. *Viewpoints Dig Dis* 1991; 23: 7–12.

62 Suda K, Mogaki M, Oyama T, Matsumoto Y. Histopathologic and immunohistochemical studies on alcoholic pancreatitis and chronic obstructive pancreatitis: special emphasis on ductal obstruction and genesis of pancreatitis. *Am J Gastroenterol* 1990; 85: 271–6.

63 Kozarek R, Ball TJ, Patterson DJ *et al.* Endoscopic pancreatic duct sphincterotomy: indications, technique, and analysis of results. *Gastrointest Endosc* 1994; 40: 592–8.

64 Esber E, Sherman S, Earle D *et al.* Complications of major papilla pancreatic sphincterotomy: a review of 106 patients. *Gastrointest Endosc* 1995; 41: 422A.
65 Kim MH, Myung SJ, Kim YS *et al.* Routine biliary sphincterotomy may not be indispensable for endoscopic pancreatic sphincterotomy. *Endoscopy* 1998; 30: 697–701.
66 Delhaye M, Vandermeeren A, Baize M, Cremer M. Extracorporeal shockwave lithotripsy of pancreatic calculi. *Gastroenterology* 1992; 102: 610–20.
67 Sherman S, Lehman GA, Hawes RH *et al.* Pancreatic ductal stones: frequency of successful endoscopic removal and improvement in symptoms. *Gastrointest Endosc* 1991; 37: 511–17.
68 Smits ME, Rauws EA, Tytgat GNJ, Huibregtse K. Endoscopic treatment of pancreatic stones in patients with chronic pancreatitis. *Gastrointest Endosc* 1996; 43: 556–60.
69 Schneider MU, Lux G. Floating pancreatic duct concrements in chronic pancreatitis. *Endoscopy* 1985; 17: 8–10.
70 Fuji T, Amano H, Ohmura R *et al.* Endoscopic pancreatic sphincterotomy: technique and evaluation. *Endoscopy* 1989; 21: 27–30.
71 Kozarek RA, Ball TJ, Patterson DJ. Endoscopic approach to pancreatic duct calculi and obstructive pancreatitis. *Am J Gastroenterol* 1992; 87: 600–3.
72 Sauerbruch T, Holl J, Sackman M *et al.* Disintegration of a pancreatic duct stone with extracorporeal shockwaves in a patient with chronic pancreatitis. *Endoscopy* 1987; 19: 207–8.
73 Soehendra N, Grimm H, Meyer HW *et al.* Extrakorporale stobwellen lithotripsie bei chronischer pankreatitis. *Dtsch Med Wochenschr* 1989; 114: 1402–6.
74 Neuhaus H. Fragmentation of pancreatic stones by extracorporeal shock wave lithotripsy. *Endoscopy* 1989; 23: 161–5.
75 den Toom R, Nijs HG, van Blankenstein M *et al.* Extracorporeal shock wave lithotripsy of pancreatic duct stones. *Am J Gastroenterol* 1991; 86: 1033–6.
76 Sauerbruch T, Holl J, Sackmann M, Paumgartner G. Extracorporeal lithotripsy of pancreatic stones in patients with chronic pancreatitis and pain: a prospective followup study. *Gut* 1992; 33: 969–72.
77 Schneider HT, May A, Benninger J *et al.* Piezoelectric shock wave lithotripsy of pancreatic duct stones. *Am J Gastroenterol* 1994; 89: 2042–8.
78 van der Hul R, Plaiser P, Jeekel J *et al.* Extracorporeal shockwave lithotripsy of pancreatic duct stones: immediate and longterm results. *Endoscopy* 1994; 26: 573–8.
79 Dumonceau JE, Deviere J, LeMoine O *et al.* Endoscopic pancreatic drainage in chronic pancreatitis associated with ductal stones: longterm results. *Gastrointest Endosc* 1996; 43: 547–55.
80 Kozarek R, Brandabur J, Ball T *et al.* Clinical outcomes in patients who undergo extracorporeal shock wave lithotripsy for chronic pancreatitis. *Gastrointest Endosc* 2002; 56: 496–500.
81 Farnbacher M, Schoen C, Rabenstein T *et al.* Pancreatic ductal stones in chronic pancreatitis: criteria for treatment intensity success. *Gastrointest Endosc* 2002; 56: 501–6.
82 Alvarez C, Widdison AL, Reber HA. New perspectives in the surgical management of chronic pancreatitis. *Pancreas* 1991; 6 (Suppl. 1): 576–81.
83 Fogel EL, Eversman D, Jamidar P, Sherman S, Lehman GA. Sphincter of Oddi dysfunction: pancreaticobiliary sphincterotomy with pancreatic stent placement has a lower rate of pancreatitis than biliary sphincterotomy alone. *Endoscopy* 2002; 34: 325–9.
84 Neuhaus H, Hoffman W, Classen M. Laser lithotripsy of pancreatic and biliary stones via 3.4 mm and 3.7 mm miniscopes: first clinical results. *Endoscopy* 1992; 24: 208–14.
85 Sahel J, Sarles H. (1981) Citrate therapy in chronic calcifying pancreatitis: preliminary results. In: Mitchell, CJ, Keelleheer, J, eds. *Pancreatic Disease in Clinical Practice.* London: Pitman, 346–53.
86 Berger Z, Topa L, Takacs T, Pap A. Nasopancreatic drainage for chronic calcifying pancreatitis (CCP). *Digestion* 1992; 52: 70A.
87 Noda A, Shibata T, Ogawa Y *et al.* Dissolution of pancreatic stones by oral trimethadione in a dog experimental model. *Gastroenterology* 1987; 93: 1002–8.
88 Lehman GA, Sherman S. Pancreatic stones: to treat or not to treat? *Gastrointest Endosc* 1996; 43: 625–6.
89 Grace PA, Williamson RCN. Modern management of pancreatic pseudocysts. *Br J Surg* 1993; 80: 573–81.

90 Gumaste VV, Pitchumoni CS. Pancreatic pseudocysts. *Gastroenterologist* 1996; 4: 33–43.

91 Smits ME, Rauws EAJ, Tytgat GNJ, Huibregtse K. The efficacy of endoscopic treatment of pancreatic pseudocysts. *Gastrointest Endosc* 1995; 42: 202–7.

92 Barthet M, Sahel J, BodiouBertel C, Bernard JP. Endoscopic transpapillary drainage of pancreatic pseudocysts. *Gastrointest Endosc* 1995; 42: 208–13.

93 Catalano MF, Geenen JE, Schmalz MJ *et al.* Treatment of pancreatic pseudocysts with ductal communication by transpapillary pancreatic duct endoprosthesis. *Gastrointest Endosc* 1995; 42: 214–18.

94 Binmoeller KF, Seifert H, Walter A, Soehendra N. Transpapillary and transmural drainage of pancreatic pseudocysts. *Gastrointest Endosc* 1995; 42: 219–24.

95 Lehman GA. Endoscopic management of pancreatic pseudocysts continues to evolve. *Gastrointest Endosc* 1995; 42: 273–5.

96 Howell DA, Lehman GA, Baron TH *et al.* Endoscopic treatment of pancreatic pseudocysts: a retrospective multicenter analysis. *Gastrointest Endosc* 1995; 41: 424A.

97 Howell DA, Lehman GA, Baron TH *et al.* Recurrent pseudocyst formation in patients managed with endoscopic drainage: predrainage features and management. *Gastrointest Endosc* 1996; 43: 407A.

98 Sahel J. Endoscopic drainage of pancreatic cysts. *Endoscopy* 1991; 23: 181–4.

99 Cremer M, Deviere J, Engelholm L. Endoscopic management of cysts and pseudocysts in chronic pancreatitis: long term followup after 7 years' experience. *Gastrointest Endosc* 1989; 35: 1–9.

100 Kozarek RA, Ball TJ, Patterson DJ *et al.* Endoscopic transpapillary therapy for disrupted pancreatic duct and parapancreatic fluid collection. *Gastroenterology* 1991; 100: 1362–70.

101 Deviere J, Buseo H, Baize M *et al.* Complete disruption of the main pancreatic duct: endoscopic management. *Gastrointest Endosc* 1995; 42: 445–51.

102 Espinel J, Jorquera F, Fernandez-Gundin MJ, Munoz F, Herrera A, Olcoz JL. Endoscopic transpapillary drainage of an infected pancreatic fluid collection in pancreas divisum. *Dig Dis Sci* 2000; 45: 237–41.

103 Kozarek RA, Jiranek G, Traverso LW. Endoscopic treatment of pancreatic ascites. *Am J Surg* 1994; 168: 223–8.

104 Kim HS, Lee DK, Kim IW *et al.* The role of endoscopic retrograde pancreatography in the treatment of traumatic pancreatic duct injury. *Gastrointest Endosc* 2001; 54: 49–55.

105 Costamagna G, Mutignani M, Igrosso M *et al.* Endoscopic treatment of postsurgical external pancreatic fistulas. *Endoscopy* 2001; 33: 317–22.

106 Lau ST, Simchuk EJ, Kozarek RA, Traverso LW. A pancreatic ductal leak should be sought to direct treatment in patients with acute pancreatitis. *Am J Surg* 2001; 181: 411–15.

107 Frey CF, Suzuki M, Isaji S. Treatment of chronic pancreatitis complicated by obstruction of the common bile duct or duodenum. *World J Surg* 1990; 14: 59–69.

108 Deviere J, Devaere S, Baize M, Cremer M. Endoscopic biliary drainage in chronic pancreatitis. *Gastrointest Endosc* 1990; 36: 96–100.

109 Davids PHP, Rauws EAJ, Coene PPLO *et al.* Endoscopic stenting for postoperative biliary strictures. *Gastrointest Endosc* 1992; 38: 12–18.

110 Barthet M, Bernard JP, Duval JL *et al.* Biliary stenting in benign biliary stenosis complicating chronic calcifying pancreatitis. *Endoscopy* 1994; 26: 569–72.

111 Haber G, Freeman M, Bedford R *et al.* A prospective multi-center study of a bioabsorbable biliary Wallstent in 50 patients with malignant obstructive jaundice. *Am J Gastroenterol* 1997; 9: A200.

112 Deviere J, Cremer M, Love J *et al.* Management of common bile duct strictures caused by chronic pancreatitis with metal mesh self-expandable stents. *Gut* 1994; 35: 122–6.

113 Kuo W-H, Pasricha P, Kalloo AN. The role of sphincter of Oddi manometry in the diagnosis and therapy of pancreatic disease. *Gastrointest Endosc Clin N Am* 1998; 8: 79–85.

114 Guelrud M. How good is sphincter of Oddi manometry for chronic pancreatitis? *Endoscopy* 1994; 26: 265–7.

115 Pirola RC, Davis E. Effects of ethyl alcohol on sphincter resistance at the choledochoduodenal junction in man. *Gut* 1968; 9: 447–560.

116 Guelrud M, Mendoza S, Rossiter G *et al*. Effect of local instillation of alcohol on sphincter of Oddi motor activity: combined ERCP and manometry study. *Gastrointest Endosc* 1991; 37: 428–32.

117 Viceconte G. Effects of ethanol on the sphincter of Oddi: an endoscopic manometry study. *Gut* 1983; 24: 20–7.

118 Morita M, Okazaki K, Yamasaki K *et al*. Effects of long term administration of ethanol on the papillary sphincter and exocrine pancreas in the monkey. *Gastroenterology* 1994; 106: 309A.

119 Vestergaard H, Krause A, Rokkjaer M *et al*. Endoscopic manometry of the sphincter of Oddi and the pancreatic and biliary ducts in patients with chronic pancreatitis. *Scand J Gastroenterol* 1994; 29: 188–92.

120 Ugljesic M, Bulajic M, Milosavljevic T, Stimec B. Endoscopic manometry of the sphincter of Oddi and pancreatic duct in patients with chronic pancreatitis. *Int J Pancreatol* 1996; 19: 191–5.

121 Sherman S, Hawes RH, Madura JA, Lehman GA. Comparison of intraoperative and endoscopic manometry of the sphincter of Oddi. *Surg Gynecol Obstet* 1992; 175: 410–18.

122 Williamson RCN. Pancreatic sphincteroplasty: indications and outcome. *Ann R Coll Surg* 1988; 70: 205–11.

123 Bagley FH, Braasch JW, Taylor RH, Warren KW. Sphincterotomy or sphincteroplasty in the treatment of pathologically mild chronic pancreatitis. *Am J Surg* 1981; 141: 418–22.

124 Lehman GA, Sherman S. Pancreas divisum: diagnosis, clinical significance, and management alternatives. *Gastrointest Endosc Clin North Am* 1995; 5: 145–70.

125 Cotton PB. Congenital anomaly of pancreas divisum as cause of obstructive pain and pancreatitis. *Gut* 1980; 21: 105–14.

126 Soehendra N, Kempeneers I, Nam VC, Grimm H. Endoscopic dilation and papillotomy of the accessory papilla and internal drainage in pancreas divisum. *Endoscopy* 1986; 18: 129–32.

127 Ligoury C, Lefebvre JF, Canard JM *et al*. Le pancreas divisum: etude clinique et therapeutique chez l'homme: a propos de 87 cas. *Gastroenterol Clin Biol* 1986; 10: 820–5.

128 Lans JI, Geenen JE, Johanson JF, Hogan WJ. Endoscopic therapy in patients with pancreas divisum and acute pancreatitis: a prospective, randomized, controlled clinical trial. *Gastrointest Endosc* 1992; 38: 430–4.

129 Coleman SD, Eisen GM, Troughton AB, Cotton PB. Endoscopic treatment in pancreas divisum. *Am J Gastroenterol* 1994; 89: 1152–5.

130 Sherman S, Hawes R, Nisi R *et al*. Randomized controlled trial of minor papilla sphincterotomy (MiES) in pancreas divisum (PDiv) patients with pain only. *Gastrointest Endosc* 1994; 40: 125A.

131 Kozarek RA, Ball TJ, Patterson DJ *et al*. Endoscopic approach to pancreas divisum. *Dig Dis Sci* 1995; 40: 1974–81.

132 Ertan A. Long term results after endoscopic pancreatic stent placement without pancreatic papillotomy in acute recurrent pancreatitis due to pancreas divisum. *Gastrointest Endosc* 2000; 52: 9–14.

133 Wehrmann T, Schmitt T, Seifert H. Endoscopic botulinum toxin injection into the minor papilla for treatment of idiopathic recurrent pancreatitis in patients with pancreas divisum. *Gastrointest Endosc* 1999; 50: 545–8.

134 Farrell RJ, Noonan N, Mahmud N, Morrin MM, Kelleher D, Keeling PWN. Potential impact of magnetic resonance cholangiopancreatography on endoscopic retrograde cholangiopancreatography workload and complication rate in patients referred because of abdominal pain. *Endoscopy* 2001; 33: 668–75.

135 Sahel J, Devonshire D, Yeoh KG *et al*. The decision making value of magnetic resonance cholangiopancreatography in patients seen in a referral center for suspected biliary and pancreatic disease. *Am J Gastroenterol* 2001; 96: 2074–80.

136 Van Berkel AM, Van Westerloo D, Cahen D *et al*. Efficacy of wallstents in benign biliary strictures due to chronic pancreatitis. *Gastrointest Endosc* 2003; 57: AB198.

137 Okolo PI, Pasricha PJ, Kalloo AN. What are the long-term results of endoscopic pancreatic sphincterotomy? *Gastrointest Endosc* 2000; 52: 15–19.

CHAPTER 11

Complications of Pancreatitis

DOUGLAS A. HOWELL

Synopsis

Complications of acute and chronic pancreatitis are varied, often complex, and potentially fatal. This chapter attempts to summarize all of these feared developments, address their causation, and review current and potential future approaches.

The first section deals with the toxic and metabolic complications. Early death from pancreatitis most frequently follows shock, a poorly understood but dramatic occurrence seen, fortunately, in a small minority. All organ systems may be affected, in a fashion that can range from mild to very severe, resulting in renal failure, respiratory failure, disseminated intravascular coagulation, and severe gastrointestinal bleeding. Prolonged septic-like systemic inflammatory response syndrome may result in coma and a profound catabolic state untreatable by total parenteral nutrition.

Recent clinical experience has recognized the major difference in clinical course and treatment when pancreatic necrosis complicates the early phase of acute pancreatitis. Diagnosis, treatment, and predictors of outcome are addressed.

The chapter closes with a comprehensive review of the main miscellaneous complications which are often recognized during the later phase of pancreatitis. Patients who appear to be recovering may experience fistula formation, producing acute pancreatic hydrothorax or enteric fistulas. Percutaneous or surgical drainage is a frequent cause of cutaneous fistulas, a particularly difficult and debilitating complication. Finally, dramatic and potentially fatal vascular complication can occur very abruptly, taxing the diagnostic and interventional skills of the treating team.

Throughout this review, up-to-date reports of successful approaches to all of these events are addressed. It is emphasized that since controlled trials of newer treatment modalities have, in general, not been directly compared to traditional surgical therapy, a multidisciplinary approach with gastroenterology, interventional radiology, and surgery is vital.

281

Toxic and metabolic complications

Few diseases can produce more varied and severe diffuse metabolic complications than acute pancreatitis. Although the organ weighs only 90 g in the adult, when inflamed, the pancreas can produce such profound systemic effects that respiratory, renal, and circulatory failure can rapidly ensue, producing multiorgan system death within a few days. In patients with severe acute pancreatitis, the likely sequence is peripancreatic leakage of proteolytic juice, activation of proinflammatory cytokines, third space loss secondary to retroperitoneal injury, hypoperfusion, and finally, rapid progression to frank pancreatic necrosis.

This sequence is variable and may appear as partial individual organ compromise or full-blown multiorgan failure. The recognition of these end organ complications served as the basis for the famous 'Ranson's criteria', which have for nearly 30 years remained the most popular clinical measure of the severity of acute pancreatitis (Table 11.1) [1].

A principal drawback to Ranson's scoring system has been the need to reassess the patient at 48 h before a final score can be calculated. In an effort to predict severity as early as possible to help triage patients to the most appropriate level of care, several other clinical scoring systems have been advocated [2–4]. The Acute Physiologic and Chronic Health Evaluation scoring system (APACHE II and III) permits a more comprehensive initial assessment of severity. Khan *et al.* pointed out recently that since the natural history of pancreatitis varies considerably depending upon underlying etiology, patient responses, and presence of comorbidity, APACHE scoring, when repeated at 48 h, as in Ranson's criteria, more accurately predicts outcome [4].

Table 11.1 Ranson's criteria. Clinical features significantly related to the severity of an episode of pancreatitis.

On admission	Within first 48 h
1 Age > 55 years	1 Ca < 8 mg %
2 Glucose > 200 mg %	2 P_aO_2 < 65 mmHg
3 WBC > 16 000 mm^3	3 Base deficit > 4 mEq/liter
4 LDL > 700 IU	4 BUN increase > 5 mg %
5 SGOT > 250 SFU	5 Hct fall > 10 points
	6 Fluid sequestration > 6 liter
Mortality and morbidity	
Less than three clinical features	*Three or more clinical features*
Mortality 3%	Mortality 62%
Serious illness 11%	Serious illness 33%

After Ranson JH, Rifkind KM, Turner JW. *Surg Gynecol Obstet* 1976; **143**: 209–19.

The modified Glasgow Coma/Imrie score has also been used to predict severity and thus the development of complications. One direct comparison of these three scoring systems recently reported that APACHE III and modified Glasgow/Imrie had a greater magnitude of correlation with length of hospital stay as a measure of severity than did Ranson's traditional criteria [2]. However, death was equally predicted, with fatal cases uniformly having > 5 Ranson's criteria, APACHE III scores > 30 at 96 h, and modified Glasgow/Imrie scores > 4.

Alternatively, in a slightly smaller but contemporary study, Ranson's criteria, particularly at 48 h, remained a valid scoring system for severity of pancreatitis when compared to the newest APACHE III scoring [5]. Because of its inherit simplicity, the authors advocated the continued use of the venerable Ranson's criteria and emphasized that elevated BUN, low calcium, base deficit, and third space loss predicted mortality.

In clinical practice currently, a CT-based measure of severity has proved valuable when added to clinical scoring [6]. Robert *et al.* recently analyzed all available clinical scoring systems plus a CT scan score of severity in 130 patients [7]. Multivariate analysis revealed that low serum albumin plus extrapancreatic fluid collections on initial CT scanning within the first 24 h was the best predictor of severe pancreatitis overall.

Although some concern has been raised as to the potential for renal toxicity of contrast-enhanced early CT scanning in acute pancreatitis, the general consensus suggests that the value of the information gained remains worthwhile [8].

Shock and renal failure have traditionally been the most frequent and perhaps the most feared of the potential toxic and metabolic complications of acute pancreatitis. In the mid-1990s, Frey and Brody reported a 22% rate of shock and renal failure in their series of 490 patients [9]. At that time mortality followed in nearly 80% of these complications.

Although shock and renal failure are associated in most patients, oliguria and even anuria requiring prolonged dialysis can be seen in euvolemic patients with normal blood pressures throughout their early illness. This dramatic systemic complication is attributed to profound renal cortical vasoconstriction due to poorly understood nephrotoxic vasoactive circulating factors produced by the acute inflammatory response. Permanent renal failure eventuating in renal transplantation rarely occurs.

Respiratory complications occur in a variable percentage and often in a stepwise fashion, with hypoxemia with a normal chest X-ray being the most frequently recognized. Pulmonary infiltrates, atelectasis with elevated diaphragms, and pleural effusions may then ensue and progress to full-blown acute respiratory distress syndrome (ARDS), often requiring ventilatory support. This sequence is again poorly understood but appears to be precipitated by circulating proinflammatory cytokines due to the retroperitoneal proteolytic injury, producing an alveolar capillary leak. The flood of protein-rich fluid can, at times, produce such complete consolidation that mechanical ventilation cannot compensate, resulting in a respiratory death [10].

Disseminated intravascular coagulation (DIC) is a less frequent complication of acute pancreatitis [1]. DIC may produce severe bleeding since extensive retroperitoneal injury is present. The consequence of such hemorrhage can greatly worsen the above outlined systemic complications.

A more recently described toxic reaction to pancreatitis has been termed systemic inflammatory response syndrome (SIRS) [11]. High fever, tachycardia, and delirium may persist for days or even weeks and may be difficult to distinguish from bacterial sepsis. This syndrome can produce a profoundly catabolic state that cannot be adequately reversed with total parenteral nutrition (TPN) [12–14].

In patients with severe SIRS, fine-needle radiologically guided aspiration of retroperitoneal fluid collections has proved to be valuable for distinguishing this syndrome from complicating retroperitoneal infection. To avoid potential contamination of otherwise sterile fluid, a fastidious technique to avoid traversing bowel, particularly colon, and with adequate skin preparation, is mandatory [15,16].

In patients with a less severe form of SIRS, TPN can be switched to enteral feeding to further minimize pancreatic stimulation; Takacs et al. demonstrated that adding octreotide to enteric feedings reduces gastrointestinal hormone release (CCK, glucagon, gastrin, and glucose) to baseline [17]. Windsor et al. have provided evidence that this change to the enteral route for nutrition can actually diminish the inflammatory response and lead to more rapid improvement compared to continuing TPN [18]. Tube placement, duodenal edema, and prolonged ileus may all hamper the initiation of enteral feeding in sicker patients, however.

Platelet activating factor (PAF) has been implicated in the pathogenesis of SIRS, possibly by amplifying mediators of inflammation. Unfortunately, an attempt to block this effect by the infusion of lexiphant, a potent inhibitor of PAF, was demonstrated to have no clinical benefit in a placebo-controlled trial [19].

Death due to acute pancreatitis follows two patterns: early (within 1, or in some series, 2 weeks) and late. Early death is secondary to these incompletely understood severe metabolic inflammatory responses leading to multiorgan system failure. Death later than 2 weeks is generally secondary to sepsis and represents about one-half of fatal cases [20]. Death rates in various recent series with variable etiologies range from 2 to 9%, which represents a marked improvement compared to the pre-TPN era [21].

Factors which may be important in the sequence of rapid onset multiorgan system failure are under active research. Ethridge *et al.* recently studied the impact of cyclo-oxygenase (COX) on pancreatitis severity, especially with regard to lung injury [22]. In their mouse model, inhibition of COX-2 or deletion of the COX gene profoundly decreased the severity of pancreatitis and protected against ARDS.

Host response may prove to be a critical determinate of the severity of pancreatitis and the resulting complications [23,24]. A defect in interleukin-10 function has been identified in some patients with severe acute pancreatitis [25]. This defect might result in a failure to down-regulate the initial acute inflammatory reaction once the patients have been maximally stimulated. If confirmed, this finding would help us to understand why these seemingly unpredictable complications may be seen even after rather trivial injury, such as after simple cannulation or unremarkable sphincterotomy at ERCP.

In an attempt to prevent post-ERCP pancreatitis, an initial randomized trial of a single bolus of interleukin-10 (8 µg/kg) was given to patients 15 min prior to ERCP and compared to a placebo group [26]. Unfortunately, both groups experienced an identical rate of pancreatitis and, furthermore, the severity as measured by length of stay was the same. Nevertheless, a full understanding of the role of pro- and anti-inflammatory cytokines may be the best hope of preventing or at least attenuating the severity of acute pancreatitis.

Pancreatic fluid collections

In the setting of pancreatitis, fluid collections are frequent and have been used as a measure of severity to create a CT-based score as previously discussed [6]. When combined with extent of non-perfusion (equivalent to necrosis) and detection of retroperitoneal complications, CT becomes a vital tool in predicting severity [27].

Fluid collections are at first sterile, amylase rich, and unorganized. They are seen early, often within 24 h, and may persist. Unencapsulated and younger than 4 weeks from the onset of pancreatitis, they are properly watched expectantly (Fig. 11.1a). If necrosis is not present, infection is rare. Whether they will persist, organize, and encapsulate beyond 4 weeks into a true pseudocyst largely depends on pancreatic ductal anatomy and the presence of necrosis. Normal ductal and sphincter anatomy predicts spontaneous resolution, whereas fistula, ductal obstruction, or disruption predict persistence and pseudocyst formation [28]. Finally, necrosis will organize slowly and an associated fluid collection will usually become a complex pseudocyst; this might be better termed an area of 'organizing necrosis' to distinguish them [29].

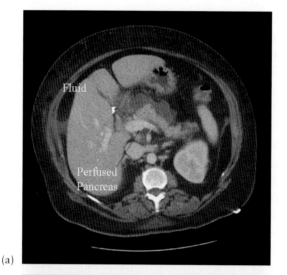

(a)

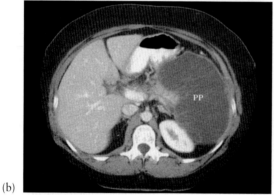

(b)

Fig. 11.1 (a) Peripancreatic fluid with a well-perfused duct predicts probable resolution. A good case to 'wait and see'. (b) Pancreatic pseudocyst. Typical well-matured pseudocysts in the lesser sac elevating and displacing the stomach which contains oral contrast. The viable well-perfused pancreatic tail is seen in the medial aspect of the pseudocysts.

Pseudocysts and abscesses

A pseudocyst of the pancreas is a maturing fluid collection surrounded by granulation tissue which occurs as a consequence of acute or chronic leakage of pancreatic juice (Fig. 11.1b). In distinction, acute fluid collections may be wholly inflammatory and will frequently resolve. Alternatively, severe ductal disruption with a consequent large fistula will virtually always result in pseudocyst formation [30,31].

Prior to any decision regarding management, a pancreatic pseudocyst must be carefully distinguished from other cystic or fluid-filled collections in the retroperitoneum [32–35]. In the absence of a definite attack of pancreatitis, some pseudocysts may be exceedingly difficult to differentiate from true cystic neoplasms [36,37]. Inadvertent endoscopic or surgical drainage of true neoplasms is ineffective and occasionally disastrous. Be aware that obstructing neoplasms, usually malignant, can produce acute or chronic pancreatitis and result in a pseudocyst. These combination cases can be extremely challenging to diagnose and treat [38]. In most cases, careful clinical history, dynamic CT, and pancreatography are necessary prior to establishing a complete diagnosis. In atypical cases, endoscopic ultrasound (EUS) adds important diagnostic information, especially if a small obstructing tumor or a cystic neoplasm is present [39–42].

The evolving pseudocyst requires time to develop a complete encircling wall which, of course, lacks an epithelial lining (Fig. 11.1b). By recent consensus, 4 weeks has been chosen as a minimal time from the onset of acute pancreatitis until this process is reasonably complete and the collection can be termed a pseudocyst [43]. The development of a pseudocyst in chronic pancreatitis is often more difficult to precisely age. These collections often occur more gradually as a consequence of ductal obstruction by stones or fibrotic strictures and are frequently mature upon discovery. Once a secure diagnosis of a mature or maturing pseudocyst is established, the clinician must remember that many pseudocysts will still resolve. Early authors emphasized that pseudocysts larger than 6 cm rarely resolve, but size alone does not always warrant intervention [30]. Etiology remains important since pseudocysts complicating acute pancreatitis are much more likely to resolve than those due to chronic pancreatitis [44]. Clinicians were formerly hesitant to follow pseudocysts for fear of the spontaneous development of complications, especially infection and hemorrhage. However, several authors have reported a surprisingly low incidence of adverse events during follow-ups in asymptomatic patients with stable or slowly resolving pseudocysts [45,46].

In general, patients with continued ductal leakage communicating with the pseudocyst will not stabilize and permit resumption of a diet (Fig. 11.2). Clinicians should be suspicious if, after initial improvement with symptom resolution on IV therapy (with or without TPN and octreotide), pain returns upon oral feeding. A serious ductal injury or leak is often present in this setting [47].

Unchecked, continued leakage with resulting expansion can produce a series of additional complications. Progressive enlargement in the usual retrogastric position will produce gastric compression resulting in early satiety, nausea, vomiting, pain, and weight loss. Frank outlet obstruction usually occurs at the pylorus or in the duodenal sweep (Fig. 11.3). When the ampullary area and pancreatic head are involved, obstructive jaundice often occurs.

The accumulating fresh enzyme-rich pancreatic juice from a ductal leak can lead to damage and digestion of additional retroperitoneal structures such as blood vessels, or adjacent hollow organs such as the duodenum or colon, or lead to spontaneous perforation into the peritoneal cavity resulting in pancreatic ascites.

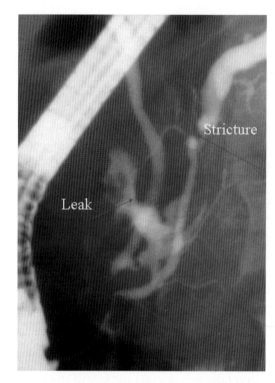

Fig. 11.2 ERCP pancreatography with obvious leakage of contrast into a communicating pseudocyst from a side branch above a stricture.

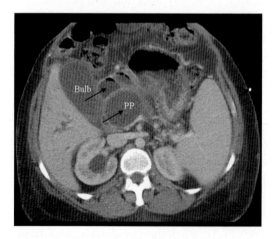

Fig. 11.3 Pseudocyst compressing the duodenum, producing gastric outlet obstruction.

Spontaneous infection of a pseudocyst is a feared late complication. Formerly termed infected pseudocyst, the preferred term now is pancreatic abscess [43]. The source of the infecting organism is often unknown, presumably from transmigration of nearby colonic bacteria or from transient bacteremia, but may follow line sepsis or fine-needle aspiration. Gas-producing organisms produce

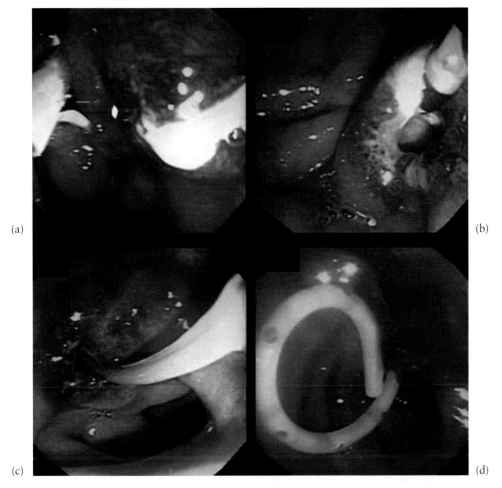

(a)

(b)

(c)

(d)

Fig. 11.4 Endoscopic view of spontaneous fistulization of a pseudocyst of the pancreatic head into the duodenum with resulting infection. This resolved with endoscopic lavage and stent placement. (a) Spontaneous fistula with pus anterior to bile duct stent. (b) View into abscess cavity. (c) Guidewire placement into deepest aspect of abscess. (d) 10 Fr silicone pigtail stent in place.

multiple small air bubbles in the pseudocyst, but the presence of gross air within the cavity is often due to fistulization to the duodenum or colon (Fig. 11.4) [48].

Gaining an understanding of the pancreatic ductal anatomy earlier in the course of pseudocyst patients holds the promise of allowing earlier necessary intervention in pancreatitis patients [28,49]. Traditionally, diagnostic ERCP has been the major test for defining pancreatic ductal anatomy, but most clinicians would not perform early ERCP due to the fear of introducing potentially catastrophic infection. Magnetic resonance pancreatography (MRP) is proving

Table 11.2 Indications for
pseudocyst intervention.

Continuing symptoms on medical Rx
Progressive expansion on serial imaging
Obstructive jaundice
Duodenal obstruction
Pseudoaneurysm formation
Rupture with pancreatic ascites
Abscess formation
Gross ductal disruption (usually)

useful in detecting major disruption and predicting the need for intervention without this risk. In our experience, MRP does not permit reliable ductal anatomy in lesser leaks since communicating fistulas may contain very little of the static fluid upon which MRP depends for imaging.

Once the need for intervention has become apparent, the choice of drainage has gradually yielded to endoscopic transmural and transpapillary techniques [50,51]. Clear indications for intervention in well-defined pseudocysts are summarized in Table 11.2. Radiological drainage remains popular in some centers but risks include prolonged drainage, introducing infection, and establishing a fistula when ductal obstruction or disruption is present [30,52].

The detailed techniques of endoscopic drainage have been outlined completely in several recent comprehensive reviews [53,54]. To summarize, transmural endoscopic puncture begins with the identification of the appropriate site, and then proceeds to needle localization with injection of contrast, puncture (Fig. 11.5), 10 mm balloon dilation of the tract, and, finally, multiple stent placement (Fig. 11.6).

Transpapillary therapy involves pancreatic stent placement with or without pancreatic sphincterotomy [55–57]. We have employed pancreatic sphincterotomy alone when the anatomy suggests that complete decompression of the duct by transecting the sphincter muscle should be adequate, thus avoiding the risks of pancreatic stent placement.

A recent long-term follow-up of such endoscopically treated pseudocysts reported excellent results with 15% (6 of 38) recurrence, all in alcohol-induced and therefore chronic pancreatitis [58]. Complications of endoscopic drainage include perforation when the true lumen of the pseudocyst is missed or the pseudocyst is not adherent or sufficiently organized. Severe bleeding, especially from the gastric wall, was a former frequent complication when simple diathermic puncture was followed by extension of the entry point using a sphincterotome [59]. A recently described technique of drainage to avoid any cautery advocated placing a guidewire through a special needle used for the initial localizing puncture. Once the guidewire is within the cavity, balloon dilation alone is used to create the endoscopic cystenterostomy drainage site [60].

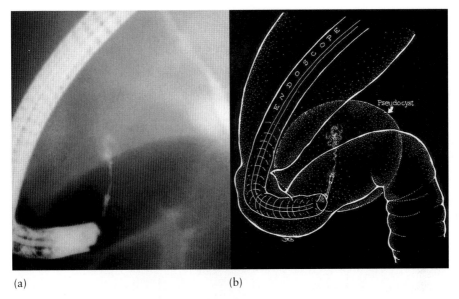

(a)   (b)

Fig. 11.5 22-gauge needle puncture before transmural pseudocyst drainage to select an optimal site for entry. (a) Endoscopic needle localization (ENL) aids by aligning the entry, confirming a shallow depth, checking for integrity by injecting contrast, and aspirating to be sure there is no blood. This is the fluoroscopic view during ENL. (b) Artist's drawing of ENL.

Overall, the success rates for endoscopic pseudocyst drainage are summarized in Table 11.3 and approach 80%. The complication risk and recurrence rates stated in these studies are included in Table 11.4 and were 12% and 16%, respectively. Finally, recurrences could be retreated endosurgically about 50% of the time, relegating surgery to only eight patients out of the 141 cases selected and reported.

The role of EUS pseudocyst management remains in evolution (Fig. 11.7). Some authors report rarely needing or using EUS but others consider EUS valuable in selecting appropriate drainage sites, excluding intervening blood vessels, and determining depth of puncture [53,61]. However, when collected in the diagnostic setting, this information may be difficult to transfer to actual therapy, which is generally performed with larger channel therapeutic endoscopes whose angle of view and therefore alignment for puncture is different from EUS [62,63]. Direct EUS therapeutic drainage by placing 7 Fr stents has been reported, but results are unlikely to equal 10 Fr drainage [63]. Finally, the development of a therapeutic 4.2 channel EUS endoscope has permitted complete therapy, including 10 Fr stent placement, in pseudocyst patients [64]. As EUS becomes a more available therapeutic technique, this approach may compete well with our current endoscopic transmural drainage procedure.

Finally, laparoscopically directed pseudocyst drainage has been reported but

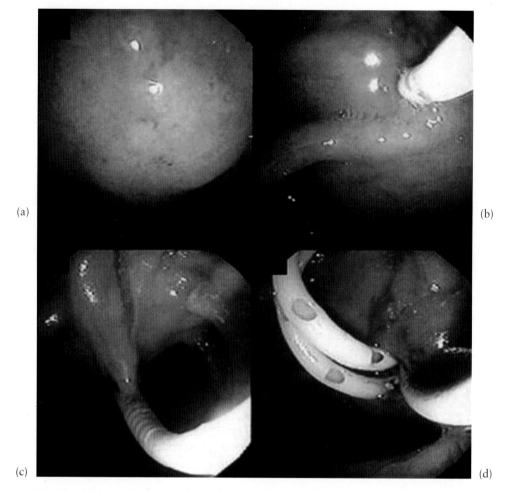

(a)

(b)

(c)

(d)

Fig. 11.6 Endoscopic transmural pseudocyst puncture and drainage. (a) Identification of bulge into the duodenal bulb. (b) Puncture for localization with injection of contrast and aspiration. (c) 10 mm balloon dilation after guidewire placement. (d) Stents in place—two 10 Fr silicone pigtails and a 7 Fr nasocystic drain.

appears to be more invasive, more costly, and does not show a superior outcome [65].

Pancreatic necrosis

Necrosis of pancreatic tissue complicates acute pancreatitis in a variable percentage of cases, is seen less often in acute exacerbations of chronic pancreatitis, and accounts for many of the complications and much of the mortality (Fig. 11.8). Etiologies may have an impact on severity with the pancreatitis

Table 11.3 Methods of drainage and success rates in recent studies of endoscopic pseudocyst drainage.

Reference	All patients		Cystgastrostomy alone		Cystduodenostomy alone		Pancreatic duct stent alone		Combined procedure	
	Patients	Resolution	Patients	Resolution	Patients	Resolution	Patients	Resolution	Patients	Resolution
Barthet et al. [55]	30	23 (77%)	0		0		20	16 (80%)	10	7 (70%)
Grimm et al. [62]	53	47 (89%)	20 total (site not specified)[a]		16 (80%)		29	27 (93%)	4	4 (100%)[b]
Catalano et al. [56]	21	17 (81%)	0		0		21	17 (81%)	0	
Smits et al. [51]	37	24 (65%)	10	3 (30%)	7	7 (100%)	12	7 (58%)	8	7 (88%)
Total	141	111 (79%)	Of a total of 37 patients, 26 (70%) had resolution				82	67 (82%)	22	18 (82%)

[a]Resolution refers to initial, complete drainage of a pseudocyst.
[b]These results are not explicitly given in the study, but are inferred.

Table 11.4 Complications, recurrence rates, and types of retreatment in recent studies of endoscopic pseudocyst drainage.

Reference	Patients	Complications according to drainage type[a]			Initial resolution	Recurrence	Retreatment after recurrence	
		Total	Transmural	Transpapillary			Endoscopic	Surgical
Barthet et al. [55]	30	4 (13%)	1 (3%)[b]	4 (13%)[b]	23 (77%)	3 (13%)	0	3
Grimm et al. [62]	53	6 (11%)	5 (9%)	1 (2%)	47 (89%)	11 (23%)	7[c]	2[c]
Catalano et al. [56]	21	1 (5%)	N/A	1 (5%)	17 (81%)	1 (6%)	Unclear	Unclear
Smits et al. [51]	37	6 (16%)	5 (14%)	1 (3%)	24 (65%)	3 (13%)	0	3
Total	141	17 (12%)	11 (8%)[b]	7 (5%)[b]	111 (79%)	18 (16%)	7	8

N/A = not applicable; all patients in this study underwent transpapillary drainage.
[a]Excludes stent migration. Percentages refer to the proportions of the total number of patients who underwent this type of treatment, including those who had combined therapy.
[b]One complication occurred in a patient undergoing combined treatment, and is listed under both headings.
[c]Two patients in this study declined further treatment after recurrence.

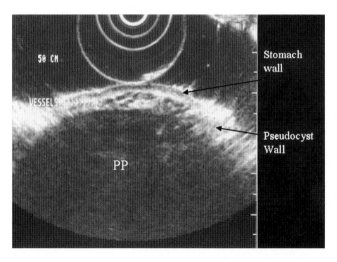

Fig. 11.7 EUS of pseudocyst behind the gastric wall showing intervening vessels consistent with varices.

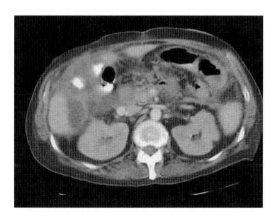

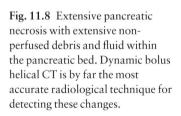

Fig. 11.8 Extensive pancreatic necrosis with extensive non-perfused debris and fluid within the pancreatic bed. Dynamic bolus helical CT is by far the most accurate radiological technique for detecting these changes.

caused by hypertriglyceridemia producing necrosis in perhaps the highest percentage of at-risk cases [66].

In a large single institutional review, Blum *et al.* [21] reported a respectably low overall mortality rate of 5% amongst 368 cases of acute pancreatitis, again with about half being earlier than 2 weeks and the remainder later. To emphasize the importance of necrosis, only 36 cases (10%) had documented necrosis but accounted for nine of the overall 17 deaths. Thus, the presence of necrosis resulted in an eventual death rate of 25%. Finally, the authors noted that late deaths in the absence of necrosis were seen in only four of 212 patients at risk (2%).

At present, the exact mechanism of necrosis is unknown but ischemic infarction is held as most likely. Poor perfusion secondary to rapid third space loss has been postulated but recent data suggest that the process of necrosis may be underway very rapidly before perfusion is affected. In a retrospective case analysis, patients with necrosis presented earlier but had a similar incidence of hemoconcentration compared to patients with interstitial pancreatitis [67]. Resuscitation volumes were similar retrospectively in both groups. However, patients whose hematocrits continued to rise despite large volumes of fluid resuscitation were all subsequently proven to have necrosis. A cause and effect of inadequate resuscitation could not be established.

The consequence of necrosis is a high likelihood of developing infection in the devitalized tissue, and the loss of a functioning pancreas with consequent diabetes, fistula formation, and various vascular injuries. Many of these complications result in the need for operative and, more recently, endoscopic management.

Since pancreatic necrosis produces significant morbidity and a large proportion of the late mortality caused by acute pancreatitis, a search for necrosis using dynamic CT is generally felt justified [68].

Management of necrosis initially is conservative, with the expectation of most patients who do not develop infection eventually spontaneously resolving [69]. However, once the necrotic tissue becomes infected, intervention is almost always required. At present, the majority of these patients are still best managed with surgical debridement and drainage, almost always externally [15]. Prolonged hospitalization with multiple procedures often follows, with surgical centers favoring either closed drainage with subsequent radiologically assisted catheter drainage or open drainage with surgically placed abdominal mesh to permit planned repeated debridements [70].

A few cases of attempted retroperitoneal laparoscopic necrosectomy have been reported [71,72]. At present this experience is anecdotal and no comparative trials have yet been reported. The risk of sudden and severe bleeding and the need for multiple repeat interventions have prevented wide adoption of the technique.

In an attempt to prevent the development of infection in the setting of necrosis, the use of broad-spectrum antibiotics, especially imipenem, has reached a consensus. All eight recently reviewed trials demonstrated benefit in the patients receiving broad-spectrum antibiotics [73]. Many questions remain as to the use of newer antibiotics, the duration of therapy, the timing of onset of use, and the need for fungal coverage [74,75].

Organizing necrosis

As stated earlier, persistent necrotic material organizes and encapsulates into a complex collection containing a mixture of solid and semisolid debris and fluid. Simple catheter drainage will be insufficient to evacuate this material and infec-

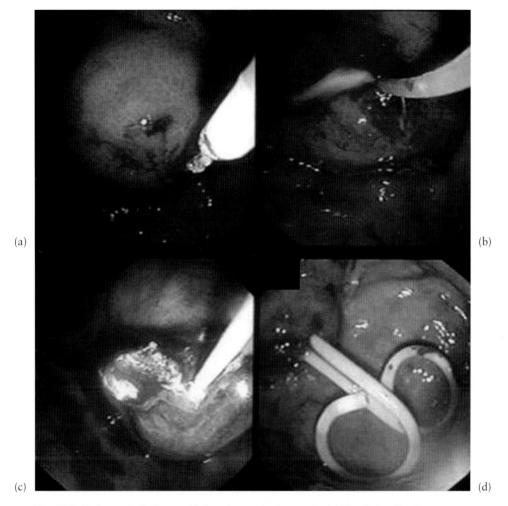

(a)

(b)

(c)

(d)

Fig. 11.9 Endoscopic drainage of infected organized necrosis. (a) Needle localization. (b) Purulent drainage noted upon puncture. (c) Endoscopic view of necrotic material coming through an endoscopically created cystogastrostomy during endoscopic drainage of organizing necrosis. (d) Following 10 mm balloon dilation, two 10 Fr stents are positioned. A nasocystic lavage catheter was then placed.

tion will often complicate such efforts. When approaching apparent pseudocyst patients, it is of paramount importance to assess for necrosis, and then plan and treat patients appropriately [76]. Endoscopic treatment of organizing necrosis is possible but demands techniques of wider drainage such as the placement of multiple stents, creation of a large cyst gastrostomy, and at times nasocystic lavage [29] (Fig. 11.9).

Repeated endoscopic procedures should be anticipated since cavity infections will occur in greater than 50%. When prompt reintervention is performed, these infections can usually be managed with lavage and repeat or additional stent placement. Nevertheless, a multidisciplinary approach to these cases is mandatory for optimal patient outcome. The interventional disciplines of surgery, gastroenterology, and radiology all have roles to play in specific situations [66].

Miscellaneous complications

Pancreatic fistulas

These occur in both interstitial and necrotizing pancreatitis. In the presence of an intact pancreatic sphincter or a ductal stricture, the initial leak continues and, as discussed earlier, is often the etiology of pseudocyst formation. At times and for unclear reasons, some collections do not wall-off and the fistula may track throughout the retroperitoneum. Fistulous communication under the diaphragmatic cruri can result in amylase-rich pleural effusions, broncho-pleural fistulas, or even pericardial tamponade [77,78]. Cases of inguinal, scrotal, femoral, and other hernias developing with amylase-rich fluid tracking down these potential spaces have been reported.

Internal fistulas adjacent to hollow organs are perhaps the most frequently recognized. Fistulization to the duodenum may result in resolution of an otherwise expanding pseudocyst as mentioned earlier [48]. Communication between a pseudocyst and the colon will be complicated by sepsis and generally will require surgery. However, Howell *et al.* reported successful endoscopic treatment of two such cases without requiring surgery [79].

Perhaps the most dramatic consequence of a pancreatic ductal fistula is pancreatic ascites. Easily diagnosed by routine testing of paracentesis fluid for amylase, these rather rare cases are often overlooked and treated mistakenly as cirrhotic ascites since liver and pancreatic disease often coexist in the alcoholic.

Finally, cutaneous pancreatic fistulas occur after attempts at external drainage have been performed. Although these very severe, disabling fistulas are occasionally unavoidable, they are often a consequence of imprecise knowledge of the true diagnosis or the lack of appreciation of the importance of ductal anatomy (Fig. 11.10).

Currently, many of these complex fistulas can be managed endoscopically providing the duct is intact to the papilla. Various authors advocate pancreatic stent placement or nasopancreatic drainage with or without pancreatic sphincterotomy. Rapid closure of these fistulas can be expected with effective endoscopic transpapillary drainage. If no infection is present, endoscopic management is often definitive and should be attempted before external drainage establishes a cutaneous fistula [80].

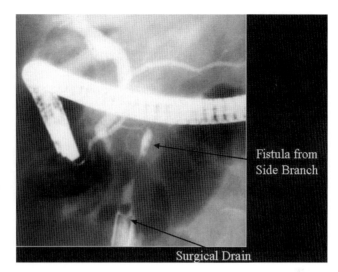

Fig. 11.10 Pancreatic fistula from a small side branch with a persistent fistula for over 3 months to a surgically placed drain. This fistula closed promptly following endoscopic pancreatic sphincterotomy and stent placement.

Ductal disruption

Severe ductal disruption is the rule in necrosis cases but can be seen in well-perfused interstitial pancreatitis. To define the term, disruption occurs when the main pancreatic duct has been transected by the inflammatory process of pancreatitis, most likely by direct proteolytic digestion or ischemic infarction. Ductal disruption greatly complicates the approach to treatment and worsens outcome in both acute and chronic pancreatitis. Spontaneous resolution without intervention is very unlikely to occur. External cutaneous fistulas usually follow a percutaneous or surgical drainage approach due to the presence of a viable but disconnected gland. Although the downstream pancreas can be drained and diverted endoscopically by transpapillary therapy, the upstream pancreas continues to contribute to persistence of the fistula. This so-called 'disconnected tail syndrome' often results in pseudocyst recurrence after internal transmural endoscopic or surgical internal cystgastrostomy drainage [51] (Fig. 11.11). A few authors have reported successful endoscopic drainage by bridging the disruption to reconnect the tail, but the long-term outcome of these efforts remains unclear. More often these patients will experience a long illness with TPN and repeated interventions until the disconnected tail eventually autolyses, atrophies due to stricturing, or is surgically resected [81].

Vascular complications

Venous thrombosis

A frequent vascular complication of acute pancreatitis is thrombosis of the

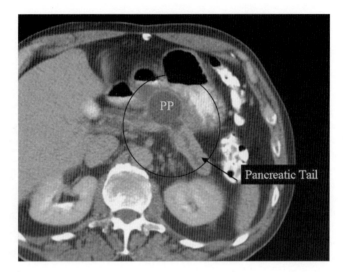

Fig. 11.11 CT scan revealing an obvious disconnected tail as the cause of a pseudocyst recurrence, 3 months after successful endoscopic cystgastrostomy. Note the dilated duct within the free tail.

splenic vein and, less frequently, of the portal vein [82]. The cause is an intense inflammatory response surrounding these venous structures, often with compression by the resulting edematous reaction. Stasis and activation of clotting factors then produce acute thrombosis with resulting left-sided portal hypertension. Because the obstruction to portal inflow to the liver is usually partial, esophageal varices usually do not occur. Nonetheless, bleeding from gastric varices can be severe, especially when coagulopathy coexists (Fig. 11.12).

During the period of convalescence, where often surgical debridement or pseudocyst drainage must be undertaken, a secondary venous thrombosis may be a major determinant in treatment selection. Furthermore, the failure to recognize this form of portal hypertension prior to such interventions can prove disastrous. Significant gastric wall varices often contraindicate endoscopic or even surgical pseudocyst gastrostomy. Helical dynamic contrast CT scanning should detect venous thrombosis and predict left-sided portal hypertension accurately (Fig. 11.13). EUS has proven particularly valuable in assessing for gastric varices. One or both studies should be performed near the time of any invasive intervention.

Arterial complications

Thrombotic arterial complications secondary to acute pancreatitis are less common, but when they occur they can be severe. Splenic artery thrombosis with

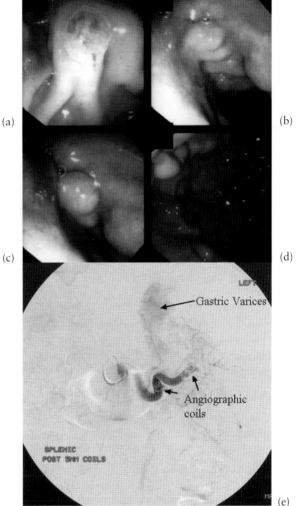

Fig. 11.12 Multiple duodenal and gastric varices which bled, detected on endoscopy, in a patient with a large pseudocyst and secondary splenic and portal vein thrombosis. (a) Ampulla with surrounding edema. (b) Duodenal varices of the second portion. (c) Duodenal bulb varices. (d) Extensive varices in the gastric fundus. (e) Angiographic embolization of the splenic artery to control gastric varices bleeding. Note that there is no flow beyond the farthest coils.

resulting splenic infarction is generally survivable with splenectomy. However, superior mesenteric artery thrombosis resulting in small and, at times, large bowel infarction is accompanied by a high mortality. The middle colic artery is perhaps the most frequent artery to thrombose, often resulting in a more limited large bowel infarction which may respond to resection and temporary surgical colostomy.

A more frequent arterial complication of pancreatitis is the formation of a pseudoaneurysm resulting in hemorrhage. Various series report this serious complication in up to 10% of cases of severe acute pancreatitis and it can complicate chronic pancreatitis as well [83,84].

If the pseudoaneurysm has formed in an expanding pseudocyst wall, sudden hypotension with syncope followed by intense pain has been termed 'pancreatic

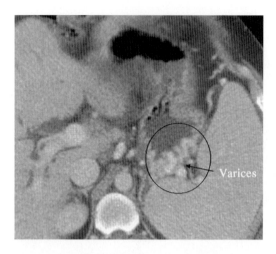

Fig. 11.13 Endoscopic view of congested ampulla gastric varices duodenum varices CT of varices in splenic hilum involving greater curvature of stomach.

apoplexy. If the pseudocyst into which the pseudoaneurysm ruptures communicates with the pancreatic duct, frank gastrointestinal bleeding can be the presenting symptom. Termed 'hemosuccus pancreaticus', such bleeding is amongst the rarest causes of gastrointestinal hemorrhage [85].

Finally, the presence of a pseudoaneurysm may be silent, only to acutely rupture during any invasive intervention where the surrounding tamponade is decompressed. This can be especially devastating in endoscopic pseudocyst drainage since prompt control of bleeding in general is not possible. Delayed rupture may also occur, resulting in exsanguinating gastrointestinal bleeding if a pseudocyst enterostomy has been created or if a surgical or radiological external drain has been placed [86].

To avoid these severe bleeding complications, it is imperative that the presence of a pseudoaneurysm is carefully searched for before intervention. All drainage procedures are strictly contraindicated until such a vascular lesion can be addressed and resolved. Dynamic, arterial phase, thin-section helical CT scanning through the pancreatic region is likely the best diagnostic study [87] (Fig. 11.14). Doppler ultrasound can be confirmatory but does not have the comprehensive screening power of CT. MRI with an arteriography protocol has been little reported but would likely visualize these lesions [8].

Once detected, preoperative angiography with embolization of the pseudoaneurysm has become a popular approach [88] (Fig. 11.15). These procedures can be technically challenging if the pancreatico-duodenal artery is the affected vessel since embolization may be necessary from both the celiac trunk and the superior mesenteric artery. Pseudoaneurysm of the celiac trunk can present a nearly insurmountable problem since gallbladder, gastric, and even hepatic infarction may follow embolization. If portal vein thrombosis is also present,

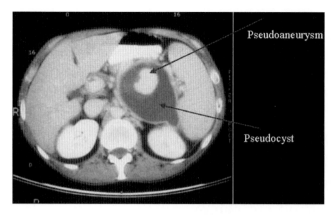

Fig. 11.14 Pseudoaneurysm of the splenic artery complicating chronic pancreatitis within a pseudocyst. This has not yet ruptured.

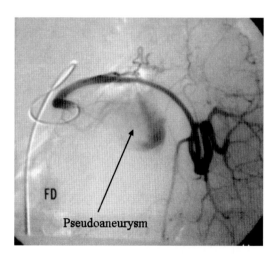

Fig. 11.15 Pseudoaneurysm within a pseudocyst filled with contrast on dynamic bolus helical CT scan. The same pseudoaneurysm on angiography is of the splenic artery. This was successfully embolized.

the risk of hepatic infarction increases dramatically. Successful treatment of hemosuccus pancreaticus radiological embolization at angiography is the preferred approach as well [89].

Once the pseudoaneurysm has been thoroughly embolized and thrombosed, interventions can then be safely carried out [84]. Elton *et al.* reported successful endoscopic pseudoaneurysm/pseudocyst drainage following radiological embolization in three such cases [90]. In all three patients, thrombosis following embolization was documented by repeat dynamic contrast CT or Doppler ultrasound prior to endoscopic intervention. Successful endoscopic drainage of the obstructing pseudocyst, stent management of strictures, and clearance of obstructing clots within the pancreatic duct resulted in symptom resolution and avoided surgery in these cases.

Finally, massive diffuse retroperitoneal bleeding may be seen in the setting of necrotizing pancreatitis, often with coincident coagulopathy. This so-called 'hemorrhagic pancreatitis' is less often reported since better radiology more often identifies a focal arterial source. However, when true diffuse hemorrhagic pancreatitis does occur, mortality rates exceed 35%, even in the modern era [88].

Summary

Complications of pancreatitis vary widely, are of complex etiology, and involve multiple organ systems. Avoiding these complications remains the basic goal for all treating physicians, but, once present, their expert detection and appropriate management are the key to optimizing patient outcome [91]. Great progress has been made in treating these supremely ill patients but early and specific treatments to prevent complications are still lacking. Prolonged hospitalizations, TPN, dialysis, ventilatory support, antibiotic therapy, and radiological, endoscopic, and surgical treatments all have had a role in reducing mortality to less than 10% of afflicted patients. However, much needs to be discovered [92].

Outstanding issues and future trends

The major need in pancreatology remains a full understanding of the pathophysiology of acute pancreatitis that results in the dramatic cascade of events outlined in this chapter. Once the earliest events are identified, specific medical interventions, possibly extremely specific pharmacological agents, can be developed that can prevent progression to shock, end organ compromise, necrosis, and the other late complications outlined. More basic research is needed.

Lacking this knowledge, research will continue to look for methods of preventing the complications of pancreatitis once severe disease has been established. A major need is an effective way to prevent progression to necrosis, beyond aggressive fluid resuscitation.

Trends in the future will continue to be innovations in minimally invasive therapies. Debridement of infected necrosis, intervention prior to infection, and management of ductal disruption resulting in a disconnected tail are all areas of considerable confusion and often subjects of interdisciplinary debate. Therapeutic, endoscopic, percutaneous laparoscopic debridement, and transgastric endoscopic therapy are the newest players on a seemingly crowded field.

References

1 Ranson JHC, Rifkind KM, Roses DF *et al*. Prognostic signs and the role of operative management in acute pancreatitis. *Surg Gynecol Obstet* 1974; 139: 69–81.

2 Williams M, Simms HH. Prognostic usefulness of scoring systems in critically ill patients with severe acute pancreatitis. *Crit Care Med* 1999; 27: 901–7.

3 Halonen KI, Pettila V, Leppaniemi AK, Kemppainen EA, Puolakkainen PA, Haapiainen RK. Multiple organ dysfunction associated with severe acute pancreatitis. *Crit Care Med* 2002; 30: 1274–9.

4 Khan AA, Parekh D, Cho Y *et al*. Improved prediction of outcome in patients with severe acute pancreatitis by the APACHE II score at 48 hours after hospital admission compared with the APACHE II score at admission: acute physiology and chronic health evaluation. *Arch Surg* 2002; 137: 1136–40.

5 Eachempati SR, Hydo LJ, Barie PS. Severity scoring for prognostication in patients with severe acute pancreatitis. *Arch Surg* 2002; 17: 730–6.

6 Balthazar EJ, Fisher LA. Hemorrhagic complications of pancreatitis: radiologic evaluation with emphasis on CT imaging. *Pancreatology* 2001; 1: 306–13.

7 Robert JH, Frossard JL, Mermillod B *et al*. Early prediction of acute pancreatitis: prospective study comparing computed tomography scans, Ranson, Glasgow, acute physiology and chronic health evaluation II scores, and various serum markers. *World J Surg* 2002; 26: 612–19.

8 Robinson PJ, Sheridan MB. Pancreatitis: computed tomography and magnetic resonance imaging. *Eur Radiol* 2000; 10: 401–8.

9 Frey CF, Brody GL. Relationship of azotemia and survival in bile pancreatitis in the dog. *Arch Surg* 1996; 93: 295–300.

10 Salomone T, Tosi P, Di Battista N *et al*. Impaired alveolar gas exchange in acute pancreatitis. *Dig Dis Sci* 2002; 47: 2025–8.

11 Hietaranta A, Kemppainen E, Puolakkainen P *et al*. Extracellular phospholipases A2 in relation to systemic inflammatory response syndrome (SIRS) and systemic complications in severe acute pancreatitis. *Pancreas* 1999; 18: 385–91.

12 Kingsnorth A. The role of cytokines in the pathogenesis of acute pancreatitis. *Am J Surg* 1997; 40: 1–4.

13 Norman J. The role of cytokines in the pathogenesis of acute pancreatitis. *Am J Surg* 1998; 175: 76–83.

14 Brivet F, Emilie D, Galanaud P *et al*. Pro- and anti-inflammatory cytokines during acute severe pancreatitis: an early and sustained response, although unpredictable of death. Parisian Study Group on Acute Pancreatitis. *Crit Care Med* 1999; 27: 749–55.

15 Hartwig W, Werner J, Uhl W, Buchler MW. Management of infection in acute pancreatitis. *J Hepatobiliary Pancreat Surg* 2002; 9: 423–8.

16 Banks PA, Gerzof SG, Langevin RE *et al*. CT-guided aspiration of suspected pancreatic infection: bacteriology and clinical outcome. *Int J Pancreatol* 1995; 18: 256–70.

17 Takacs T, Hajnal F, Nemeth J *et al*. Stimulated gastrointestinal hormone release and gallbladder contraction during continuous jejunal feeding in patients with pancreatic pseudocyst is inhibited by octreotide. *Int J Pancreatol* 2000; 28: 215–20.

18 Windsor ACJ, Kanwar S, Li AGK *et al*. Compared with parenteral nutrition, enteral feeding attenuates the acute phase response and improves disease severity in acute pancreatitis. *Gut* 1998; 42: 431–5.

19 Johnson CD, Imrie CW, McMahon MJ *et al*. Double blind, randomized, placebo controlled study of a platelet activating factor antagonist, lexipafant, in the treatment and prevention of organ failure in predicted severe acute pancreatitis. *Gut* 2001; 48: 62–9.

20 Isenmann R, Schwarz M, Rau B, Trautmann M, Schobr W, Beger HG. Characteristics of infection with candida species in patients with necrotizing pancreatitis. *World J Surg* 2002; 26: 372–6.

21 Blum T, Maisonneuve P, Lowenfels AB, Lankisch PG. Fatal outcome in acute pancreatitis: its occurrence and early prediction. *Pancreatology* 2001; 1: 237–41.

22 Ethridge RT, Chung DH, Slogoff M *et al*. Cyclooxygenase-2 gene disruption attenuates the severity of acute pancreatitis and pancreatitis-associated lung injury. *Gastroenterology* 2002; 123: 1311–22.

23 Pezzilli R, Billi P, Miniero R, Barakat B. Serum interleukin-10 in human acute pancreatitis. *Dig Dis Sci* 1997; 42: 1469–72.

24 Chen CC, Wang SS, Lu RH, Chang FY, Lee SP. Serum interleukin 10 and interleukin 11 in patients with acute pancreatitis. *Gut* 1999; 45: 895–9.

25 Eskdale J, Peat J, Gallagher GE, Imrie CW, McKay CJ. Fine genomic mapping implicates IL-10 as a severity gene in acute pancreatitis. *Gastroenterology* 2001; 120: A24.

26 Dumot JA, Conwell DL, Zuccaro C *et al*. A randomized, double blind study of interleukin 10 for the prevention of ERCP-induced pancreatitis. *Am J Gastroenterol* 2001; 96: 2098–102.

27 Balthazar EJ. Staging of acute pancreatitis. *Radiol Clin North Am* 2002; 40: 1199–209.

28 Lau ST, Simchuk EJ, Kozarek RA, Traverso LW. A pancreatic ductal leak should be sought to direct treatment in patients with acute pancreatitis. *Am J Surg* 2001; 181: 411–15.

29 Baron TH, Harewood GC, Morgan DE, Yates MR. Outcome differences after endoscopic drainage of pancreatic necrosis, acute pancreatic pseudocysts, and chronic pancreatic pseudocysts. *Gastrointest Endosc* 2002; 56: 7–17.

30 Bradley EL III, Clements JL Jr, Gonzales AC. The natural history of pancreatic pseudocysts: a unified concept of management. *Am J Surg* 1979; 137: 135–41.

31 D'Edogo A, Schein M. Pancreatic pseudocysts: a proposed classification and its management implications. *Br J Surg* 1991; 78: 981–4.

32 Warshaw AL, Compton CC, Lewandrowski K *et al*. Cystic tumors of the pancreas: new clinical, radiologic, and pathogenic observations in 67 patients. *Am Surg* 1990; 212: 432–45.

33 Levin MF, Vellet AD, Bach DB *et al*. Peripancreatic fluid collections: vascular structures masquerading as pseudocysts. *Can Assoc Radiol J* 1992; 43: 267–72.

34 Sorgman JA, Langevin E, Banks PA. Urinoma masquerading as pancreatic pseudocyst. *Int J Pancreatol* 1992; 11: 195–6.

35 Sperti C, Cappellazzo F, Pasquali C *et al*. Cystic neoplasms of the pancreas: problems in differential diagnosis. *Am Surg* 1993; 59: 740–5.

36 Warshaw AL, Rutledge PL. Cystic tumors mistaken for pancreatic pseudocysts. *Am Surg* 1987; 205: 393–8.

37 Hammond N, Miller FH, Sica GT, Gore RM. Imaging of cystic diseases of the pancreas. *Radiol Clin North Am* 2002; 40: 1243–62.

38 Hsieh CH, Tseng JH, Huang SF. Co-existence of a huge pseudocyst and mucinous cystadenoma: report of a case and the value of magnetic resonance imaging for differential diagnosis. *Eur J Gastroenterol Hepatol* 2002; 14: 191–4.

39 Fockens P, Johnson TG, van Dulleman HM *et al*. Endosonography is a prerequisite before endoscopic drainage of pancreatic pseudocysts. *Gastrointest Endosc* 1996; 43: 516 (A).

40 Brugge WR. Role of endoscopic ultrasound in the diagnosis of cystic lesions of the pancreas. *Pancreatology* 2001; 1 (6): 637–40 [Review].

41 Kloppel G, Kosmahl M. Cystic lesions and neoplasms of the pancreas: the features are becoming clearer. *Pancreatology* 2001; 1 (6): 648–55 [Review].

42 Sedlack R, Affi A, Vazquez-Sequeiros E, Norton ID, Clain JE, Wiersema MJ. Utility of EUS in the evaluation of cystic pancreatic lesions. *Gastrointest Endosc* 2002; 56 (4): 543–7.

43 Banks PA. Practice guidelines in acute pancreatitis. *Am J Gastroenterol* 1997; 3: 377–86.

44 O'Malley VP, Cannon JP, Postie RG. Pancreatic pseudocysts: cause, therapy, and results. *Am J Surg* 1985; 150: 680–2.

45 Yeo CJ, Bastidas JA, Lynch-Nyhan A *et al*. The natural history of pancreatic pseudocysts documented by computed tomography. *Surg Gynecol Obstet* 1990; 170: 411–17.

46 Vitas GJ, Sarr MG. Selected management of pancreatic pseudocysts: operative versus expectant management. *Surgery* 1992; 111: 123–30.

47 Kozarek RA, Ball TJ, Patterson DJ, Freeny PC, Ryan JA, Traverso LW. Endoscopic transpapillary therapy for disrupted pancreatic duct and peripancreatic fluid collections. *Gastroenterology* 1996; 100 (5 Part 1): 1362–70.

48 Urakami A, Tsunoda T, Hayashi J, Oka Y, Mizuno M. Spontaneous fistulization of a pancreatic pseudocyst into the colon and duodenum. *Gastrointest Endosc* 2002; 55: 949–51.

49 Nealon W, Walser E. Main pancreatic ductal anatomy can direct choice of modality for treating pancreatic pseudocysts (surgery versus percutaneous drainage). *Ann Surg* 2002; 235: 751–8.

50 Grace PA, Williamson RCN. Modern management of pancreatic pseudocysts. *Br J Surg* 1993; 80: 573–81.

51 Smits ME, Rauws EA, Tytgat GN *et al.* The efficacy of endoscopic treatment of pancreatic pseu-docysts. *Gastrointest Endosc* 1995; 42: 202–7.

52 VanSonnenberg E, Wittich GR, Casola G. Complicated pancreatic inflammatory disease: diag-nostic and therapeutic role of interventional radiology. *Radiology* 1985; 155: 355–40.

53 Howell DA, Elton E, Parsons WG. Endoscopic management of pseudocysts of the pancreas. *Gastrointest Endosc Clin N Am* 1998; 8 (1): 143–62 [Review].

54 Parsons WG, Howell DA. (1998). Endoscopic management of pancreatic pseudocysts. In: *ERCP and its Applications* (ed. Jacobson IM), pp. 193–207. Lippincott-Raven, Philadelphia.

55 Barthet M, Sahel J, Bodlou-Bertel C *et al.* Endoscopic transpapillary drainage of pancreatic pseudocysts. *Gastrointest Endosc* 1995; 42: 208–13.

56 Catalano MF, Geenen JE, Schmalz MJ. Treatment of pancreatic pseudocysts ductal communica-tion by transpapillary pancreatic duct endoprosthesis. *Gastrointest Endosc* 1995; 42: 214–18.

57 Mallavarapu R, Habib TH, Elton E, Goldberg MJ. Resolution of mediastinal pancreatic pseu-docysts with transpapillary stent placement. *Gastrointest Endosc* 2001; 53: 367–70.

58 Sharma SS, Bhargawa N, Govil A. Endoscopic management of pancreatic pseudocyst: a long-term follow-up. *Endoscopy* 2002; 34: 203–7.

59 Cremer M, Deviere J, Engelholm L. Endoscopic management of cysts and pseudocysts in chronic pancreatitis: long-term follow-up after 7 years of experience. *Gastrointest Endosc* 1989; 35: 1–9.

60 Monkemuller KE, Baron TH, Morgan DE. Transmural drainage of pancreatic fluid collections without electrocautery using the Seldinger technique. *Gastrointest Endosc* 1998; 48: 195–200.

61 Chak A. Endosonographic-guided therapy of pancreatic pseudocysts. *Gastrointest Endosc* 2000; 52: S23–S27.

62 Grimm H, Binmoeller KE, Soehendra N. Endosonography-guided drainage of a pancreatic pseudocyst. *Gastrointest Endosc* 1992; 38: 170–1.

63 Brand B, Penaloza-Ramirez A, Gupta R *et al.* New mechanical puncture video echoendoscope: one-step transmural drainage of a pseudocyst. *Dig Liver Dis* 2002; 34: 133–6.

64 Wiersema MJ. Endosonography-guided cystduodenostomy with a therapeutic ultrasound endo-scope. *Gastrointest Endosc* 1996; 44: 614–17.

65 Trias M, Targarona EM, Balague C *et al.* Intraluminal stapled laparoscopic cystogastrostomy for treatment of pancreatic pseudocysts. *Br J Surg* 1995; 82: 403.

66 Baron TH, Morgan DE. Endoscopic transgastric irrigation tube placement via PEG for debride-ment of organized pancreatic necrosis. *Gastrointest Endosc* 1999; 50 (4): 574–7.

67 Brown A, Baillargeon JD, Hughes MD, Banks PA. Can fluid resuscitation prevent pancreatic necrosis in severe acute pancreatitis? *Pancreatology* 2002; 2: 104–7.

68 Lankisch PG, Struckmann K, Assmus C, Lehnick D, Maisonneuve P, Lowenfels AB. Do we need a computed tomography examination in all patients with acute pancreatitis within 72 h after admission to hospital for the detection of pancreatic necrosis? *Scand J Gastroenterol* 2002; 36: 432–6.

69 Ashley SW, Perez A, Pierce EA *et al.* Necrotizing pancreatitis: contemporary analysis of 99 con-secutive cases. *Ann Surg* 2001; 234: 572–9.

70 Uhl W, Warshaw A, Imrie C *et al.* IAP guidelines for the surgical management of acute pancre-atitis. *Pancreatology* 2002; 2: 565–73.

71 Horvath KD, Kao LS, Wherry KL, Pellegrini CA, Sinanan MN. A technique for laparoscopic-assisted percutaneous drainage of infected pancreatic necrosis and pancreatic abscess. *Surg Endosc* 2001; 15: 1221–5.

72 Castellanos G, Pinero A, Serrano A, Parrilla P. Infected pancreatic necrosis: translumbar approach and management with retroperitoneoscopy. *Arch Surg* 2002; 13: 1060–3.

73 Bassi C. Infections in pancreatic inflammatory disease: clinical trials for antibiotic prophylaxis. *Pancreatology* 2001; 1: 210–12.

74 Isenmann R, Rau B, Beger HG. Early severe acute pancreatitis: characteristics of a new sub-group. *Pancreas* 2001; 22: 274–8.

75 Howard TJ, Temple MB. Prophylactic antibiotics alter the bacteriology of infected necrosis in severe acute pancreatitis. *J Am Coll Surg* 2002; 195: 759–67.

76 Hariri M, Slivka A, Carr-Locke DL *et al.* Pseudocyst drainage predisposes to infection when pancreatic necrosis is unrecognized. *Am J Gastroenterol* 1994; 89: 1781–4.

77 Mahlke R, Warnecke B, Lankisch PG, Elbrechtz F, Busch C. A sudden coughing up of foul-smelling sputum: a first sign of a pancreaticobronchial fistula, a severe pulmonary complication in acute pancreatitis. *Am J Gastroenterol* 2001; 96: 1952–3.

78 Olah A, Jagy AS, Racz I, Gamal ME. Cardiac tamponade as a complication of pseudocyst in chronic pancreatitis. *Hepatogastroenterology* 2002; 49: 594–6.

79 Howell DA, Dy RM, Gerstein WH, Hanson BL, Biber BP. Infected pancreatic pseudocysts with colonic fistula formation successfully managed by endoscopic drainage alone: report of two cases. *Am J Gastroenterol* 2000; 95: 1822–3.

80 Costamagna G, Mutignani M, Ingrosso M *et al.* Endoscopic treatment of postsurgical external pancreatic fistulas. *Endoscopy* 2001; 33: 317–22.

81 Kozarek RA. Endoscopic therapy of complete and partial pancreatic duct disruptions. *Gastrointest Endosc Clin N Am* 1998; 8: 39–53 [Review].

82 Isbicki JR, Yekebas EF, Strate T *et al.* Extrahepatic portal hypertension in chronic pancreatitis. *Ann Surg* 2002; 236: 82–9.

83 Sawlani V, Phadke RV, Baijal SS *et al.* Arterial complications of pancreatitis and their radiological management. *Australas Radiol* 1996; 40 (4): 381–6 [Review].

84 Marshall GT, Howell DA, Hansen BL *et al.* Multidisciplinary approach to pseudoaneurysms complicating pancreatic pseudocysts: impact of pretreatment diagnosis. *Arch Surg* 1996; 131: 278–83.

85 Koizumi J, Inoue S, Yonekawa H, Kunieda T. Hemosuccus pancreaticus: diagnosis with CT and MRI and treatment with transcatheter embolization. *Abdom Imaging* 2002; 27: 77–81.

86 Born LJ, Madura JA, Lehman GA. Endoscopic diagnosis of a pancreatic pseudoaneurysm after lateral pancreaticojejunostomy. *Gastrointest Endosc* 1999; 49: 382–3.

87 Balthazar EJ. Acute pancreatitis: assessment of severity with clinical and CT evaluation. *Radiology* 2002; 223: 603–13.

88 Flati G, Andren-Sandberg A, La Pinta M, Porowska B, Carboni M. Potentially fatal bleeding in acute pancreatitis: pathophysiology, prevention, and treatment. *Pancreas* 2003; 26: 8–14.

89 Dasgupta R, Davies MJ, Williamson RC, Jackson JE. Haemosuccus pancreaticus: treatment by arterial embolization. *Clin Radiol* 2002; 57: 1021–7.

90 Elton EDA, Howell SM, Amberson Dykes TA. Combined angiographic and endoscopic management of bleeding pancreatic pseudoaneurysms. *Gastrointest Endosc* 1997; 46: 544–9.

91 Beger HG, Rau B, Isenmann R. Prevention of severe change in acute pancreatitis: prediction and prevention. *J Hepatobiliary Pancreat Surg* 2001; 8: 140–7.

92 Bank S, Singh P, Pooran N, Stark B. Evaluation of factors that have reduced mortality from acute pancreatitis over the past 20 years. *J Clin Gastroenterol* 2002; 35: 50–60.

CHAPTER 12

ERCP in Children

MOISES GUELRUD

Synopsis

ERCP has substantially influenced the evaluation and treatment of adult patients with suspected pancreatic and biliary disease. The first reports of ERCP in infants and children were chiefly from adult gastroenterologists experienced with such techniques. The growth in number and availability of skilled endoscopists has resulted in more frequent performance of ERCP in children. Moreover, the acquired ability to perform therapeutic endoscopic procedures is also applicable to children and adolescents. Techniques such as endoscopic sphincterotomy, biliary drainage, extraction of common bile duct and pancreatic duct stones, implantation of endoprostheses, and drainage of pancreatic pseudocysts are beginning to be used in children with an overall success rate similar to that reported for adult patients. In this chapter, the technique, indications, complications, and diagnostic and therapeutic applications of ERCP in children are defined.

Introduction

Endoscopic retrograde cholangiopancreatography (ERCP) is the most demanding endoscopic procedure in children. It is the most sensitive and specific technique in the evaluation and treatment of children with suspected disorders of the pancreas and the biliary tract. The disadvantage is that it is an invasive procedure that frequently needs general anesthesia. The use of this technique in children has been limited. This may be due to the relatively low incidence of diseases, low incidence of clinical suspicion, limited availability of pediatric duodenoscopes, lack of pediatric gastroenterologists well trained in ERCP due to little exposure to the procedure, impression that ERCP in children is technically difficult to accomplish, difficulty in the effective evaluation of the therapeutic result, and because the indications and safety of ERCP in children have not been well defined. Since the procedure is frequently performed by experienced adult endoscopists, it is important to have a close working collaboration between them and pediatric gastroenterologists.

309

Patient preparation

Sedation for ERCP in children

The preparation and sedation of a child undergoing ERCP are similar to those used for upper gastrointestinal endoscopy. Since young children and some adolescents are unable to fully cooperate with procedures under conscious sedation, a state of deep sedation from which the patient is not easily aroused is often required. The endoscopist must choose between conscious sedation and general anesthesia after considering the pertinent risks and taking into account personal skill and experience, expected complexity of the procedure, and lastly, cost.

Most children can be adequately sedated with a combination of meperidine (2–4 mg/kg, maximum 100 mg) and diazepam (0.1–0.3 mg/kg, maximum 15 mg) or midazolam (0.1–0.3 mg/kg, maximum 15 mg). To obtain adequate sedation, children frequently require much higher doses of midazolam on a milligram per kilogram basis than adults. Post-procedure monitoring is the same as for other endoscopic procedures requiring sedation.

Antibiotic prophylaxis

There are no data to guide antibiotic prophylaxis for ERCP in children. In our experience, routine antibiotic prophylaxis is unnecessary in neonates with cholestasis. Prophylactic antibiotics should be used to prevent endocarditis in susceptible patients in the same manner as for upper gastrointestinal endoscopy. Special situations that require a valvular prosthesis, vascular graft material, indwelling catheters, or transplanted organ in an immunosuppressed patient need individual consideration.

Other medication

Additional medications, which may be useful during ERCP, include glucagon and Buscopan (hyoscine-*N*-butyl bromide) to reduce duodenal motility, and secretin to facilitate identification and cannulation of the minor papilla.

Instruments

In neonates and infants younger than 12 months, ERCP is performed with a special Olympus pediatric duodenoscope PJF [1] (Olympus America Inc., Melville, NY) which has an insertion tube diameter of 7.5 mm, a channel of 2.0 mm, and an elevator. A standard adult duodenoscope (insertion tube diameter approximately 11 mm) can be used for older children and adolescents. Therapeutic maneuvers, such as placement of endoprostheses and passage of some dilators and retrieval baskets, require instruments with a larger (3.2 mm) channel.

Technique

ERCP is performed in a radiology suite. Pediatric endoscopy assistants and specially trained nurses can help reduce pre-procedure anxiety, monitor the clinical status of the patient, and assist in holding and reassuring, administering medication, handling catheters, and injecting contrast material. The heart rate and oxygen saturation must be continuously monitored. Resuscitation medications and appropriate equipment should be available. ERCP is performed on an ambulatory basis. A recovery area equipped with monitors and specialized pediatric nurses familiar with the needs of children is necessary.

The principles of cannulation are those used in adult patients, with the additional limitations of space within the duodenum that depend on age. In young infants, such as those undergoing investigation for neonatal cholestasis, it is important to minimize the procedure time to avoid abdominal overdistension and respiratory compromise.

Indications

In general, children with suspected biliary and pancreatic disease should undergo MRCP nowadays before considering ERCP (which is more often used for therapy).

Biliary indications

The only indication for ERCP in neonates and young infants is cholestasis. Biliary indications for ERCP in children older than 1 year and in adolescents are:
- obstructive jaundice
- known or suspected choledocholithiasis
- abnormal liver enzymes in children with inflammatory bowel diseases
- evaluation of biliary ductal leaks after cholecystectomy or liver transplantation
- evaluation of abnormal scans (ultrasound, computerized tomography (CT), or MRCP)
- therapeutic ERCP.

Pancreatic indications

Pancreatic indications for ERCP in children are:
- non-resolving acute pancreatitis
- idiopathic recurrent pancreatitis, chronic pancreatitis

- evaluation of persistent elevation of pancreatic enzymes
- evaluation of abnormal scans (ultrasound, CT, or MRCP)
- evaluation of pancreatic pseudocysts and pancreatic ascites
- evaluation of pancreatic ductal leaks from blunt abdominal trauma
- therapeutic ERCP.

Success rates for ERCP in children

Successful cannulation of the common bile duct in neonates and young infants is lower than that in adults. It varies from 27% to 95% according to the endoscopist's experience [1–7] (Table 12.1). In our unpublished experience with 184 neonates and young infants with neonatal cholestasis, the procedure was successful technically in 93% of cases. Failure was due to duodenal malrotation in two cases and inability to cannulate in six.

In older children, the success rate for cannulation of the desired duct is comparable to that achieved in adults [8–24] (Table 12.2). Our ERCP success in 220 children older than 1 year was 98%.

Complications

The incidence of complications in pediatric patients is not well established. In neonates and young infants with neonatal cholestasis, there were no major complications in the series reported in the literature [1–7]. In our unpublished experience with 184 neonates and young infants, minor complications without clinical significance occurred in 24 patients (13%). Two neonates had transient narcotic-induced respiratory depression and four young infants had non-narcotic respiratory depression, which resolved with oxygen administration. In

Table 12.1 Success of ERCP in infants with neonatal cholestasis.

Author, year	No. of patients	Success
Guelrud et al. 1987 [1]	22	19 (86%)
Heyman et al. 1988 [3]	11	3 (27%)
Wilkinson et al. 1991 [7]	9	4 (45%)
Derkx et al. 1994 [2]	20	18 (90%)
Mitchell and Wilkinson 1994 [5]	40	36 (95%)
Ohnuma et al. 1997 [6]	75	66 (88%)
Iinuma et al. 2000 [4]	50	43 (86%)
Guelrud 2000 (unpublished)	184	172 (93%)
Total	411	361 (88%)

Table 12.2 Successful cannulation during ERCP in children older than 1 year.

Author, year	Number of patients	Success
Cotton and Laage 1982 [12]	25	24 (96%)
Kunitomo et al. 1988 [17]	16	14 (88%)
Buckley and Connon 1990 [11]	42	41 (98%)
Putnam et al. 1991 [21]	42	39 (93%)
Dite et al. 1992 [13]	19	19 (100%)
Brown et al. 1993 [9]	121	116 (96%)
Brown and Goldschmiedt 1993 [56]	25	25 (100%)
Lemmel et al. 1994 [18]	55	54 (98%)
Portwood et al. 1995 [20]	26	26 (100%)
Abu-Khalaf 1995 [8]	16	16 (100%)
Manegold et al. 1996 [19]	38	36 (94%)
Su et al. 1996 [22]	162	157 (97%)
Tagge et al. 1997 [23]	26	25 (96%)
Graham et al. 1998 [14]	17	16 (94%)
Guitron et al. 1998 [15]	50	49 (98%)
Hsu et al. 2000 [16]	22	22 (100%)
Poddar et al. 2001 [24]	72	70 (97%)
Guelrud 2000 (unpublished)	220	215 (98%)
Total	922	904 (98%)

17 patients, minor acute duodenal erosions were observed without clinical consequences. One neonate had abdominal distension for 10 h after completion of ERCP, which resolved without treatment. There were no major complications.

Complications in children older than 1 year vary according to the system studied, biliary or pancreatic. The overall incidence is approximately 4.7% [8–24]. In our unpublished experience with 220 ERCPs in children older than 1 year, ERCP was performed for diagnostic purposes in 108 cases with two (1.8%) complications. In 112 therapeutic ERCPs, complications occurred in 12 (10.7%).

Biliary findings (Table 12.3)

Biliary atresia vs. neonatal hepatitis

The differential diagnosis of neonatal cholestasis is critical in the first 2 months of life. In approximately 30% of patients, a specific metabolic or infectious disease can be recognized. In the remaining 70% of neonates, the key differentiation is between biliary atresia and neonatal hepatitis. Discriminating analysis using duodenal drainage, ultrasound, scintigraphy, and liver biopsy permitted

Table 12.3 Biliary findings in ERCP in neonates and children.

Congenital anomalies
   Biliary atresia vs. neonatal hepatitis
   Alagille syndrome and paucity syndrome
   Congenital hepatic fibrosis
   Caroli's disease and Caroli's syndrome
   Biliary strictures due to cystic fibrosis
   Choledochal cyst
   Benign biliary strictures

Acquired diseases
   Bile plug syndrome
   Primary sclerosing cholangitis
   Biliary obstruction due to parasitic infestation
   Choledocholithiasis
   Benign biliary strictures
   Malignant biliary strictures
   Common bile duct complications after liver transplantation

---

accurate diagnosis of either biliary atresia or neonatal hepatitis in 80–90% of patients [25]. Thus, 10–20% of neonates required laparotomy to establish the diagnosis. In these patients, visualization of a patent biliary tree by ERCP may help.

Clearly, the success of ERCP in this context depends upon the experience of the endoscopist, who must have confidence that non-visualization of the common bile duct is not related to technical problems and to positioning of the catheter. ERCP is the most direct method of establishing a diagnosis in the hands of skilled endoscopists, and may be appropriate as the first-line test when expertise and equipment are available.

ERCP findings

Three types of ERCP findings have been described in patients with biliary atresia [26] (Fig. 12.1): Type 1, no visualization of the biliary tree (Fig. 12.2); Type 2, visualization of the distal common duct and gallbladder (Fig. 12.3); Type 3 is divided into two subtypes: Type 3a, visualization of the gallbladder and the complete common duct with biliary lakes at the porta hepatis (Fig. 12.4), and Type 3b, in which both hepatic ducts are seen with biliary lakes.

Several authors [2,4–6,27] have shown that in half of the patients in whom extensive investigations failed to distinguish intra- from extrahepatic cholestasis, the biliary tree was opacified, thus avoiding surgery. When the biliary tree was partially visualized (Type 2 and Type 3), the diagnosis of biliary atresia was made and confirmed by surgery. When the biliary tree was not opacified and

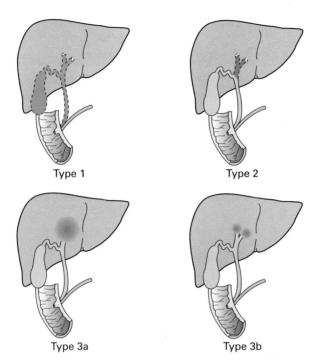

Type 1

Type 2

Type 3a

Type 3b

Fig. 12.1 Variants of biliary atresia.

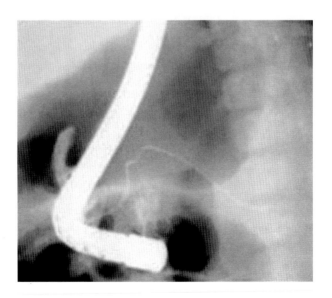

Fig. 12.2 Biliary atresia Type 1. No visualization of biliary tree. Opacification of normal pancreatic duct.

only the pancreatic duct was visualized (Type 1), the diagnosis of biliary atresia was suspected and exploratory laparotomy was indicated. Of the 310 infants with neonatal cholestasis reported in the literature (Table 12.4), the diagnosis by ERCP was incorrect in only five (1.6%) patients.

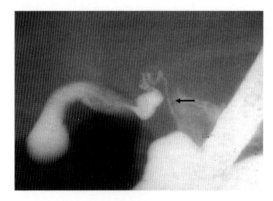

Fig. 12.3 Biliary atresia Type 2. Visualization of a narrow and irregular distal common bile duct (*arrow*). Normal cystic duct and gallbladder.

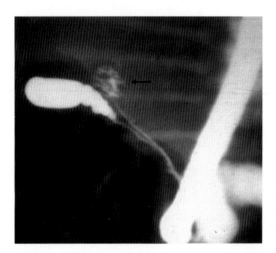

Fig. 12.4 Biliary atresia Type 3a in a 25-day-old neonate. Visualization of narrow and irregular distal common bile duct and common hepatic duct with biliary lakes (*arrow*) at the porta hepatis.

Table 12.4 ERCP findings in patients with neonatal cholestasis.

Author, year	No. patients	Visualization of the biliary tree		Visualization of only the PD
		Complete	Partial	
Derkx *et al.* 1994 [2]	18	5 (28%)	6 (33%)	7 (39%)
Mitchell and Wilkinson 1994 [5]	36	21 (58%)	10 (28%)	5 (14%)
Ohnuma *et al.* 1997 [6]	66	20 (30%)	11 (17%)	35 (53%)
Guelrud *et al.* 1997 [27]	147	85 (58%)	41 (28%)	21 (14%)
Iinuma *et al.* 2000 [4]	43	14 (33%)	5 (12%)	24 (56%)
Total	310	145 (47%)	73 (23%)	92 (30%)

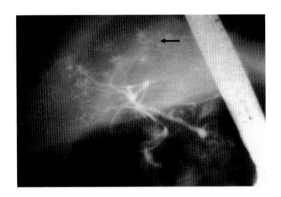

Fig. 12.5 Congenital hepatic fibrosis in a 38-day-old infant. Normal extrahepatic ducts. Irregular intrahepatic ducts with multiple small cysts (*arrow*).

Miscellaneous genetic cholestatic diseases

In Alagille syndrome, the extrahepatic ducts are normal. ERCP shows marked and diffuse narrowing of the intrahepatic duct and reduced arborization [27,28]. Congenital hepatic fibrosis is characterized by disordered terminal interlobular bile ducts, which form multiple macroscopic and microscopic cysts (Fig. 12.5) that can be demonstrated by ERCP [27]. In Caroli's disease, there are multiple segmental cylindrical or saccular dilatations of small biliary radicles with a normal common bile duct that can be demonstrated by ERCP [27]. Diagnosis of these conditions is necessary in order to avoid needless surgery.

Bile plug syndrome

Bile plug syndrome represents a correctable cause of obstruction of the extrahepatic bile ducts by bile sludge in patients with a normal biliary tract. The diagnosis is suspected by ultrasonography and confirmed by ERCP, which offers therapeutic possibility. Improvements of patients after ERCP suggest that simple irrigation with contrast material may be helpful [27].

Choledochal cyst

Choledochal cyst is a congenital malformation of the biliary tract characterized by saccular dilatation of the biliary tree. Choledochal cyst is primarily a disease of children and young adults, and 60% of reported cases are diagnosed before age 10 [29]. The diagnosis of this congenital malformation of the biliary tract is made by abdominal ultrasound, CT, or MRCP. ERCP confirms the diagnosis and helps surgical planning.

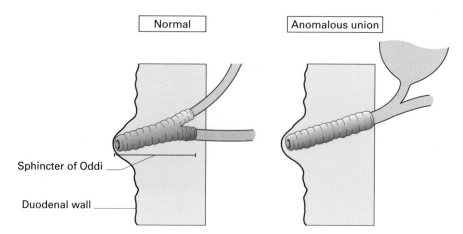

Fig. 12.6 The normal pancreatico-biliary union is located within the duodenal wall. The anomalous pancreatico-biliary union is located outside the duodenal wall and is not under the influence of the sphincter of Oddi mechanism.

Pathogenesis of choledochal cyst

Many theories have been proposed to explain the development of choledochal cysts. The more generally accepted theory proposes that cysts are acquired. The majority of patients with choledochal cysts have an anomalous pancreatico-biliary union [30–34] located outside the duodenal wall (Fig. 12.6) and are not under the influence of the sphincter of Oddi mechanism. According to this theory, there is reflux of pancreatic juice upward into the biliary system that can produce damage to the common duct lining resulting in saccular dilatation of the duct [35].

The maximum normal length of the common channel in neonates and infants younger than 1 year is 3 mm. It increases with age to a maximum of 5 mm in children and adolescents between 13 and 15 years of age [36].

Classification of anomalous ductal union   There are three types of anomalous ductal union [37]. If it appears that the pancreatic duct is joining the common bile duct, it is denoted as P–B type. If the common bile duct appears to join the main pancreatic duct, it is denoted as B–P type, and if there is only a long common channel, it is denoted as Long Y type (Fig. 12.7).

Classification of choledochal cysts

The anatomical classification by Todani *et al.* [38] of bile duct cysts is most often used (Fig. 12.8).

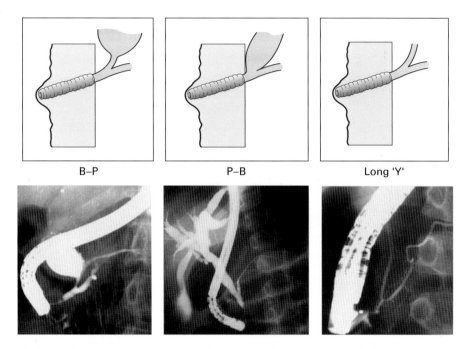

B–P

P–B

Long 'Y'

Fig. 12.7 There are three types of anomalous pancreatico-biliary union. Type B–P: the common bile duct appears to join the main pancreatic duct. Type P–B: the pancreatic duct is joining the common bile duct. Long Y type: there is only a long common channel.

Type I The Type I cyst is the most common and accounts for 80–90% of all choledochal cysts [29]. Type I is subdivided into: Type A, a typical cyst dilatation of the choledochus; Type B, segmental choledochal dilatation; and Type C, diffuse or fusiform dilatation (Figs 12.9 and 12.10).

Type II Type II is a diverticulum anywhere in the extrahepatic duct.

Type III Type III, a choledochocele, involves only the intraduodenal duct.

Type IV Type IV represents multiple intrahepatic and extrahepatic cysts (Fig. 12.11).

Type V Type V (Caroli's disease) includes single or multiple intrahepatic cysts.

Choledochocele Although classified as one of the forms of choledochal cysts, choledochocele is probably not related. It is a rare cause of obstructive jaundice. The diagnosis is established with certainty by ERCP, and it may be effectively treated with endoscopic sphincterotomy [39].

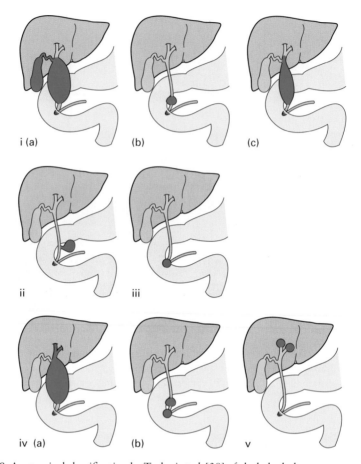

Fig. 12.8 Anatomical classification by Todani *et al.* [38] of choledochal cysts.

The presence of a distal bile duct stricture at its point of connection with the pancreatic duct is frequently observed (Fig. 12.11). Primary cystolithiasis occurs in 8% of patients and usually is multiple (Fig. 12.10), involving intrahepatic and extrahepatic ducts [29].

Treatment of choledochal cysts

The anomalous anatomical configuration of the pancreatico-biliary ductal system observed in most patients with choledochal cysts has certain technical implications with regard to management. In most patients, endoscopic sphincterotomy is probably not indicated, and endoscopic access to the biliary system for removal of stones or sludge is therefore not possible. In selected cases, with fusiform bile duct dilatation and widely dilated common channel, endoscopic sphincterotomy has been attempted, with encouraging results [40].

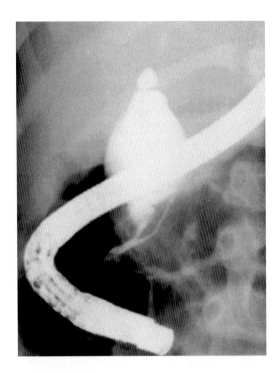

Fig. 12.9 Choledochal cyst Type I-C in a 3-year-old female. Note an anomalous Type B–P union.

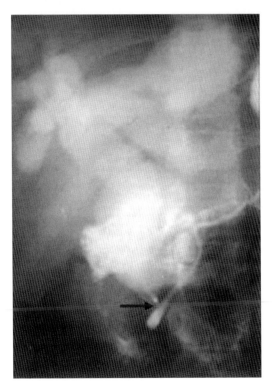

Fig. 12.10 Choledochal cyst Type I-C with cystolithiasis (*arrow*).

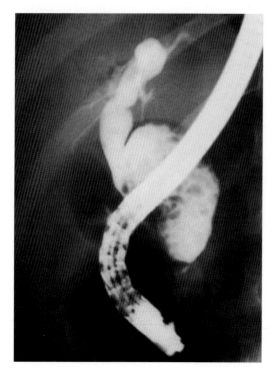

Fig. 12.11 Choledochal cyst Type IV-A in a 12-year-old female. Note an anomalous Type B–P union.

Fusiform choledochal dilatation and carcinoma

Fusiform choledochal dilatation, as opposed to cystic dilatation, has been observed to be more commonly associated with low-grade, short strictures located at or distal to the pancreatico-biliary junction [41]. Moreover, carcinoma seldom, if ever, develops in fusiform dilatation [42].

Primary sclerosing cholangitis

In children, primary sclerosing cholangitis is associated with histiocytosis X [43], immune deficiency states [44], and, less frequently, in patients with reticular cell sarcoma [45] and sickle cell anemia [46]. The association with inflammatory bowel disease is relatively uncommon (14%), suggesting that genetic and immunological features are the most important factors [47,48].

Most benign biliary strictures in children are due to sclerosing cholangitis. ERCP provides an accurate and sensitive method of diagnosing sclerosing cholangitis. Recently, MRCP has been shown to be a useful non-invasive diagnostic technique [49]. The cholangiogram will show pruning of the peripheral biliary tree and areas of stenosis and ectasia [27,48]. Patients with major ductal strictures are candidates for endoscopic treatment with sphincterotomy and

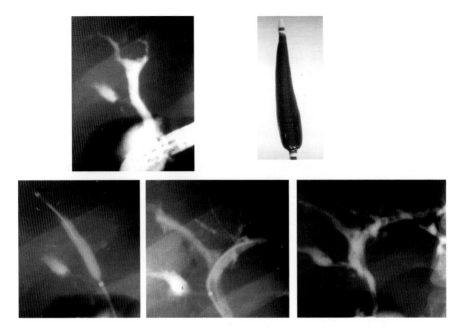

Fig. 12.12 Primary sclerosing cholangitis in a 16-year-old male. Severe narrowing of both right and left hepatic ducts without opacification of intrahepatic ducts. A guidewire is introduced into both hepatic ducts. A tapered hydrophilic balloon is fully inflated. Cholangiogram obtained immediately after dilatation shows visualization of irregular areas of stenosis and ectasia of intrahepatic ducts.

balloon dilatation to relieve the obstruction in order to delay the progression to cirrhosis [50]. Hydrostatic balloon dilatation has been used to dilate biliary strictures [51]. We developed a tapered hydrophilic balloon to dilate hepatic duct strictures and to avoid small intrahepatic duct rupture (Fig. 12.12) [52].

Parasitic infestation

Ascaris infestation can produce acute biliary obstruction with cholangitis. The worm can be seen with ERCP and can be removed with a tripod basket [27].

Choledocholithiasis

Choledocholithiasis occurs rarely in both infants and children [53]. Conditions associated with the presence of stones include biliary tract malformations such as choledochal cyst, chronic liver disease, hemolysis, and infection. The diagnostic approach is more difficult, and identification of the cause of obstruction by ultrasonography is often impossible. MRCP is the best non-invasive technique in demonstrating common bile duct stones and is clearly superior to ultrasonography [54].

ERCP for stones

The role and value of ERCP and endoscopic sphincterotomy in children with choledocholithiasis are not well established. Sphincterotomy with common bile duct stone removal has been successfully performed in young infants [55], and in children and adolescents [11,56–60]. Endoscopic papillary balloon dilatation with stone extraction is an alternative technique for stone removal [61]. However, pancreatitis can occur in 7% of cases. In children, published experience with this technique is limited [59].

Most infants with asymptomatic gallstones and no factors that would make them susceptible to stone formation can be managed conservatively [62]. However, larger stones are less likely to resolve, whereas smaller stones, sludge, and mucus should be able to pass in response to oral feeding without symptoms or complications. In children, sphincterotomy should be reserved for symptomatic patients or those with underlying lithogenic disorders.

A combined endoscopic sphincterotomy with common stone extraction followed by laparoscopic cholecystectomy has been successfully reported in children [63]. Although the combined procedure seems to be safe, additional experience is awaited so that the true advantages, limitations, and complications of this approach can be placed into clinical perspective.

Biliary strictures and leaks

Primary stricture

Primary stricture of the common hepatic duct has been reported [64]. Hydrostatic balloon dilatation may be used in the treatment of dominant common duct strictures [27].

Malignant strictures

Malignant strictures of the common bile duct are uncommon in children and have been successfully treated by placement of stents [65,66].

Liver transplantation

In patients whose liver is transplanted, the integrity of the anastomosis can be studied. ERCP is an alternative to percutaneous transhepatic cholangiography, and is the procedure of choice in patients with coagulopathy when the biliary tree must be imaged. When a stricture is found, the area may be dilated and a stent may be placed for a limited period of time.

Bile leaks

Bile leaks may be found and can be treated by endoscopic sphincterotomy or with stent placement [67].

Pancreatic findings (Table 12.5)

Recurrent pancreatitis

ERCP has been found to be useful in the identification of treatable causes in approximately 75% of children with recurrent pancreatitis [10–14,18,21,24,68–70]. Whatever the etiology of pancreatitis, the possibility of an anatomical abnormality amenable to endoscopic therapy or surgery should always be considered.

The timing of performance of an ERCP in children is controversial. In children with idiopathic pancreatitis in whom recovery has occurred with standard

Table 12.5 Pancreatic findings in ERCP in children.

Recurrent pancreatitis
Congenital disorders
  Biliary anomalies
    Choledochal cyst
    Anomalous pancreatico-biliary union
  Pancreatic anomalies
    Pancreas divisum
    Annular pancreas
    Short pancreas
    Cystic dilatation of the pancreatic duct
     (pancreatocele)
  Duodenal anomalies
    Duodenal or gastric duplication cysts
    Duodenal diverticulum

Acquired disorders
  Parasitic infestation: *Ascaris*
  Sphincter of Oddi dysfunction
  Pancreatic trauma
  Acquired immunodeficiency syndrome

Chronic pancreatitis

Pseudocysts

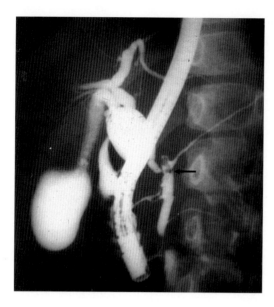

Fig. 12.13 Choledochal cyst Type I-A and pancreas divisum in a 5-year-old male with recurrent pancreatitis. A long common channel is observed with pancreatic stones (*arrow*).

medical treatment, there is no consensus as to when an ERCP to look for an obstructive cause is indicated. The potential benefit of proceeding with ERCP after the first episode as opposed to waiting for a second attack of pancreatitis is, of course, in preventing that second episode with its associated morbidity and mortality. No randomized controlled clinical trials have been performed that directly address this issue. Although not reported in the literature, it is the experience of the author that children with normal MRCP after the first episode of pancreatitis should not be studied.

Choledochal cyst and anomalous pancreatico-biliary union

Choledochal cysts have been associated with recurrent pancreatitis in 6–18% of cases [9–13,18,21,69,70]. An anomalous pancreatico-biliary union has been observed in most children with choledochal cysts and recurrent pancreatitis (Fig. 12.13) [37,71,72]. In this subgroup of patients, sphincter of Oddi dysfunction has been demonstrated, suggesting that this motor abnormality might be related to the development of recurrent pancreatitis [72]. Moreover, because the sphincter of Oddi muscular segment is located within the duodenal wall, endoscopic sphincterotomy prior to surgery has been performed with excellent results, supporting this theory [72]. Occasionally, pancreatic stones or protein plugs may be endoscopically removed (Fig. 12.14) [27]. Choledochoceles have been reported in patients with recurrent pancreatitis [27,73,74]. Treatment by endoscopic sphincterotomy provides excellent results [70,75].

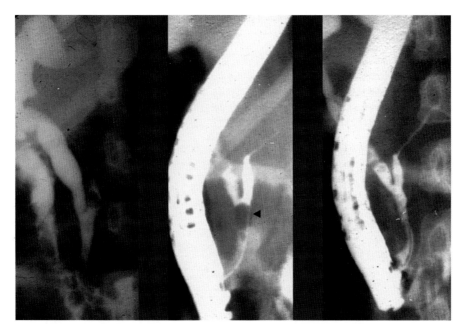

Fig. 12.14 Choledochal cyst Type IV-A in a 6-year-old female with recurrent pancreatitis. An anomalous pancreatico-biliary union, Long Y type. Stone in the pancreatic duct (*arrow*). After endoscopic sphincterotomy the pancreatic stone is removed with an occlusion balloon (*arrowhead*).

Pancreas divisum Pancreas divisum is a congenital anomaly caused by failure of fusion of the dorsal and ventral endodermal buds. Each duct drains via its own separate orifice, the major papilla of Vater for the ventral duct of Wirsung, and the minor accessory papilla for the dorsal duct of Santorini.

Prevalence of pancreas divisum
Pancreas divisum is the most common congenital anomaly of the pancreas. In adults, it has been found in 5–14% of autopsy series and 0.3–8% of ERCP studies [76,77].

The prevalence of pancreas divisum in children is not known. In our experience with 272 consecutive cases of successful ERCP performed in children, pancreas divisum was found in nine (3.3%) children [78]. Two patient groups were identified on the basis of the age at which ERCP was performed. Group 1 included 147 neonates or young infants in whom ERCP was performed to evaluate neonatal cholestasis. Two (1.4%) neonates had pancreas divisum, one with neonatal hepatitis and the other with biliary atresia. Group 2 included 125 children older than 1 year in whom ERCP was performed to evaluate pancreatic and biliary disorders. Seven (5.6%) children had pancreas divisum.

Table 12.6 Frequency of pancreas divisum in children with recurrent pancreatitis.

Author, year	No. of patients	No. of patients with pancreas divisum
Forbes *et al.* 1984 [69]	25	4 (16%)
Buckley and Connon 1990 [11]	18	1 (5%)
Putnam *et al.* 1991 [21]	12	0
Dite *et al.* 1992 [13]	16	1 (6%)
Brown and Goldschmiedt 1994 [10]	9	2 (22%)
Lemmel *et al.* 1994 [18]	29	2 (7%)
Guelrud *et al.* 1994 [70]	50	6 (12%)
Portwood *et al.* 1995 [20]	26	3 (11%)
Manegold *et al.* 1996 [19]	38	3 (8%)
Graham *et al.* 1998 [14]	23	1 (4%)
Hsu *et al.* 2000 [16]	22	6 (27%)
Poddar *et al.* 2001 [24]	28	3 (11%)
Total	296	32 (10.8%)

Significance of pancreas divisum

The clinical significance of pancreas divisum is controversial. An association between pancreas divisum and pancreatitis has been suggested [76,79–83]. However, others [84–86] have considered it to be a coincidental finding. It appears that the combination of pancreas divisum with accessory papilla stenosis would lead to a real functional obstruction. In 296 children with recurrent pancreatitis, pancreas divisum has been found in 10.8% of patients (Table 12.6).

ERCP diagnosis of pancreas divisum

ERCP is mandatory in the diagnosis of pancreas divisum. Cannulation of the major papilla shows a short duct of Wirsung (ventral pancreas) that quickly tapers and undergoes arborization (Fig. 12.15). To confirm the diagnosis, it is most important to cannulate the minor papilla to demonstrate the dorsal pancreas. Interventional treatment in patients with pancreas divisum is applied to those whose symptoms are disabling.

Treatment of pancreas divisum

Surgical minor papilla sphincteroplasty used to be the treatment of choice, with a 70% improvement [87]. Endoscopic treatment has been utilized to decompress the dorsal duct by a variety of methods, including endoscopic minor papilla sphincterotomy with or without insertion of an endoprosthesis.

Endoscopic sphincterotomy of the minor papilla is indicated in patients with disabling symptoms. It has been attempted in conjunction with temporary stent

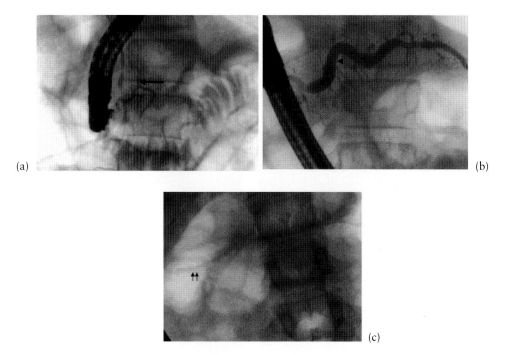

Fig. 12.15 Pancreas divisum and chronic pancreatitis in a 12-year-old male. (a) Cannulation of the major papilla shows a normal common duct and a small ventral pancreatic duct (*arrow*). (b) Cannulation of the minor papilla shows a dilated dorsal pancreatic duct (*arrowhead*) with dilated primary and secondary branches. (c) After minor papilla sphincterotomy, a 5 Fr pancreatic stent (*two arrows*) without proximal flaps was left in place for 5 days.

placement in the dorsal pancreatic duct (Fig. 12.16), and has led to improvement in approximately 75% of children [16,18,70]. Overall, these results indicate that in certain children with recurrent pain or pancreatitis and pancreas divisum, endoscopic therapy can offer relief or improvement of symptoms.

Other pancreatic congenital anomalies

Annular pancreas has been associated with recurrent pancreatitis in children [70,88–90]. However, the relationship with pancreatitis is unclear. In 14 cases of annular pancreas reported in the English literature, there were five with coexistent pancreas divisum, suggesting that pancreas divisum occurs more often in the presence of annular pancreas than in the general population [89]. This associ-ation may explain pancreatitis in some patients.

Other pancreatic congenital anomalies found to cause pancreatitis include short pancreas [70,91] and cystic dilatation or pancreatocele of the distal pancreatic duct [60].

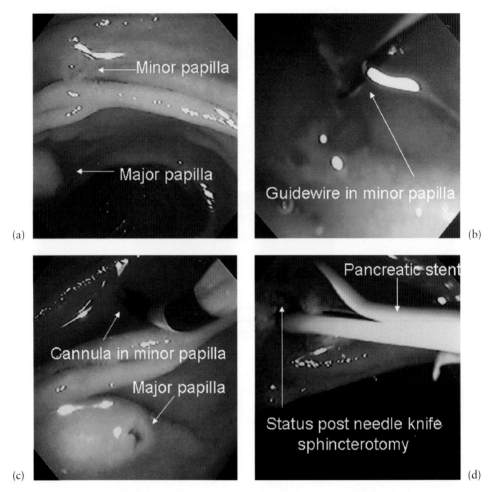

Fig. 12.16 Endoscopic view of the major and minor papilla. (a) A tapered balloon (3 Fr) is used to cannulate the minor papilla. (b) A guidewire is introduced into the dorsal pancreas. (c) A 5 Fr pancreatic stent is introduced into the dorsal pancreas. (d) A sphincterotomy of the minor papilla is performed with a needle-knife sphincterotome over the pancreatic stent.

Duodenal duplication cyst

Duodenal duplication cyst is a congenital anomaly which has been associated with recurrent pancreatitis due to intermittent obstruction of the pancreatic duct [92,93]. ERCP has been shown to be useful in the diagnosis as well as for definitive treatment [92]. If the cyst is bulging into the intestinal lumen, a wide cysto-duodenostomy can be endoscopically performed, with excellent results [94].

Sphincter of Oddi dysfunction

Sphincter of Oddi manometry is the diagnostic procedure of choice for this functional motor disorder. It was found in 17 out of 139 (12.2%) children with recurrent pancreatitis [9,16,18,70]. These patients are generally treated by standard biliary sphincterotomy and, in general, they do not respond well [16], presumably because the pancreatic sphincter is not transected. Recurrent attacks of pancreatitis may be attributed to an affected pancreatic sphincter [95]. Dual endoscopic sphincterotomy of the pancreatic and common duct sphincters may be necessary to improve outcome [70]. However, the safety and efficacy of sphincter of Oddi manometry and sphincterotomy in the pediatric population await further study.

Pancreatic trauma

Recent evidence has suggested that it is safe to perform ERCP during non-resolving traumatic pancreatitis and it may be helpful in identifying the need for endoscopic therapy or surgery [96–98]. Early ERCP may identify the presence and location of duct leakage. Patients with normal ductograms are treated conservatively. Successful treatment by placement of an intrapancreatic ductal stent may be possible at the same time [98]. Surgical resection or reconstruction can then be reserved for cases in which stenting is impossible or fails.

Acquired immunodeficiency syndrome (AIDS)

Little has been written regarding pancreatic involvement in children with AIDS. Opportunistic infections may involve the pancreas, just as they do the other digestive organs in children with AIDS [99]. Most common are cytomegalovirus and *Cryptosporidium*, followed by *Pneumocystis carinii*, *Toxoplasma gondii*, and *Mycobacterium avium*. Drug-induced pancreatitis is a common complication of pentamidine [99] and dideoxyinosine [100]. ERCP has been shown to be useful in the evaluation and treatment of children with AIDS [101,102]. Pancreatic duct dilatation in two children with pancreatic duct stricture produced significant clinical improvement of pain.

Chronic pancreatitis

ERCP has been found to be useful in the identification of chronic pancreatitis in 14–69% of children with recurrent pancreatitis [9–22,69,70]. Two major morphological patterns can be demonstrated: (1) chronic calcifying pancreatitis, most often due to hereditary pancreatitis, fibrosing pancreatitis, or juvenile tropical pancreatitis; (2) chronic obstructive pancreatitis, which is associated with congenital or acquired lesions of the pancreatic duct or biliary tree, similar to those etiological factors found in recurrent pancreatitis.

In children with chronic pancreatitis, debilitating pain and recurrent attacks may be caused by strictures of the main duct, pancreatic stones, or pseudocysts

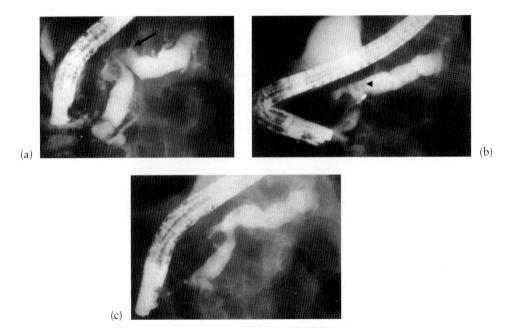

Fig. 12.17 Chronic pancreatitis in a 14-year-old female with hereditary pancreatitis.
(a) Big pancreatic stones at the junction of the head and body of the pancreatic duct (*arrow*).
(b) Two days after pancreatic sphincterotomy, followed by extracorporeal shock-wave lithotripsy, multiple small residual stones (*arrowhead*) are retrieved with a Dormia basket.
(c) After a month, a follow-up ERCP showed a dilated pancreatic duct without stones.

that impair the normal outflow of pancreatic juice. ERCP demonstrates evidence of these abnormalities that can be treated endoscopically [10,14–16,18,24,70,103].

Endoscopic treatment of chronic pancreatitis in children   The aim of endoscopic therapy is based on the concept of pancreatic duct decompression. Pancreatic sphincterotomy has been performed to improve pancreatic drainage and to allow intraductal therapeutic maneuvers, severe stenosis has been dilated and bypassed with stents, and obstructing ductal stones have been removed after destruction by electrohydraulic lithotripter or extracorporeal shock-wave lithotripter (Fig. 12.17). These endoscopic techniques constitute an excellent alternative to relieve recurrent abdominal pain and to avoid progressive parenchymal damage to the gland.

Pancreatic endotherapy has been reported in children in abstract form in five different centers [18–20,22,88], demonstrating that endoscopic pancreatic therapy in childhood is well tolerated, safe, and likely to be technically successful in experienced hands. Overall, there is an 80% short-term symptomatic

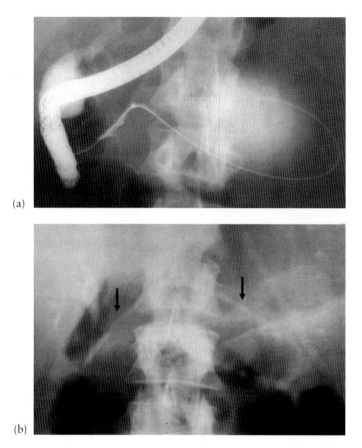

(a)

(b)

Fig. 12.18 Pancreatic pseudocyst with ductal communication treated by transpapillary pancreatic duct endoprosthesis in a 13-year-old female. (a) After endoscopic sphincterotomy of the biliary and pancreatic sphincters, a guidewire is introduced into the cystic cavity. (b) A 7 Fr stent (*arrows*) is placed beyond the stricture.

improvement after pancreatic endoscopic therapy in children with chronic pancreatitis [10,18,70,103]. A longer follow-up period will be necessary to determine whether endoscopic success produces long-standing clinical improvement.

Pancreatic pseudocysts

Pancreatic pseudocysts are common consequences of acute and chronic pancreatitis. Most of the pseudocysts resolve spontaneously. Symptomatic, large (> 4 cm), or persistent pseudocysts beyond 6 weeks are unlikely to resolve and are at risk of complication [104]. In these cases treatment is indicated. Recently, there has been increased interest in non-operative management of pancreatic pseudocysts. Endoscopic methods have been developed as an alternative to surgical treatment and percutaneous drainage of pseudocysts. These endoscopic methods include endoscopic cystogastrostomy, cystoduodenostomy, and transpapillary drainage (Fig. 12.18). In adults, successful pseudocyst resolution has been reported in approximately 80% of cases [105–107]. As with other therapeutic interventions, pediatric experience is limited to a few case reports [9,18,70,103].

Outstanding issues and future trends

ERCP is an established procedure in children. Even though there is an increased number of pediatric gastroenterologists performing ERCP, there is not enough volume for them to gain proficiency. This has become more apparent since, nowadays, ERCP is less diagnostic and more therapeutic. It is my belief that, in future, ERCP in children will be performed by highly trained endoscopists working in tertiary care facilities, which maintain a high volume of such activity. Further studies should be directed to assess the usefulness of MRCP in the diagnosis of biliopancreatic diseases in children. In general, children with suspected biliary and pancreatic disease should undergo MRCP before ERCP is considered, with the latter increasingly being reserved for therapy.

References

1 Guelrud M, Jaen D, Torres P et al. Endoscopic cholangiopancreatography in the infant: evaluation of a new prototype pediatric duodenoscope. *Gastrointest Endosc* 1987; 33: 4–8.
2 Derkx HH, Huibregtse K, Taminiau JA. The role of endoscopic retrograde cholangiopancreatography in cholestatic infants. *Endoscopy* 1994; 26: 724–8.
3 Heyman MB, Shapiro HA, Thaler MM. Endoscopic retrograde cholangiography in the diagnosis of biliary malformations in infants. *Gastrointest Endosc* 1988; 34: 449–53.
4 Iinuma Y, Narisawa R, Iwafuchi M et al. The role of endoscopic retrograde cholangiopancreatography in infants with cholestasis. *J Pediatr Surg* 2000; 35: 545–9.
5 Mitchell SA, Wilkinson ML. The role of ERCP in the diagnosis of neonatal conjugated hyperbilirubinemia. *Gastrointest Endosc* 1994; 40: A55.
6 Ohnuma N, Takahashi T, Tanabe M et al. The role of ERCP in biliary atresia. *Gastrointest Endosc* 1997; 45: 365–70.
7 Wilkinson ML, Mieli-Vergani G, Ball C et al. Endoscopic retrograde cholangiopancreatography in infantile cholestasis. *Arch Dis Child* 1991; 66: 121–3.
8 Abu-Khalaf A. The role of endoscopic retrograde cholangiopancreatography in small children and adolescents. *Surg Laparosc Endosc* 1995; 5: 296–300.
9 Brown CW, Werlin SL, Geenen JE et al. The diagnostic and therapeutic role of endoscopic retrograde cholangiopancreatography in children. *J Pediatr Gastroenterol Nutr* 1993; 17: 19–23.
10 Brown KO, Goldschmiedt M. Endoscopic therapy of biliary and pancreatic disorders in children. *Endoscopy* 1994; 26: 719–23.
11 Buckley A, Connon JJ. The role of ERCP in children and adolescents. *Gastrointest Endosc* 1990; 36: 369–72.
12 Cotton PB, Laage NJ. Endoscopic retrograde cholangiopancreatography in children. *Arch Dis Child* 1982; 57: 131–6.
13 Dite P, Vacek E, Stefan H et al. Endoscopic retrograde cholangiopancreatography in childhood. *Hepatogastroenterology* 1992; 39: 291–3.

14 Graham KS, Ingram JD, Steinberg SE *et al.* ERCP in the management of pediatric pancreatitis. *Gastrointest Endosc* 1998; 47: 492–5.

15 Guitron A, Adalid R, Barinagarrementeria R *et al.* Endoscopic cholangiopancreatography (ERCP) in pediatric patients. *Rev Gastroenterol Mex* 1998; 63: 211–16.

16 Hsu RK, Draganov P, Leung JW *et al.* Therapeutic ERCP in the management of pancreatitis in children. *Gastrointest Endosc* 2000; 51: 396–400.

17 Kunitomo K, Ming L, Urakami Y *et al.* Endoscopic retrograde cholangiopancreatography in pediatric surgical biliary diseases. *Tokushima J Exp Med* 1988; 35: 57–62.

18 Lemmel T, Hawes R, Sherman S *et al.* Endoscopic evaluation and therapy of recurrent pancreatitis and pancreaticobiliary pain in the pediatric population. *Gastrointest Endosc* 1994; 40: A54.

19 Manegold BC, Gottstein T, Pescatore P. Diagnostic and therapeutic ERCP in children under 14 years. *Gastrointest Endosc* 1996; 43: A328.

20 Portwood G, Maniatis A, Jowell PS *et al.* Diagnostic and therapeutic ERCP in children: safe with a high success rate in experienced hands. *Gastrointest Endosc* 1995; 41: A342.

21 Putnam PE, Kocoshis SA, Orenstein SR *et al.* Pediatric endoscopic retrograde cholangiopancreatography. *Am J Gastroenterol* 1991; 86: 824–30.

22 Su AY, Hernandez EJ, Brown K *et al.* Therapeutic endoscopic retrograde cholangiopancreatography in children. *Gastrointest Endosc* 1996; 43: A330.

23 Tagge EP, Tarnasky PR, Chandler J *et al.* Multidisciplinary approach to the treatment of pediatric pancreaticobiliary disorders. *J Pediatr Surg* 1997; 32: 158–64.

24 Poddar U, Thapa BR, Bhasin DK *et al.* Endoscopic retrograde cholangiopancreatography in the management of pancreaticobiliary disorders in children. *J Gastroenterol Hepatol* 2001; 16: 927–31.

25 Balistreri WF. Neonatal cholestasis. *J Pediatr* 1985; 106: 171–84.

26 Guelrud M, Jaen D, Mendoza S *et al.* ERCP in the diagnosis of extrahepatic biliary atresia. *Gastrointest Endosc* 1991; 37: 522–6.

27 Guelrud M, Carr-Locke D, Fox VL. *ERCP in Pediatric Practice. Diagnosis and Treatment.* Oxford: Isis Medical Media Ltd, 1997.

28 Morelli A, Pelli MA, Vedovelli A *et al.* Endoscopic retrograde cholangiopancreatography study in Alagille's syndrome: first report. *Am J Gastroenterol* 1983; 78: 241–4.

29 Yamaguchi M. Congenital choledochal cyst: analysis of 1433 patients in the Japanese literature. *Am J Surg* 1980; 140: 653–7.

30 Guelrud M, Jaen D, Mendoza S *et al.* Usefulness of endoscopic retrograde cholangiopancreatography in diagnosis of choledochal cysts in children. *G E N* 1989; 43: 9–12.

31 Kimura K, Ohto M, Ono T *et al.* Congenital cystic dilatation of the common bile duct: relationship to anomalous pancreaticobiliary ductal union. *Am J Roentgenol* 1977; 928: 571–7.

32 Arima E, Akita H. Congenital biliary tract dilatation and anomalous junction of the pancreaticobiliary system. *J Pediatr Surg* 1979; 14: 9–15.

33 Oguchi Y, Okada A, Nakamura T *et al.* Histopathologic studies of congenital dilatation of the bile duct as related to an anomalous junction of the pancreaticobiliary ductal system: clinical and experimental studies. *Surgery* 1988; 103: 168–73.

34 Ikada A, Nakamura T, Higaki J *et al.* Congenital dilatation of the bile duct in 100 instances and its relationship with anomalous junction. *Surg Gynecol Obstet* 1990; 171: 291–8.

35 Babbitt DP. Congenital choledochal cysts: new etiological concept based on anomalous relationship of common bile duct and pancreatic bulb. *Ann Radiol* 1969; 12: 231–40.

36 Guelrud M, Morera C, Rodriguez M *et al.* Normal and anomalous pancreaticobiliary union in children and adolescents. *Gastrointest Endosc* 1999; 50: 189–93.

37 Misra SP, Dwivedi M. Pancreaticobiliary ductal union. *Gut* 1990; 31: 1144–9.

38 Todani T, Watanabe Y, Narusue M. Congenital bile duct cyst. *Am J Surg* 1977; 134: 263–9.

39 Venu RP, Geenen JE, Hogan WJ *et al.* Role of endoscopic retrograde cholangiopancreatography in the diagnosis and treatment of choledochocele. *Gastroenterology* 1984; 87: 1144–9.

40 Ng WD, Liu K, Wong MK *et al.* Endoscopic sphincterotomy in young patients with choledochal dilatation and a long common channel: a preliminary report. *Br J Surg* 1992; 79: 550–2.

41 Ito T, Ando M, Nagaya T, Sugito T. Congenital dilatation of the common bile duct in children: the etiologic significance of the narrow segment distal to the dilated common bile duct. *Z Kinderchir* 1984; 30: 40–5.

42 Todani T, Watanabe Y, Fujii T *et al.* Cylindrical dilatation of the choledochus: a special type of congenital bile duct dilatation. *Surgery* 1985; 98: 964–8.

43 Leblanc A, Hadchouel M, Jehan P *et al.* Obstructive jaundice in children with histiocytosis X. *Gastroenterology* 1981; 80: 134–9.

44 DiPalma JA, Strobel CT, Farrow JG. Primary sclerosing cholangitis associated with hyper-immunoglobulin M immunodeficiency (dysgammaglobulinemia). *Gastroenterology* 1986; 91: 464–8.

45 Alpert LI, Jindrak K. Idiopathic retroperitoneal fibrosis and sclerosing cholangitis associated with a reticulum cell sarcoma. *Gastroenterology* 1972; 62: 111–17.

46 Werlin LS, Glicklich M, Jona J *et al.* Sclerosing cholangitis in childhood. *J Pediatr* 1980; 96: 433–5.

47 Debray D, Pariente D, Urroas E *et al.* Sclerosing cholangitis in children. *J Pediatr* 1994; 124: 49–56.

48 Classen M, Golze H, Richter HJ *et al.* Primary sclerosing cholangitis in children. *J Pediatr Gastroenterol Nutr* 1987; 6: 197–202.

49 Ferrara C, Valeri G, Salvolini L *et al.* Magnetic resonance cholangiopancreatography in primary sclerosing cholangitis in children. *Pediatr Radiol* 2002; 32: 413–17.

50 Stoker J, Lameris JS, Robben SG *et al.* Primary sclerosing cholangitis in a child treated by non-surgical balloon dilatation and stenting. *J Pediatr Gastroenterol Nutr* 1993; 17: 303–6.

51 Siegel JH, Guelrud M. Endoscopic cholangiopancreatoplasty: hydrostatic balloon dilation in the bile duct and pancreas. *Gastrointest Endosc* 1983; 29: 99–103.

52 Guelrud M, Mendoza S, Guelrud A. A tapered balloon with hydrophilic coating to dilate difficult hilar biliary strictures. *Gastrointest Endosc* 1995; 41: 246–9.

53 Shaw PJ, Spitz L, Watson JG. Extrahepatic biliary obstruction due to stone. *Arch Dis Child* 1984; 59: 896–7.

54 Arcement CM, Meza MP, Arumania S *et al.* MRCP in the evaluation of pancreaticobiliary disease in children. *Pediatr Radiol* 2001; 31: 92–7.

55 Guelrud M, Daoud G, Mendoza S *et al.* Endoscopic sphincterotomy in a 6-month-old infant with choledocholithiasis and double gallbladder. *Am J Gastroenterol* 1994; 89: 1587–9.

56 Brown KO, Goldschmiedt M. Use of ERCP with pancreatic and biliary sphincterotomy for treatment of familial pancreatitis in a 2 year old pediatric patient. *Gastrointest Endosc* 1993; 39: A309.

57 Guelrud M, Mendoza S, Jaen D *et al.* ERCP and endoscopic sphincterotomy in infants and children with jaundice due to common bile duct stones. *Gastrointest Endosc* 1992; 38: 450–3.

58 Man DW, Spitz L. Choledocholithiasis in infancy. *J Pediatr Surg* 1985; 20: 65–8.

59 Tarnasky PR, Tagge EP, Hebra A *et al.* Minimally invasive therapy for choledocholithiasis in children. *Gastrointest Endosc* 1998; 47: 189–92.

60 Sandoval C, Stringel G, Ozkaynak MF *et al.* Perioperative management in children with sickle cell disease undergoing laparoscopic surgery. *JSLS* 2002; 6: 29–33.

61 Komatsu Y, Kawabe T, Toda N *et al.* Endoscopic papillary balloon dilation for the management of common bile duct stones: experience of 226 cases. *Endoscopy* 1998; 30: 12–17.

62 Wesdorp I, Bosman D, de Graaff A *et al.* Clinical presentations and predisposing factors of cholelithiasis and sludge in children. *Pediatr Gastroenterol Nutr* 2000; 31: 411–17.

63 Guelrud M, Zambrano V, Jaen D *et al.* Endoscopic sphincterotomy and laparoscopic cholecystectomy in a jaundiced infant. *Gastrointest Endosc* 1994; 40: 99–102.

64 Chapoy PR, Kendall RS, Fonkalsrud E *et al.* Congenital stricture of the common hepatic duct: an unusual case without jaundice. *Gastroenterology* 1981; 80: 380–3.

65 Bickerstaff KI, Britton BJ, Gough MH. Endoscopic palliation of malignant biliary obstruction in a child. *Br J Surg* 1989; 76: 1092–3.

66 Guelrud M, Mendoza S, Zager A *et al.* Biliary stenting in an infant with malignant obstructive jaundice. *Gastrointest Endosc* 1989; 35: 259–61.

67 Pfau PR, Kochman ML, Lewis JD *et al.* Endoscopic management of postoperative biliary com-
    plications in orthotopic liver transplantation. *Gastrointest Endosc* 2000; 52: 55–63.
68 Blustein PK, Gaskin K, Filler R *et al.* Endoscopic retrograde cholangiopancreatography in pan-
    creatitis in children and adolescents. *Pediatrics* 1981; 68: 387–93.
69 Forbes A, Leung JW, Cotton PB. Relapsing acute and chronic pancreatitis. *Arch Dis Child*
    1984; 59: 927–34.
70 Guelrud M, Mujica C, Jaen D *et al.* The role of ERCP in the diagnosis and treatment of idio-
    pathic recurrent pancreatitis in children and adolescents. *Gastrointest Endosc* 1994; 40:
    428–36.
71 Mori K, Nagakawa T, Ohta T *et al.* Pancreatitis and anomalous union of the pancreaticobili-
    ary ductal system in childhood. *J Pediatr Surg* 1993; 28: 67–71.
72 Guelrud M, Morera C, Rodriguez M *et al.* Sphincter of Oddi dysfunction in children with
    recurrent pancreatitis and anomalous pancreaticobiliary union: an etiologic concept. *Gastro-
    intest Endosc* 1999; 50: 194–9.
73 Greene FL, Brown JJ, Rubinstein P *et al.* Choledochocele and recurrent pancreatitis. Diagnosis
    and surgical management. *Am J Surg* 1985; 149: 306–9.
74 Weisser M, Bennek J, Hormann D. Choledochocele—a rare cause of necrotizing pancreatitis in
    childhood. *Eur J Pediatr Surg* 2000; 10: 258–64.
75 Siegel JH, Harding GT, Chateau F. Endoscopic incision of choledochal cysts (choledochocele).
    Endoscopy 1981; 13: 200–2.
76 Cotton PB. Congenital anomaly of pancreas divisum as a cause of obstructive pain and pancre-
    atitis. *Gut* 1980; 21: 105.
77 Bernard JP, Sahel J, Giovanni M *et al.* Pancreas divisum is a probable cause of acute pancre-
    atitis: a report of 137 cases. *Pancreas* 1990; 5: 248.
78 Guelrud M. The incidence of pancreas divisum in children [letter]. *Gastrointest Endosc* 1996;
    43: 83–4.
79 Cotton PB. Pancreas divisum. Curiosity or culprit? *Gastroenterology* 1985; 89: 1431.
80 Gregg JA. Pancreas divisum: its association with pancreatitis. *Am J Surg* 1977; 1 (34): 539.
81 Heiss FN, Shea JA. Association of pancreatitis and various ductal anatomy: dominant drainage
    of the duct of Santorini. *Am J Gastroenterol* 1978; 70: 158.
82 Richter JM, Shapiro RH, Mulley AG *et al.* Association of pancreas divisum and pancreatitis,
    and its treatment by sphincterotomy of the accessory ampulla. *Gastroenterology* 1981; 81:
    1104.
83 Neblett WW, O'Neill JA. Surgical management of recurrent pancreatitis in children with pan-
    creas divisum. *Ann Surg* 2000; 231: 899.
84 Delhaye M, Engelholm L, Cremer M. Pancreas divisum: congenital anatomic variant or
    anomaly? Contribution of endoscopic retrograde dorsal pancreatography. *Gastroenterology*
    1985; 89: 951.
85 Mitchell CJ, Lintott DJ, Ruddell WSJ *et al.* Clinical relevance of an unfused pancreatic duct
    system. *Gut* 1979; 20: 1066.
86 Rosch W, Koch H, Schaffner O *et al.* The clinical significance of pancreas divisum. *Gastro-
    intest Endosc* 1976; 22: 206.
87 Warshaw AL, Simeone JF, Schapiro RH *et al.* Evaluation and treatment of the dominant dorsal
    duct syndrome (pancreas divisum redefined). *Am J Surg* 1990; 159: 59.
88 Fox VL, Lichtenstein DR, Carr-Locke DL. Incomplete pancreas divisum in children with recur-
    rent pancreatitis (Abstract). *Gastrointest Endosc* 1995; 41: A337.
89 Lehman GA, O'Connor KW. Coexistence of annular pancreas and pancreas divisum – ERCP
    diagnosis. *Gastrointest Endosc* 1985; 31: 25–8.
90 Yogi Y, Shibue T, Hashimoto S. Annular pancreas detected in adults, diagnosed by endoscopic
    retrograde cholangiopancreatography: report of four cases. *Gastroenterol Jpn* 1987; 22: 92.
91 Rosenstock F, Achkar E. A 'short pancreas'. *Gastrointest Endosc* 1986; 32: 296.
92 Holstege A, Barner S, Brambs HJ *et al.* Relapsing pancreatitis associated with duodenal wall
    cysts. Diagnostic approach and treatment. *Gastroenterology* 1985; 88: 814.
93 Lavine JE, Harrison M, Heyman MB. Gastrointestinal duplications causing relapsing pancre-
    atitis in children. *Gastroenterology* 1989; 97: 1556.

94 Johanson JF, Geenen JE, Hogan WJ *et al.* Endoscopic therapy of a duodenal duplication cyst. *Gastrointest Endosc* 1992; 38: 60.

95 Guelrud M, Siegel JH. Hypertensive pancreatic duct sphincter as a cause of pancreatitis. Successful treatment with hydrostatic balloon dilatation. *Dig Dis Sci* 1984; 29: 225–31.

96 Hall RI, Lavelle MI, Venables CW. Use of ERCP to identify the site of traumatic injuries of the main pancreatic duct in children. *Br J Surg* 1986; 73: 411–2.

97 Rescorla FJ, Plumley DA, Sherman S *et al.* The efficacy of early ERCP in pediatric pancreatic trauma. *J Pediatr Surg* 1995; 30: 336–40.

98 Canty TG, Weinman D. Treatment of pancreatic duct disruption in children by an endoscopically placed stent. *J Pediatr Surg* 2001; 36: 345–8.

99 Miller TL, Winter HS, Luginbuhl LM *et al.* Pancreatitis in pediatric human immunodeficiency virus infection. *J Pediatr* 1992; 120: 223.

100 Butler KM, Venzon D, Henry N *et al.* Pancreatitis in human immunodeficiency virus-infected children receiving dideoxyinosine. *Pediatrics* 1993; 91: 747.

101 Naon H, Shelton M, Thomas D *et al.* Retrograde-cholangio-pancreatic videoendoscopy (ERCP) findings in pediatric patients with acquired immunodeficiency syndrome (AIDS). *Gastrointest Endosc* 1995; 41: A430.

102 Yabut B, Werlin SL, Havens P *et al.* Endoscopic retrograde cholangiopancreatography in children with HIV infection. *J Pediatr Gastroenterol Nutr* 1996; 23: 624.

103 Kozarek RA, Christie D, Barclay G. Endoscopic therapy of pancreatitis in the pediatric population. *Gastrointest Endosc* 1993; 39: 665.

104 Beebe DS, Bubrick MP, Onstad GR *et al.* Management of pancreatic pseudocysts. *Surg Gynecol Obstet* 1984; 159: 562–4.

105 Binmoeller KF, Seifert H, Walter A *et al.* Transpapillary and transmural drainage of pancreatic pseudocysts. *Gastrointest Endosc* 1995; 42: 219–24.

106 Cremer M, Deviere J, Engelholm L. Endoscopic management of cysts and pseudocysts in chronic pancreatitis: long-term follow-up after 7 years of experience. *Gastrointest Endosc* 1989; 35: 1–9.

107 Smits ME, Rauws EA, Tytgat GN *et al.* The efficacy of endoscopic treatment of pancreatic pseudocysts. *Gastrointest Endosc* 1995; 42: 202–7.

CHAPTER 13

ERCP: Risks, Prevention, and Management

PETER B. COTTON

Synopsis

ERCP is the most risky procedure that endoscopists perform on a regular basis. There is the potential for technical and clinical failure, for misdiagnosis, and some small risk to staff, but the main interest is in the risk for adverse clinical events. A consensus definition of complications and their severity, and a series of careful prospective studies, have clarified the degree of risk in different circumstances, and the relevant risk factors. This process has allowed a clearer picture to emerge of the risk–benefit ratios in different clinical scenarios, and a greater ability to advise patients about their options. Also, the extensive experience of the last 30 years has permitted authoritative statements on how to minimize the likelihood of complications, and how to deal with difficult situations when they arise.

Introduction

ERCP has become popular worldwide because it can provide significant benefit in many clinical contexts. Sadly, it has also caused considerable harm in a small number of patients. Thus, it is crucial for practitioners and potential patients to understand the predictors of benefit and of risk. Defining positive and negative outcomes has been a significant challenge [1–4], but much useful information has been gathered from increasingly sophisticated outcomes studies over the last two decades.

This chapter concentrates on the risks and risk factors, emphasizes ways to reduce them, and provides guidance about management when adverse events occur.

The risks of ERCP

The concept of 'risk' indicates that something can 'go wrong', and is therefore best defined as a deviation from the plan. This assumes that a plan has been clearly formulated. The patient's perspective and understanding of the plan is enshrined in the process of informed consent. Deviations are best described generically as 'unplanned events' [4].

Unplanned events of ERCP are of four types:
- risks to staff;
- technical failure;
- clinical failure;
- unplanned adverse events—complications.

Risks for endoscopists and staff

The endoscopy unit is not a dangerous place, but there are a few risks for the ERCP endoscopist and staff.

The possibility of transmission of infection exists, but should be entirely preventable with standard precautions (gowns, gloves, and eye protection) and assiduous disinfection protocols.

Certain immunizations are also appropriate. Rarely, staff may become sensitive to materials used in the ERCP process, such as glutaraldehyde, or latex gloves.

The risks of radiation are minimized by appropriate education, shielding, and exposure monitoring [5].

Many older endoscopists have neck problems caused by looking down fiberscopes, a situation aggravated by ERCP rooms where the video and X-ray monitors are not side by side. Busy ERCP practitioners sometimes complain also of 'elevator thumb'. A Canadian survey found that more than half of 114 endoscopists performing ERCP had some attributable musculo-skeletal problem [6].

Technical failure

Not all ERCP procedures are successful technically. It may prove impossible to reach the papilla, to gain access to the duct of interest, or to complete the necessary therapeutic maneuvers. The chance of failure depends upon several factors.

Expertise

An important determinant of the chance of success is the level of expertise (of the endoscopist and team). There are now good data to show that more active ERCP endoscopists have better results [7], as applies in surgery [8].

Complexity

The risk of technical failure increases with the complexity of the problem. Any

Table 13.1 Degrees of difficulty in ERCP. (Modified from [9].)

	Diagnostic	Therapeutic
Grade 1 Standard	Selective deep cannulation Biopsy and cytology	Biliary sphincterotomy Stones < 10 mm Stents for biliary leaks Stents for low tumors
Grade 2 Advanced	Billroth II diagnostics Minor papilla cannulation	Stones > 10 mm Hilar tumor stent placement
Grade 3 Tertiary	Sphincter manometry Whipple Roux-en-Y Intraductal endoscopy	Benign biliary strictures Billroth II therapeutics Intrahepatic stones Pancreatic therapies

procedure can turn out to be technically challenging (e.g. when the papilla is hiding within a diverticulum), but some can be expected to be difficult beforehand (e.g. in patients who have previously undergone Billroth II gastrectomy). The concept of a scale of difficulty was first published by Schutz and Abbott [9]. Modifications led to a scale with three levels [4].

Degree of difficulty scale for ERCP procedures (Table 13.1)

Level 1 Standard procedures which any endoscopist providing ERCP services should be able to complete to a reasonable level of competence (say 90%). This includes deep selective cannulation, diagnostic sampling, standard biliary sphincterotomy, removal of stones (up to 10 mm in diameter), and the management of low biliary obstruction and postoperative leaks.

Level 2 Advanced procedures which require technical expertise beyond standard training, for example cannulation of the minor papilla, diagnostic ERCP after Billroth II gastrectomy, large stones (needing lithotripsy), and the management of benign biliary strictures and hilar tumors.

Level 3 Tertiary procedures which are normally offered only in a few referral centers, such as Billroth II therapeutics, intrahepatic stones, complex pancreatic treatments, and sphincter manometry. Manometry is included at the tertiary level, not because it is technically challenging, but because the overall management of patients with suspected sphincter dysfunction is particularly difficult (and the risks are greater).

Defining intent

A confounding issue when trying to assess technical success or failure is how well the goal of the procedure is, or can be, defined beforehand [1,4]. When the intent is obvious, e.g. to remove a known stone, the resulting outcome is unequivocal. However, ERCP is often used to make or confirm a diagnosis, and then to perform treatment 'if appropriate', so that defining intent, and thus 'success' and 'failure', may be more subjective. Also, endoscopists have different thresholds for attempting therapy. Some may back away from a large stone, and count the case as a success for good judgement rather than as a technical failure. Treatment will not even be considered if the diagnosis is not made (e.g. if cannulation fails and a stone is missed), but such a case usually will not be counted as a failure of stone treatment [10,11]. Thus, the success literature should be viewed with some skepticism.

Risk consequences of technical failure

There are good data showing that failed procedures carry more complications than successful ones. Failure usually necessitates repeat ERCP, or a percutaneous or surgical procedure, which brings additional and significant costs and risks [12]. Strictly speaking, on an 'intention to treat basis', any complications of these subsequent procedures should be attributed to the initial ERCP attempt.

Clinical failure

Clinical success is dependent upon technical success, but the reverse is not necessarily true. A procedure may be completed technically in an exemplary fashion, but with no resulting benefit. This would be true certainly when the indication is not appropriate.

Our aim is to make patients 'better', but defining precisely what that means can also be a challenge [1,4,13]. In some contexts (e.g. stone extraction, biliary stenting for low tumors), it is reasonable to assume that technical success will almost guarantee clinical success, at least in the short to medium term. However, some of those patients will have recurrent problems (e.g. new stones and stent occlusion), as detailed later, so that the time frame of measurement is relevant to success. It may be helpful to distinguish between initial 'primary' failure and 'secondary' failure, which means a relapse of the same problem.

It is also difficult to measure the success or failure of interventions in patients who have intermittent problems such as recurrent pancreatitis or episodes of pain suspected to be due to sphincter dysfunction. The true outcome in these cases can be measured only after months or years. Furthermore, the clinical response may be incomplete, with a reduction, but not elimination, of attacks of pancreatitis, or some diminution in the overall burden of pain. The question then is how precisely to measure this 'pain burden' (which may fluctuate from day to day, or week to week), and how much of a reduction constitutes 'success'? Progress in this area will come only if we have carefully defined outcome metrics, good baseline evaluation, and structured objective follow-up [13]. Quality of life assessment should feature in these contexts. We are developing a 'pain-burden' scoring tool. This is used to follow patients sequentially, and incorporates our validated digestive quality of life instrument, the DDQ-15 [14].

Unplanned adverse clinical events—complications

Unplanned events are deviations from the expectations of the endoscopist and of the patient (as defined by the process of informed consent). Rarely, the outcome of a procedure may be better than anticipated, for example, finding a treatable benign lesion (such as a stone) in a jaundiced patient with suspected malignancy. However, most unplanned clinical events associated with procedures are unwelcome, and are often called 'adverse events'. Some are significant enough to be called 'complications' [4].

When does an event become a complication?

Some adverse events are relatively trivial (such as brief hypoxia easily managed with supplemental oxygen, or transient bleeding which stops or is stopped during the procedure). The word 'complication' is not appropriate for these events, not least because of the medico-legal connotations. However, all unexpected and adverse events should be documented and tracked for quality improvement purposes.

The level of severity at which an adverse clinical event becomes a 'complication' is an arbitrary decision, but an important one, since definitions are essential if meaningful data are to be collected and compared. A consensus workshop defined the complications of ERCP in 1991 [15]. Whilst the document focused on the complications of sphincterotomy, the principles and definitions apply to all aspects of ERCP.

Complication definition

- An adverse event.
- Attributable to the procedure.
- Requiring treatment in hospital.

The workshop also recommended working definitions of the commonest complications (Table 13.2).

Table 13.2 Definitions and grading system for the major complications of ERCP and therapy. (From [15].)

	Mild	Moderate	Severe[a]
Bleeding	Clinical (i.e. not just endoscopic) bleeding; hemoglobin drop < 3 g/dl, and no need for transfusion	Transfusion (4 units or less), no angiographic intervention or surgery	Transfusion 5 units or more, or intervention (angiographic or surgical)
Perforation	Possible or only very slight leak of fluid or contrast, treatable by fluids and suction for 3 days or less	Any definite perforation treated medically for 4–10 days	Medical treatment for more than 10 days, or intervention (percutaneous or surgical)
Pancreatitis	Clinical pancreatitis, amylase at least three times normal at more than 24 h after the procedure, requiring admission or prolongation of planned admission to 2–3 days	Pancreatitis requiring hospitalization of 4–10 days	Hospitalization for more than 10 days, or hemorrhagic pancreatitis, phlegmon, or pseudocyst, or intervention (percutaneous drainage or surgery)
Infection (cholangitis)	> 38°C for 24–48 h	Febrile or septic illness requiring more than 3 days of hospital treatment or endoscopic or percutaneous intervention	Septic shock or surgery
Basket impaction	Basket released spontaneously or by repeat endoscopy	Percutaneous intervention	Surgery

A complication is (1) an adverse, unplanned event; (2) attributable to the procedure (including preparation); (3) of a severity requiring hospital admission or prolongation of planned/actual admission.
[a]Any event requiring ICU admission, or unplanned surgery, is deemed 'severe'.

Not all complications are of equal significance, and so the workshop also recommended an arbitrary scale of severity, based mainly on the length of hospitalization required and the need for intensive care and/or surgery (Table 13.2).

Severity criteria

- Mild: 1–3 nights in hospital.
- Moderate: 4–9 nights.

- Severe: 10 nights or more, or surgery, or ICU admission.
- Fatal: death attributable to the procedure.

These concepts and definitions have been adopted widely, and have been used in many subsequent studies of ERCP outcomes. This has helped considerably in the attempt to better understand the predictors of good and bad outcomes. If surgeons and interventional radiologists used a similar lexicon, it would be easier to compare their outcomes outside the context of formal randomized trials [13].

Types of adverse clinical event

Unplanned adverse events can be categorized broadly into four groups.
- Equipment malfunction.
- Medication and sedation issues.
- Direct events: those which occur at sites which have been traversed or treated during the endoscopic procedure (e.g. perforation, bleeding, or pancreatitis).
- Indirect events: those which occur in other organs (e.g. heart, lungs, and kidneys) as a result of the procedure. Indirect events are more difficult to recognize and document because they may not become apparent until several days after the procedure, when the patient has returned home or to other clinical supervision.

Timing of events and attribution

Most adverse events are recognized during or shortly after procedures, but some happen beforehand (e.g. as a result of some aspect of preparation), and some are apparent only later (e.g. delayed bleeding after sphincterotomy).

For adverse events which occur before and during procedures, it is important to note whether the examination had to be terminated early or could be completed.

The 1991 consensus definition of complications [15] includes the phrase 'attributable to the procedure'. Attribution is not always clear-cut, especially when there is a delay. Is a cardiopulmonary event counted if it occurs a week or two after ERCP, or only if there is some other linking factor (e.g. some important medication was stopped for the procedure)?

To cover this point, the consensus workshop suggested that direct events (as defined above) are always attributable, even if they do not occur or become apparent for several weeks (e.g. delayed bleeding). However, we agreed an arbitrary time limit of 3 days for indirect events, such as cardiopulmonary problems.

As mentioned above, there is also the issue of how to report the complications of other procedures (e.g. percutaneous interventions) which become necessary when ERCP fails [12].

A dataset for unplanned events

This is shown in Table 13.3.

Table 13.3 Dataset of unplanned events.

1   **Nature of unplanned event**
    Medication/sedation/anesthesia
    - Allergic reaction
    - Drug interaction
    - Neuropsychiatric reaction
    - IV site problems
    - Cardiac event
    - Pulmonary event
    - Other

    Equipment malfunction
    - Endoscope
    - Radiology equipment
    - Accessories
    - Diathermy
    - Implanted devices
    - Other

    Direct events
    - Endoscopic perforation
    - Sphincterotomy perforation
    - Snare/diathermy perforation
    - Dilator perforation
    - Duct penetration/dissection
    - Bleeding
    - Pancreatitis
    - Cholangitis
    - Cholecystitis
    - Infection
    - Pseudocyst infection
    - Basket impaction
    - Peritonitis
    - Other

    Indirect (non-GI) events
    - Pain, cause unclear
    - Fever, cause unclear
    - Renal impairment
    - Neurological
    - Musculo-skeletal

Continued

Table 13.3 (*cont'd*)

- Pregnancy-related
- Other

2 Timing (event first appears)
- Preprocedure (from starting prep, i.e. npo or bowel prep, to entering endoscopy room)
- Procedure (in room)
- Early recovery (< 4 h)
- Late recovery (4–24 h)
- Delayed (1–30 days)
- Late (> 30 days)

3 Procedure
- Not started
- Stopped prematurely
- Completed

4 Changes in care plan
- None
- Unplanned specialty consultation
- Unplanned admission (days)
- Prolonged admission (days)
- ICU admission (days)

5 Treatment needed for unplanned events
Medical
- Naloxone
- Flumazenil
- Atropine
- Oxygen
- Transfusion
- Ventilation assistance
- Emergency code called
- Other medical care

Interventions
- Endoscopy
- Radiology imaging
- Radiology intervention
- Surgery
- Other intervention

6 Outcome
- Full recovery
- Permanent disability/loss of function
- Death (days after procedure)

7 Attribution
- Event related to endoscopy? Yes/no/probably/uncertain

8 Detail of events and comments

Overall complication rates

Rates of complications published before the 1991 consensus definitions are difficult to interpret due to a lack of consistency in reporting [15–20].

Many reviews and case series have been published subsequently [21–44]. Some of the most recent single- and multicenter data are summarized in Tables 13.4 and 13.5.

Overall, it appears that complications occur in some 5–10% of ERCP procedures. However, these global figures take no account of severity, and come from a huge variety of procedures performed on a broad spectrum of patients in different contexts. It is now clear that the risks vary considerably with the indication and setting, so that we need more focused data. Patients should be informed about the likely risk in their own precise context.

Accuracy of data collection

An important issue affecting the accuracy of reported data is the method of collection. Retrospective studies are known to underestimate complication rates, since many delayed events are missed [45–47]. This may apply particularly to

Table 13.4 Overall complications of ERCP.

First author	Loperfido	Masci	Tzovaras	Halme	Farrell	Lizcano	Vandervoort
Reference	[24]	[25]	[26]	[40]	[37]	[29]	[27]
Year	1998	2001	2000	1999	2001	2004	2002
ERCPs	3356	2444	372	813	1758	507	1223
Complications (%)	4.0	5.0	5.0	3.9	3.5	10.8	11.2
Diagnostic cases (%)	1.4			1.8	2.1	17.0	
Therapeutic cases (%)	5.4		1.3	9.1	4.6	7.4	
30 day mortality (%)			0.3		2.2		
Related mortality (%)				0.3	0.35	0.8	0.2
Pancreatitis (%)	1.3	1.8		1.8		5.5	7.2
Bleeding (%)	0.8	1.2		0.8		1.6	0.8
Perforation (%)	0.6			0.8		1.4	0.08
Infection (%)				0.7		1.6	0.8
Risk increased by							
Young age		✓					
Inexperience	✓						
Failure/difficulty		✓					✓
Sphincter dysfunction							
Precutting	✓	✓					

Table 13.5 Reported complications of biliary sphincterotomy in recent large series.

First author	Cotton[a]	Barthet	Freeman	Rabenstein
Reference	[64]	[22]	[44]	[41]
Year	1998	2002	1996	1999
Sphincterotomies	1921	658	2347	1335
Complications (%)	5.8	7.7	9.8	7.3
30 day mortality (%)	0.2	0.9	0.2	
Related mortality (%)	0.1		0.04	
Pancreatitis (%)		3.5	5.4	
Bleeding (%)		1.2	2.0	
Perforation (%)		1.8	0.3	
Infection (%)		1.2	1.5	
Risk increased by				
Young age				
Inexperience	✓			✓
Failure/difficulty			✓	
Sphincter dysfunction		✓	✓	
Precutting		✓	✓	
Cirrhosis			✓	

[a]Bile duct stones only.

the large volume centers (who publish most) since the encounters often are brief and most patients return home, often some distance away, for further care. The most reliable data come from prospective studies which include a routine 30 day follow-up visit or call [44,45], but this is labor intensive and rarely done outside of research studies.

Changes in complications over time

Bleeding, perforation, and infection were the most common complications of ERCP in the early days of ERCP and biliary sphincterotomy [15–20]; now pancreatitis dominates (Tables 13.4 and 13.5). This change appears to be due mainly to a progressive reduction in the risk of bleeding, perforation, and infection as training and techniques have improved, and may also be due to a relative increase in pancreatitis as ERCP has been used more widely for more speculative (and risky) indications, such as obscure abdominal pain, sphincter dysfunction, and recurrent pancreatitis.

Complication rates at MUSC

We have used the same definitions and database for the prospective recording of all endoscopic procedures at MUSC for more than 10 years. Delayed complications that we are aware of are reported to the group and added to the database

Table 13.6 Complications of ERCP at MUSC, 1994–2004; 9948 cases.

	Total	Percent	Percent of complications	Mild	Moderate	Severe	Fatal
Pancreatitis	270	2.7	67.5	204	53	13	0
Bleeding	34	0.34	8.5	18	9	7	0
Infection	32	0.32	8.0	24	6	2	0
Pain? cause	18	0.18	4.5	15	3	0	0
Cardiopulmonary	18	0.18	4.5	10	2	4	2
Endoscopic perforation	9	0.09	2.2	2	0	6	1
Sphincterotomy perforation	4	0.04	1.0	0	1	3	0
Medication	6	0.06	1.5	6	0	0	0
Other	13	0.13	0.3	9	1	1	2
Totals	404		100	288	75	36	5
Percent of complications				71	19	9	1
Complicate rate by severity				2.9	0.75	0.36	0.05

at a weekly pancreatico-biliary service meeting, but there has been no routine follow-up call. From studies performed by ourselves [45], and others [46,47], it is certain that some delayed complications have not been recorded, but the system has been consistent, so that trends are probably meaningful.

The overall rate of known complications in almost 10 000 procedures was 4%, with severe complications at 0.36%, and five deaths (0.05%) (Table 13.6). Pancreatitis has accounted for two-thirds of all recorded complications, occurring at a rate now of around 2%. The incidence of severe pancreatitis (more than 10 days in hospital, ICU admission, pseudocyst, or surgery) was 0.13%.

There has been a gradual reduction in the rates (and severity) of complications over the years (Table 13.7), despite an increasing proportion of complex and more risky level 3 procedures.

More details of specific complications and their management are given in the relevant later sections.

General risk issues

Endoscopists must be aware of the factors that can increase the risk of ERCP. These are both general and specific. General risks include the skill of the individual endoscopist (and team), the clinical status of the patient, and the precise nature of the procedure.

Table 13.7 ERCP complications at MUSC by year.

	Total	1995	1996	1997	1998	1999	2000	2001	2002	2003	2004
Procedures	9948	793	1013	1066	998	1035	1044	1015	1051	983	950
Complications	404	50	57	55	40	42	34	37	23	38	28
(%)	(4.1)	(6.3)	(5.6)	(5.2)	(4.0)	(4.1)	(3.3)	(3.7)	(2.2)	(3.9)	(2.9)
Mild (%)	288 (2.9)	34	38	42	25	29	27	23	21	30	19
Moderate (%)	75 (0.75)	8	13	7	11	10	7	8	2	4	5
Severe (%)	36 (0.36)	8	5	5	4	2	0	5	0	3	4
Fatal (%)	5 (0.05)	0	1	1	0	1	0	1	0	1	0
Pancreatitis	270	34	40	36	28	27	23	25	14	25	18
(%)	(2.7)	(4.3)	(4.0)	(3.5)	(2.8)	(2.6)	(2.2)	(2.5)	(1.3)	(2.5)	(1.9)

Details of the specific risks, methods to minimize them, and recommendations for management are given below. Here we document some important general points.

Operator-related issues

There are now significant data showing that more experienced endoscopists usually have higher success rates and lower rates of complications than those who are less active, even when dealing with more complex cases [7,24,28,41–43]. This fact has important implications for training, credentialing, and informed consent. Lack of experience increases the risk of technical failure. Failures carry risks also of the subsequent needed interventions. In one analysis, failed ERCPs carried three times the complication rate of successful ones (21.5% vs. 7.3%) [12]. The association between inexperience and poor outcomes has been well documented for major surgical procedures [8].

Patient-related issues; clinical status, indications, and comorbidities

Much attention has been paid to analysing the characteristics of patients which may affect the risk of performing ERCP [30,48].

Age

Age itself is not a risk factor for ERCP complications [49]. Many studies now testify to the safety of performing diagnostic and therapeutic procedures in infants [50], children [51], and the elderly [52,53].

Illness and associated conditions

Adverse events are more likely to occur in patients who are already severely ill, for example with acute cholangitis [54], and in those with substantial co-morbidities. The most important comorbidities are cardiopulmonary fragility (posing risks for sedation and anesthesia), immunosuppression, and coagulopathies (including therapeutic anticoagulation). It would be helpful if there were an agreed index or score that reflected the degree of risk, but none of the published instruments really fit the ERCP context. The American Society for Anesthesiology (ASA) score is often used in surgical practice as a guide to the risk for sedation and anesthesia, but this appears unhelpful in the context of ERCP [55]. This is because the risk is much more dependent on the indication for the procedure.

ERCP appears to be safe when needed for management of stones in pregnant patients [56].

Indication

Fortunately, it is clear that the risks of ERCP are lowest in those patients with the 'best' indications, i.e. duct stones, biliary leaks, and low tumors. Conversely, the pioneering studies by Freeman and colleagues have revealed the substantial risks involved in performing ERCP in patients with obscure abdominal pain ('suspected sphincter dysfunction') [36]. This was emphasized strongly by the NIH 'State-of-the-Science' Conference on ERCP in 2002 [57]. Sadly, it is true that 'ERCP is most dangerous for those who need it least' [58].

Anatomical factors

In some series, but not in all, the presence of a peripapillary diverticulum appears to be a risk factor [59,60]. With suitable precautions, patients with implanted pacemakers or defibrillators can be treated safely [61].

A normal-sized bile duct was earlier believed to increase the risk of post-ERCP pancreatitis [62,63], but this is a surrogate for sphincter dysfunction, and does not apply to patients with stones [64,65].

Complication-specific risk factors

Patient risk factors for specific complications are detailed below. For example, Billroth II gastrectomy carries an increased risk for afferent loop perforation, and coagulopathies and certain medications increase the risk of bleeding. Equally, patients with hilar tumors and sclerosing cholangitis are at greater risk for septic complications because it may prove difficult to provide complete drainage.

Procedure performed

Diagnostic or therapeutic?

Most people assume that therapeutic ERCP is more dangerous than diagnostic procedures. This is true in several reported series: 5.4% vs. 1.4% [24], 9.1% vs. 1.8% [40], and 4.6% vs. 2.1% [37], but not in another small series (7.4% vs. 17%) [29] (Table 13.5).

Sedation, cardiopulmonary events, and intubation carry the same risks whether the procedure is diagnostic or therapeutic. Therapeutic procedures do carry their own specific risks, e.g. bleeding and perforation after sphincterotomy, or infection after attempted pseudocyst drainage. These complications can be serious, and so it would also seem logical that the likelihood of a severe complication would be greater after therapeutic procedures. Remarkably, our own series shows very similar complication rates for diagnostic and therapeutic ERCP, and the risk of severe or fatal complications was actually slightly higher for diagnostic procedures (0.7% vs. 0.3%) (Table 13.8). It is worth noting that diagnostic ERCP in some patients may actually be riskier if not followed immediately by appropriate therapy (e.g. in a patient with malignant obstructive jaundice or proven sphincter dysfunction). Our 'diagnostic' procedures were

Table 13.8 Complications of ERCP at MUSC; therapy vs. no therapy.	Thereapeutic (%)	No therapy (%)
Total cases	8136	1812
Overall complications	339 (4.20)	68 (3.80)
Mild	242 (3.00)	52 (2.90)
Moderate	70 (0.90)	5 (0.30)
Severe	23 (0.30)	10 (0.60)
Fatal	4 (0.05)	1 (0.05)
Pancreatitis overall	222 (2.70)	48 (2.60)
Mild	165 (2.00)	39 (2.20)
Moderate	49 (0.60)	4 (0.20)
Severe	8 (0.10)	5 (0.30)
Fatal	0 (0.00)	0 (0.00)
Perforation	9 (0.11)	4 (0.20)
Bleeding	34 (0.42)	0 (0.00)

simply those that involved no therapy, and so some of them may have been technical failures. The statistics may well be different on an intention to treat basis.

The implications of the specific therapeutic procedures will be considered further when addressing the individual risks, but some details are given here.

Biliary sphincterotomy

Biliary sphincterotomy is the commonest therapeutic ERCP procedure, performed in enormous numbers throughout the world. As a result, much of the risk literature refers specifically to biliary sphincterotomy [15,17,19,20,22,31, 32,42–44,66], and mainly in the context of stones [47,66,65,67–69]. Representative series indicate an overall morbidity of 5.3–9.8%, with attributable mortality considerably below 1% (Table 13.5). Our overall complication rate for a series of 1043 biliary sphincterotomies for stone over 10 years at MUSC was 2.6%. Amongst these were only 7 (0.5%) severe complications, and one death (0.07%). In the same period there were 2021 biliary sphincterotomies performed for all other indications, with an overall complication rate of 7.5%, with 0.6% severe, and no deaths.

Pancreatic sphincterotomy

Pancreatic sphincterotomy (of the major and minor papilla) is used much less frequently than biliary sphincterotomy, but its popularity is increasing. It is performed both with a pull-type sphincterotome and with a needle-knife over a stent [70]. Few studies have analyzed its specific complications [71–73]. The overall complication rate in 1615 pancreatic sphincterotomies at MUSC (many of whom underwent biliary sphincterotomy at the same time) was 6.9%; 80% of these were pancreatitis. There was only one recorded sphincterotomy perforation, and three (0.2%) severe complications, with no related deaths.

Precut sphincterotomy

The needle-knife precut technique is useful and safe in the treatment of impacted stones [74], and is used by many as the primary method for performing pancreatic sphincterotomy (over a stent), and for biliary sphincterotomy after Billroth II gastrectomy. However, precutting used purely as a biliary access technique is contentious [75,76]. Much of the literature suggests that it is valuable and safe when used for good indications by experts [77–87], but there is ample evidence, not least from lawsuits, that it is dangerous when used by inexperienced endoscopists, especially when the indication is not strong. Several studies (including centers with considerable experience) clearly show that precutting increases substantially the risk of pancreatitis and of perforation [22,24,25,36,44]. It has been suggested that precutting has received a bad reputation only because it may be used as a last resort, after much other manipulation, and that it may be safe when used early in the cannulation process. However, it seems a poor alternative to good standard methods.

Variants of the precut technique have been described [88,89], including using a standard pull-type sphincterotome in the pancreatic duct. Despite good experience with this method reported from one center [90], this seems to be courting disaster.

The data clearly indicate that precut access techniques should be avoided by inexperienced endoscopists, especially when there is little or no evidence for biliary pathology requiring treatment.

Repeat sphincterotomy

Biliary and pancreatic sphincterotomy sometimes need to be repeated for recurrent stones or stenosis. Whether the second procedure carries increased risk clearly depends on the indication, and on the size of the prior procedure [91,92]. One study showed a significant increase in the risk of both bleeding (from 1.7% to 5%) and perforation (from 1% to 8%), but a reduction in pancreatitis (from 5.5% to 1%), when comparing repeat biliary sphincterotomies with index cases [93]. These factors are discussed further in the specific risk sections.

Balloon sphincter dilation

As endoscopic stone extraction has become more frequently used in relatively fit and young patients (after the advent of laparoscopic cholecystectomy), there has been increasing interest in trying to further reduce the (albeit small) risks of sphincterotomy by using balloon dilation of the papilla instead [94,95]. Since the main concern about this technique is the risk of provoking pancreatitis, it is discussed further in that section.

Endoscopic papillectomy

The increasing familiarity and confidence of endoscopists with polypectomy, mucosal resection, and complex ERCP has led many to perform excision of the major papilla for treatment of adenomas. The techniques (including temporary pancreatic stenting) are now fairly well established [96–99], but there is continuing concern about the precise indications [100] and the likelihood of recurrence. The immediate risks are bleeding, pancreatitis, and perforation. One large series of 70 cases reported 10 complications (14%), with bleeding in four, pancreatitis in five, and mild perforation in one, with one-third of the adenomas recurring after a median follow-up of only 7 months [101].

Stenting

Biliary stenting is widely used for the management of leaks and tumors. It carries the same general risks as any ERCP procedure, although the presence of a pancreatic tumor may protect somewhat against pancreatitis. A small biliary sphincterotomy is not necessary in most cases [102], but is wise in hilar tumors, since it may prevent pancreatitis and also facilitates the placement of two stents [103].

Biliary stenting is most risky when it fails, or when drainage is incomplete. This commonly leads to sepsis, and carries the risks of repeat procedures (whether ERCP or percutaneous). The chance of failure, and of complications, is considerably greater with lesions involving the liver hilum. The specific risks of stenting (and pancreatic stenting) are discussed later.

Pseudocyst drainage

Endoscopic drainage of pseudocysts through the stomach wall or duodenum carries a significant risk of bleeding, perforation, and infection [104].

Reducing the risks of ERCP: general issues

Methods to minimize specific risks are detailed below for each of the main complications. However, there are several general strategies which should be understood. Clearly, it is helpful to maximize the clinical and technical expertise of the endoscopist and the assisting team, and to follow accepted standards of practice. Since complications cannot be avoided completely, it is also mandatory to ensure that patients and those close to them are fully informed about the key issues.

The contract with the patient; informed consent

It is always the responsibility of endoscopists to assure themselves that the potential benefits of the proposed procedure exceed the potential risks, and to convey that information clearly to their patients [105]. Truly informed consent means that the patient really does understand the potential risks and benefits, as well as the possible limitations and any available alternative approaches. That is our contract with the patient. Signing an 'informed consent form' is a medico-legal requirement in many institutions, but this is nothing more than confirmation of the education process. It is important to 'tell it as it is'. It is in our nature as physicians to want to reassure nervous patients that 'things will go just fine', but that is neither honest nor wise.

Educational materials

Nothing can replace a detailed discussion between the endoscopist and the patient (and any accompanying persons), but this process can be enhanced with written, video- or web-based educational materials. Suitable brochures are available from national organizations, and on many websites, and can be adapted for local conditions. The document in routine use at MUSC is shown in Table 13.9. The process of informed consent must be clearly documented and witnessed. For elective procedures, this process should take place preferably at least a day beforehand to give time for review of the materials and unhurried reflection. Whatever the details of the education process, patients must be given the opportunity to ask questions of their endoscopist (and support staff) again before the procedure.

Humanity

It is appropriate also to emphasize the importance of simple courtesies and common humanity in dealing with our customers. What is familiar and routine to the endoscopist and staff may be viewed by patients as a major ordeal—especially by those unfortunate enough to experience a significant adverse event.

Care after ERCP

Admission?

Many patients are kept in hospital under observation overnight after ERCP. The advantage is that nursing staff can ensure adequate fluid intake (mainly intravenously), and can quickly detect and pay appropriate attention to symptoms which may herald important complications. However, overnight observation adds costs, and can add other burdens for patients and their families. Several studies have evaluated factors predicting the need for admission [106–110]. Admission is unnecessary in the majority of standard level 1 procedures (simple biliary stones and stents), but seems wise when the risk is predicted to be higher than average (e.g. sphincter dysfunction management), when the procedure has been difficult in some way, or when the patient is frail or has no responsible accompanying person. Staying overnight in a local hotel is an appropriate compromise option for patients who live more than an hour or two away. Attempts have been made to use serum tests early in the recovery period to predict subsequent pancreatitis [111,112], but this has not become standard practice.

Table 13.9 ERCP information sheet for patients at MUSC.

ERCP stands for Endoscopic Retrograde Cholangio Pancreatography
ERCP uses an endoscope which is a long narrow tube with a camera at the end. The doctor passes the endoscope through your mouth (under sedation/anesthesia) to get into the papilla of Vater, a small nipple in your upper intestine (duodenum). This papilla is the drainage hole for your bile duct and the pancreatic duct, which bring digestive juices from your liver, gallbladder, and pancreas. X-rays are taken to show whether there are any lesions such as stones, spasms, or blockages. If the X-ray pictures do show a problem, the doctor may be able to treat it right away. The most common treatments are:
- **Sphincterotomy.** This involves making a small cut in the papilla of Vater to enlarge the opening to the bile duct and/or pancreatic duct. This is done to improve the drainage or to remove stones in the ducts. Removed stones are usually dropped in the intestine, and pass through quickly.
- **Stenting.** A stent is a small plastic tube which is left in a blocked or narrowed duct to improve drainage. The narrowing may need to be stretched (dilated) before the stent is placed. Some stents are designed to pass out into the intestine after a few weeks when they have done their work. Other stents have to be removed or changed after 3–4 months. There are also permanent stents made out of metal.
- **Other treatments** are used occasionally. Your doctor will explain these if necessary.

Limitations and risks? There are some drawbacks to ERCP. Discuss these with your doctor
- The test and treatments are not perfect. Occasionally, important lesions may not be seen, and treatment attempts may be unsuccessful.
- The medicines may make you sick. You may have nausea, vomiting, hives, dry mouth, or a reddened face and neck. A tender lump may form where the IV was placed. Call your doctor if redness, pain, or swelling appears to be spreading.
- You will receive a low dose of radiation from the X-rays.
- Working on the pancreas can cause complications, even in the best hands. Your doctor will explain these and answer your questions. The most common complication is pancreatitis.
  - **Pancreatitis** (swelling and inflammation of the pancreas). This occurs in about 1 patient in 20, and results in the need to stay in hospital for pain medications and IV fluids. This usually lasts for 1 or 2 days, but can be much more serious.
- Other rare complications (less than 1 per 100) include, but are not limited to:
  - **Heart and lung problems.**
  - **Bleeding** (after sphincterotomy).
  - **Infection** in the bile duct (cholangitis).
  - **Perforation** (a tear in the intestine).
These may require surgery (about 1 case in 500), and prolonged stays in hospital. Fatal complications are very rare.
Alternatives? There are some different approaches. Discuss them with your doctor.
- Diagnoses can often be made by scans, such as ultrasound, CT, MRI, or nuclear medicine scans.
- ERCP is usually done only when appropriate scans have failed to provide a diagnosis, or when they have shown something that is best treated by ERCP.
- Alternative treatments include surgical operations, or, in some cases, interventional radiology.

Early refeeding?

Patients are often keen to catch up on the meals that they have missed as a result of the procedure, but it has been my practice to recommend taking fluids only until the next morning, when the main risk of pancreatitis has passed. However, a recent randomized trial suggests that early refeeding is not detrimental [113].

Pancreatitis after ERCP

Pancreatitis is now by far the most common complication of ERCP and sphincterotomy (Tables 13.4 and 13.5). Our better understanding of the risk factors in recent years is largely attributable to the seminal studies anchored by Freeman, who has published several comprehensive reviews [114,115]. This chapter focuses on the key facts.

Definitions

Serum amylase and lipase levels can be shown to rise in almost every patient if measured within a few hours of ERCP, even sometimes when the pancreatic duct has not been entered or opacified. While this indicates some irritation of the pancreas, it does not constitute clinically relevant pancreatitis. The incidence of pancreatitis clearly depends greatly on the criteria used for the diagnosis [116].

The consensus workshop suggested this working definition of post-ERCP pancreatitis [15]. 'Pancreatitis after ERCP is a clinical illness with typical pain, associated with at least a three-fold increase in serum amylase (or lipase) at 24 h, with symptoms impressive enough to require admission to hospital for treatment (or extension of an existing or planned admission).' Severity is graded as mild if hospitalization is needed for less than 3 nights, moderate if 4–9 nights, and severe if more than 10 nights, or if patients require intensive care or surgical treatment.

This definition has been widely used, despite some concern about the relevance of hospitalization, and the fact that the apparent incidence will vary according to the admission policy. It is also sometimes difficult to decide how to deal (statistically as well as clinically) with patients with long-standing pancreatic pain who linger in hospital after their procedures. We do not count this as a complication unless the patient is obviously worse afterwards.

Incidence of pancreatitis after ERCP

In addition to the major reviews and studies of ERCP complications [21–44], there is extensive literature specific to the risk of pancreatitis after ERCP

[114–123]. The reported incidence ranges widely, from less than 1% up to as high as 40%. Much of this huge variation can be attributed to different definitions, incomplete data collection, and differing case mixes. Ranges of 2–9% are representative of more recent prospective series, mostly using consensus definitions [114] (Tables 13.4 and 13.5). An innovative population-based study of 97 810 ERCPs in Canada reported a pancreatitis rate of 2.2%, with greater risk in younger patients and in women [124].

The overall pancreatitis rate in our series at MUSC is < 3%, with a gradual reduction over the years, despite an increasing number of cases with suspected sphincter dysfunction, where the risk is known to be greater (Tables 13.6 and 13.7). More than 75% of all these cases of pancreatitis after ERCP were graded as mild (Table 13.6). Mild complications are disappointing and inconvenient, but are not serious or threatening (medically or legally). Severe pancreatitis occurred in 13 cases (0.13%). They are devastating for all involved, and fatalities occur (one in our series). For these reasons, there is great interest in understanding the true risk factors, and ways to minimize them.

Risk factors for pancreatitis

Any ERCP procedure can cause pancreatitis, but certain factors are well known to increase the risk. A listing, adapted from Freeman *et al.* [115], is shown in Table 13.10. The factors are both patient- and procedure-related.

Table 13.10 Risk factors for pancreatitis after ERCP. (Adapted from [115].)

Increased risk?	Patient-related	Procedure-related
Yes	Young age	Pancreatography
	Female	Pancreatic sphincterotomy
	Suspected SOD	Balloon dilation of intact sphincter
	Recurrent pancreatitis	Difficult cannulation
	No chronic pancreatitis	Precut (access) sphincterotomy
	Prior post-ERCP pancreatitis	
Maybe	No stone	Pancreatic acinarization
	Normal bilirubin	Pancreatic brush cytology
	Low-volume endoscopist	Pain during ERCP
No	Small/normal bile duct	Therapeutic versus diagnostic
	Periampullary diverticulum	Biliary sphincterotomy
	Pancreas divisum	Sphincter manometry
	Contrast allergy	Intramural contrast injection
	Prior failed ERCP	

Patient factors increasing the risk [114,115,122,123]

It has become abundantly clear that the risk of developing pancreatitis is greater in younger patients, and in women as compared to men [114,124], and particularly when ERCP is performed for 'suspected sphincter dysfunction' in the absence of much objective evidence for biliary or pancreatic pathology. A prior history of recurrent pancreatitis, or of post-ERCP pancreatitis, also increases the risk in most studies. Contrary to earlier reports [62,63], a 'small' or normal-sized bile duct is not an independent risk factor [114,115].

Procedure factors increasing the risk

Pancreatic manipulation Pancreatitis is more likely to occur with aggressive manipulation of the pancreatic orifice [114], and with repeated injections of contrast [117], sometimes evidenced by acinarization or the appearance of a urogram [125]. The importance of increased pressure in the duct is supported by the old observation that postprocedure pancreatitis is less likely in patients who have a patent duct of Santorini. Variations on methods for cannulation have been explored [126–130], without any new consensus.

Sphincter manometry For a long time, it was believed that sphincter manometry was a potent cause of pancreatitis [131]. However, it is now clear that manometry is simply a surrogate for sphincter of Oddi dysfunction (SOD), which is the real culprit [115,133]. Several series show that the apparent increase disappears if increased sphincter pressure is treated (by pancreatic sphincterotomy or temporary stenting). It has been shown also that the risk is actually higher when suspected SOD (e.g. postcholecystectomy pain) is treated empirically by sphincterotomy than when manometry is employed [114].

Sphincterotomy Several studies now indicate that standard biliary sphincterotomy does not markedly increase the overall risk of pancreatitis (when compared with diagnostic ERCP) (Tables 13.4, 13.5 and 13.8). The suggestion that pure cutting current could reduce the risk of pancreatitis has not been proven in most of the published studies [134–139].

In the hands of experts (who publish), access precut sphincterotomy appears to be both useful and safe, at least when used for good (biliary) indications [75–87,140]. However, many series document a significantly increased risk of pancreatitis when precutting is performed [44,114,115,118,123]. In Freeman *et al*'s large prospective multicenter analysis, the complication rate was 24.3% after precutting, with 3.6% severe pancreatitis [44].

Pancreatic sphincterotomy is being performed increasingly in referral centers for many different indications. The pancreatitis rate for 1615 pancreatic sphincterotomies in our unit (performed mainly for sphincter dysfunction and with temporary stenting) was 5.6%.

Biliary sphincter dilation Balloon dilation of the biliary sphincter has been advocated as an alternative to sphincterotomy for removal of duct stones, in the hope of reducing the (small) short- and long-term risks [94,95]. Early case series gave encouraging results [94,141,142], but the technique can cause pancreatitis [143]. Many randomized studies have been performed to compare the risk with that of standard sphincterotomy [144–150]. Some involved older patients, often with dilated ducts and large stones, and showed that the short-term risks of sphincterotomy and of balloon dilation were similar [142,144]. However, the concept of sphincter preservation is most attractive in younger patients with smaller stones and relatively normal ducts. A major multicenter US study in these types of patients (in the context of laparoscopic cholecystectomy) showed a marked increase in the risk of pancreatitis, with two deaths [150]. This has led to a consensus, at least in the USA, that the balloon technique should be considered now only in special circumstances, such as coagulopathy [151] and maybe Billroth II patients [152,153]. This restrictive recommendation could change with further progress in preventing pancreatitis, e.g. by combining balloon dilation with pharmacological or stenting prophylaxis.

Biliary stenting Temporary stenting of the biliary sphincter has been used as a therapeutic trial in patients with suspected sphincter dysfunction. This technique is a potent cause of pancreatitis [154] and should be avoided.

Some endoscopists routinely perform sphincterotomy before placing biliary stents through strictures, to facilitate subsequent stent exchange and to reduce the risk of pancreatitis caused by irritating the pancreatic orifice. The latter hope has been documented only in a few patients with hilar tumors [103], where sphincterotomy is necessary anyway to place more than one stent. Sphincterotomy is not necessary or protective in other circumstances [102].

Pancreatic stenting The precise risk of causing immediate pancreatitis by placing pancreatic stents is difficult to measure, since this is done in many ways for many different indications, and often in conjunction with other manipulations such as pancreatic sphincterotomy.

Combining patient- and procedure-related factors

Many of these risk factors are additive [114]. For instance, precutting in suspected sphincter dysfunction resulted in a complication rate of 35.3%, with no fewer than 23.5% overall graded as severe [44]. In another study from the same group concerning post-ERCP pancreatitis, a woman with a normal serum bilirubin, bile duct stone, and easy cannulation had a 5% risk of pancreatitis. This increased to 16% if cannulation proved difficult, and to 42% if no stone was found (i.e. suspected SOD) [115]. These are the unfortunate patients who are still developing severe pancreatitis after ERCP, and who feature in lawsuits.

Prevention of pancreatitis after ERCP

Avoiding ERCP, especially in high-risk patients

Post-ERCP pancreatitis cannot (currently) be prevented completely, except by avoiding the procedure, which is a good strategy in many cases; sadly, it is not applicable in retrospect. The availability of sophisticated imaging techniques such as MRCP and EUS means that ERCP should be used nowadays almost exclusively for therapy. There is a less than 10% chance of finding objective pathology by ERCP in a patient with pain, normal or only slightly deranged chemistry, and normal CT/MRCP imaging. Where sphincter dysfunction is suspected, wisdom dictates referral to a center able to perform manometry, and experienced in methods (e.g. pancreatic stenting) known to reduce the risk of pancreatitis.

The consensus panel at the 2002 NIH State-of-the-Science Conference on ERCP advised strongly against the 'casual use' of ERCP in the investigation of patients with obscure abdominal pain, stating 'Diagnostic ERCP has no role in the assessment of these patients. It is precisely the typical SOD patient profile (young, healthy female) that is at the highest risk for ERCP-induced severe pancreatitis and even death. Indeed the risk of complication exceeds potential benefit in many cases. Therefore, ERCP, if performed, must be coupled with diagnostic SOM (sphincter of Oddi manometry), possible dual sphincterotomy, and possible pancreatic stent placement. ERCP with SOM and sphincterotomy should ideally be performed at specific referral centers, and in randomized controlled trials that examine the impact and timing of therapeutic maneuvers on clinical outcome' [57].

When ERCP is indicated, there are several ways to reduce the risk of the procedure [114,118,126,155].

Mechanical factors

Attention to the mechanical factors discussed above can reduce the risk. Gentle intelligent probing for the desired duct with minimal injections of contrast will help. The endoscopist who personally injects the contrast has better control of this important variable. Probing with a guidewire rather than contrast may be prudent, but reduced risk has not been proven. It is important to know when to stop. Failure to complete an ERCP may feel bad, but severe pancreatitis feels much worse, to both endoscopist and patient. Persisting, and using more dangerous approaches like precutting, can be justified only when there is a strong indication for the procedure, i.e. good evidence for biliary (or pancreatic) pathology, and a likelihood of needing endoscopic therapy.

When manometry is performed, it is clearly wise to use an aspirating catheter system [156]. In the future, microtransducer technology may be preferable and safer [157].

The type of current used for sphincterotomy does not appear to be a big factor influencing the pancreatitis rate [134–139], but it is clearly wise to avoid excessive coagulation near the pancreatic orifice.

Contrast agents

Extensive studies have not shown any consistent benefit for one or other contrast agent for ERCP [158–163].

Pharmacological prophylaxis

The list of pharmacological agents that have been proposed and tested for prophylaxis of post-ERCP pancreatitis is long and varied [114,126,155,164,165]. It includes antibiotics [166], heparin [167], corticosteroids [168–173], nifedipine [174,175], octreotide and somatostatin derivatives [176–193], trinitrin [194–196], lidocaine spray [197], gabexate [198,199], secretin, cytokine inhibitors [200–203], and a non-steroidal (rectal diclofenac) [204]. Apart from a 12 h infusion of gabexate [198], the study using diclofenac is so far the only one to show some promise. It deserves further evaluation, not least because of its simplicity, and the fact that it can be given selectively after ERCP. Preliminary data on secretin prophylaxis are encouraging [205].

None of the agents tested so far has proven to be sufficiently effective and practicable to find a place in routine practice, at least in Western countries. Reports suggest that octreotide analogs are widely used for this purpose in Japan.

Pancreatic stenting to prevent pancreatitis

There is now overwhelming evidence that temporary stenting of the pancreatic duct can reduce the risk of pancreatitis after ERCP in high-risk patients, e.g.

those with suspected or proven sphincter dysfunction, at least in expert centers [114]. This recognition is one of the most important developments in ERCP in the last 15 years. The first assessment was not convincing [206], but a randomized trial from our group in 1998 showed a dramatic benefit [207]. Eighty patients undergoing biliary sphincterotomy after manometry for suspected SOD were randomized to placement (with extraction next day) of a short 5 Fr pancreatic stent, or no stent. The pancreatitis rate fell from 26% to 7%.

The need for a second procedure to remove the stent is now obviated by the currently preferred technique of placing small stents that pass spontaneously within 1–2 weeks. We use stents of 3 Fr, with no internal flaps, and 8–12 cm long (so that the internal tip is in a straight part of the duct). Unlike larger and stiffer stents, these stents do not appear to cause any duct damage. Since mid-2000 this has been routine in all of our patients being investigated and treated for suspected sphincter dysfunction. The pancreatitis rate in these patients was 5.8% in 2002–03. We also use 3 Fr stents in other contexts when there has been extensive pancreatic manipulation.

Studies from many centers have amply confirmed the value of this technique [114,208–213]. One important caveat is that additional skills are required to pass small guidewires deeply into the pancreatic duct, so that the safety and value of the method are unproven in less experienced hands.

Feeding and monitoring

The need for postprocedure observation and possible food restriction to reduce the risks of ERCP has been discussed earlier.

Post-ERCP pancreatitis: recognition and management

Many patients experience some epigastric distress and bloating in the hour or two after ERCP. Often this is due to excessive air insufflation, which settles quickly. By contrast, pancreatitis usually becomes evident after a delay of 4–12 h, and is characterized by typical pancreatic-type pain, often associated with nausea and vomiting. Patients have tachycardia, epigastric tenderness, and absent or diminished bowel sounds. Serum levels of amylase and lipase are elevated, but leukocytosis is more predictive of severity than the enzyme levels.

Perforation is the most important alternative diagnosis, which should always be considered early if there is marked distress and abdominal tenderness (and especially if the serum levels of amylase/lipase are not impressive). Abdominal radiographs may be diagnostic in some cases, but CT is more sensitive.

The spectrum of severity and treatment of patients with pancreatitis after ERCP is the same as for pancreatitis occurring spontaneously [214]. Adequate

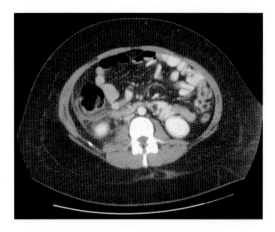

Fig. 13.1 CT scan of severe pancreatitis, taken 1 week after ERCP.

analgesia and aggressive fluid replacement are key. Some experts use octreotide analogs, but proof of benefit is anecdotal. CT scanning is indicated within 24 h if there is suspicion of perforation, and after a few days if clinical progress is slow or if fever develops (Fig. 13.1). Antibiotics are usually not given unless pancreatic infection is proven by percutaneous aspiration. The rare patient who develops a pseudocyst or pancreatic necrosis may require percutaneous or endoscopic drainage, or surgical debridement, and may require transfer to a tertiary center.

Post-ERCP pancreatitis: conclusion

Pancreatitis is now the commonest complication of ERCP, and can be devastating. It cannot yet be prevented completely, even in expert hands. It is most likely to occur when inexperienced endoscopists work on patients with minimal pathology. When the indication is not strong, wise clinicians will exhaust less invasive approaches before recommending or performing ERCP, will make sure that patients fully appreciate their individualized risk/benefit balance, and will include referral to expert centers in their consent process. Skillful technique, and the use of small pancreatic stents, will keep the risk of pancreatitis below 5% in most circumstances, but cannot yet eliminate it.

Perforation

Four different types of perforation have been described resulting from ERCP procedures [215]. They are:
• Perforation of ducts or tumors by guidewires and other instruments—perhaps better called 'penetrations'.
• Retroduodenal perforation related to sphincterotomy.

- Endoscopic perforation of the esophagus, stomach, or duodenum (away from the papilla).
- Stent-related perforation.

These types have different causes and consequences.

Duct and tumor 'penetrations'

Guidewires and occasionally accessories passed over guidewires (such as sphincterotomes, catheters, and dilators) can pass through the wall of the biliary or pancreatic ductal system (or indeed the raw area of a fresh sphincterotomy) [215,216]. This occurs perhaps most often when attempting to cannulate in a patient with a tumor involving the region of the papilla. These incidents are rarely reported, and so their frequency is unknown. They are more likely to occur with vigorous probing in difficult cases, especially when there is distortion by tumor or sharp ductal deviation for other reasons. Rigid guidewires may be more dangerous. Often it is safer to proceed with a 'flipped' tip wire, which tends to find the lumen more easily.

Ducts have also been disrupted occasionally by over-aggressive balloon dilatation of biliary (and pancreatic) strictures. The radiographic appearances may appear somewhat alarming when contrast is injected.

The risk of this event can be reduced by careful insertion of instruments whilst being aware of the potential problem. Recognition is usually straightforward, and the problem is defused satisfactorily by finding the correct lumen, and by completing the procedure (e.g. by stenting). It is very unusual indeed for a patient to have any adverse consequences.

Sphincterotomy-related perforation

Perforation occurring after sphincterotomy is always retroduodenal. It is defined by the presence of air (and/or contrast) in the retroperitoneum.

A review of more than 12 000 biliary sphincterotomies performed before 1990 showed a sphincterotomy perforation rate of 1.3%; 27% of these patients were operated on, and the overall mortality was 0.2%. Since that time, most publications show a sphincterotomy perforation rate of < 1% [24,25,44,49,62,215,217]. Three studies have reported higher perforation rates: 1.1% [218], 1.8% [22], and 2.2% [40].

Only four perforations have been recorded after 2820 biliary sphincterotomies at MUSC over the last 10 years, a rate of 0.14%: three were operated on, and none died.

Routine CT scans in asymptomatic patients after uncomplicated sphincterotomy have shown small quantities of periduodenal or retroperitoneal air in up to

10% of patients [219,220], so it may be that there are more asymptomatic 'micro-perforations' than is commonly recognized.

Risk factors for sphincterotomy perforation

It is assumed that perforation is more likely with larger and repeat biliary sphincterotomies, and that cutting beyond '1–2 o'clock' is more risky. It is not reported more frequently in patients with peripapillary diverticula [59,60]. As discussed above, precut sphincterotomy appears to be relatively safe and useful in expert hands, with restricted indications, but it is clearly more dangerous in routine practice, and when used, for instance, in patients with suspected sphincter dysfunction [44,76]. Perforation rates after precutting as high as 5% have been reported [22,75,77], and precut-related perforations feature prominently in medico-legal cases involving ERCP.

Perforation also appears to be more likely in patients with suspected SOD [44]. This may be due simply to the smaller (often normal-) sized ducts, or because patients with bile duct stones are somehow protected (due to the distorting/fibrotic effect of recurrent stone impaction or passage). It has been reported occasionally after forceful extraction of large stones, and at least once after balloon dilatation of the sphincter to remove stones without sphincterotomy [144].

Perforation after pancreatic sphincterotomy (at the main or minor papilla) is extremely rare [71]. One occurred during 1615 pancreatic sphincterotomies at MUSC over the last 10 years.

Recognition of sphincterotomy perforation

Perforation may become obvious during the procedure itself, when unusual territory is encountered (Figs 13.2 and 13.3), or when the radiographs show contrast in non-anatomical shapes around the duodenum. This is best recognized by inflating and then aspirating air to show that the odd radiographic shape does not change (which it does if the contrast is in the duodenum). Occasionally, if sufficient air has been insufflated after the perforation, fluoroscopy may show air around the right kidney and along the lower edge of the liver (Fig. 13.4) [218].

Most cases of perforation are not recognized until after the procedure, when the patient complains of epigastric pain. The differential diagnosis is pancreatitis, which is far more common. Perforation should always be considered when the pain starts soon after the procedure (pancreatitis may not develop for 4–12 h), when symptoms are more severe than anticipated, and when accompanied by guarding and tachycardia. Rarely, patients may develop subcutaneous emphysema, pneumo-mediastinum or pneumo-thoraces after a few hours [221,222]. The white blood count usually rises quickly. Finding a normal or

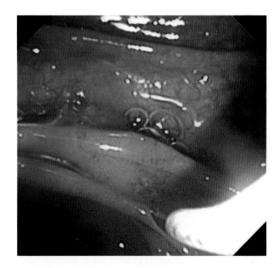

Fig. 13.2 Endoscopic view of the minor papilla before needle-knife sphincterotomy.

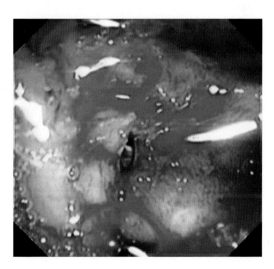

Fig. 13.3 Perforation visible after needle-knife sphincterotomy of the minor papilla.

only slightly elevated serum level of amylase or lipase in patients with impressive abdominal pain should raise suspicion of perforation.

A plain abdominal X-ray may show retroduodenal air, but CT scanning is more definitive (Fig. 13.5) [218], and should be performed within 24 h in any patient with severe abdominal symptoms after sphincterotomy.

Reducing risks of sphincterotomy perforation

Clearly, the best way to reduce the risk of causing perforation at sphincterotomy is to minimize the use of higher risk techniques, such as cutting too far, cutting 'off-line', extending prior sphincterotomies, and precutting.

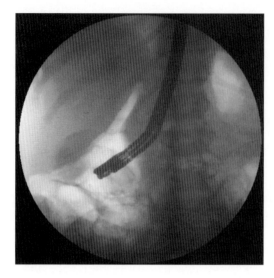

Fig. 13.4 Abdominal radiograph at ERCP showing retroperitoneal air.

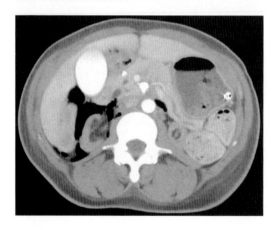

Fig. 13.5 CT scan showing retroperitoneal air after perforation.

Management of sphincterotomy perforation

Perforation is a life-threatening event; prompt recognition and efficient management are very important [215,217,223–227]. Patients should have nothing by mouth and adequate intravenous fluids (and nutrition as necessary), and are usually given antibiotics. Most experts recommend placement of a gastric or duodenal drainage tube. A few endoscopists have suggested placing a biliary stent or nasobiliary drain to reduce contamination of the retroperitoneum, but this is not proven or standard practice, and the additional manipulation may make matters worse.

Surgery? Most surgeons equate perforation with immediate operation. However, surgeons exploring cases often are unable to find the site of perforation, and end up simply leaving retroperitoneal drains. Reported experience, including surgical studies [217,226], shows that surgery is not usually necessary, and that most (reported) retroduodenal perforations have been managed conservatively. An important caveat is that conservative therapy seems to be effective only when perforation is recognized early [217].

Despite the dominance of non-operative treatment for perforation, it is wise to obtain a surgical opinion at the earliest possible stage. Patients should be managed jointly on a daily basis. I recommend immediate/early surgery only if there is remaining biliary pathology which itself requires operation. Thus, a patient with gallbladder stones can reasonably undergo immediate cholecystectomy and placement of drains. However, most perforations occur in patients with little or no remaining pathology (e.g. cleared retained stones or SOD), where there is no indication for surgery—other than the known perforation. Conservative management is usually effective if started early, but intervention (percutaneous or surgical) may be required in the ensuing days or weeks if fluid collections/abscesses develop in the right renal or pericolic areas. Operating at a later stage is often difficult because of infection; it may be necessary to perform diversionary procedures as well as multiple drains [217]. A few patients have had a very bad experience, with months in hospital and multiple operations.

One successful case of endoscopic treatment with multiple clips has been reported [228].

Perforation remote from the papilla

Endoscopic perforation can occur anywhere that endoscopes travel.

The lateral-viewing nature of the duodenoscope may perhaps increase the risk of pharyngeal perforation in elderly patients with diverticula. In the absence of pathology, it is difficult to conceive how endoscopic perforation could occur in the esophagus or stomach, but such events have been reported [215,229,230]. It has also happened rarely in the duodenum, when attempting to negotiate a stricture or marked distortion by tumor. The first therapeutic video-duodeno-scopes had a long distal tip, which caused perforations during forceful stone extraction maneuvers [231,232].

Perforation of the afferent loop is a definite risk during endoscopy of patients after Billroth II gastrectomy (and more complex bypass procedures) [232–234]. Rates as high as 6% [233] and even 20% [234] have been reported in this context.

Perforation usually occurs as a result of stretching of loops rather than penetration of the endoscopic tip. It can be avoided largely by careful endo-scopic technique, especially in patients who have undergone diversionary pro-cedures or who have known stenosing pathology.

One expert suggests that all Billroth II patients (and more complex diver-sions) should be referred to tertiary centers, because of the added difficulty and significant risk [232].

The incidence of endoscopic (as opposed to sphincterotomy) perforations is unknown, but should be extremely low. It is less than 1:1000 in our series, all of them in the afferent loop context (Table 13.6).

Recognition and management of endoscopic perforation

Diagnosis of endoscopic perforation is usually obvious, either during the pro-cedure, or because of obvious patient distress and clinical signs in the chest or abdomen. Radiographs show intraperitoneal (or mediastinal) air.

Endoscopic perforation usually requires surgical intervention, and prompt surgical consultation is mandatory. Rare episodes have been treated conservatively.

Stent migration perforation

There have been rare reports of penetration and even perforation of the duode-num, small bowel, and colon by stents which have migrated from the bile duct [235,236]. Almost all of these have been 'straight' 10 Fr gauge stents. Those that have migrated down from the bile duct and penetrated the opposite duodenal wall can sometimes be managed simply by endoscopic extraction. Others have required surgical intervention.

Infection after ERCP

Generic infection risks of all endoscopic procedures (e.g. endocarditis, viral transmission) are discussed elsewhere [237]. Preprocedure antibiotics are recommended for prophylaxis against endocarditis by standard guidelines.

ERCP differs from most other endoscopies in that it risks contaminating territory that is usually sterile. Also, when bile is infected (e.g. in patients with stones or blocked stents), biliary manipulation may disseminate the infection locally or systemically.

By consensus, infection is defined as 'an otherwise unexplained fever of greater than 38°C lasting 24–48 h after ERCP'. It is described as moderately severe if it requires more than 3 days' treatment in hospital, or further endoscopic or percutaneous intervention, and as severe if the patient develops septic shock or requires surgery [15].

The reported incidence of clinical infections after ERCP is low, ranging from 0.7 to 1.6% in various modern series [22,27,29,40,44,238–243]. However, bacteremia rates of up to 27% have been reported [237,244].

Nosocomial infection

In the early days of ERCP, before the importance of disinfection was recognized, there were several unfortunate outbreaks of nosocomial infections (usually due to *Pseudomonas*) [16,18,237,245]. Sadly, *Pseudomonas* infections are still being described after ERCP [246–249]. Almost all are due to faulty cleaning and disinfection, and should be preventable.

Cholangitis

Bacteremia and septicemia occur when the bile is infected and drainage is compromised. This can occur after ERCP in patients with stones or strictures if adequate drainage is not achieved, and when bilary stents become occluded [238–244,250]. The risk of introducing or stirring up infection when the bile is infected can be minimized by adhering to disinfection protocols, by reducing the biliary pressure (by aspirating bile before injecting much contrast), and by ensuring adequate drainage by removing all obstructing stones or placing appropriate stents. Sepsis is a particular risk after ERCP management of hilar tumors and sclerosing cholangitis, where it may prove impossible to provide complete drainage of all obstructed segments. This is a good reason for obtaining detailed anatomical imaging (by CT and/or MRCP) beforehand to assist therapeutic planning.

Cholecystitis

Cholecystitis, sometimes with odd characteristics [251,252], has occurred soon after ERCP; presumably this is more likely when there is cystic duct compromise by stone or tumor (or occasionally after stenting). It is managed by standard percutaneous or surgical techniques.

Pancreatic sepsis

This has occurred as part of severe pancreatitis after ERCP [253], and in patients with pseudocysts [104], due to inadequate disinfection or incomplete drainage.

Prophylactic antibiotics

The role of prophylactic antibiotics in the prevention of infection after ERCP is still unclear, despite a very substantial literature and much opinion [254–263]. Although one randomized study did appear to show benefit for antibiotic prophylaxis [260], this and others [258] demonstrated most clearly that biliary obstruction is the main hazard, and that effective drainage is the best treatment. The risk of serious infection is now so low that further randomized trials are unlikely to be helpful.

In earlier years, we gave intravenous antibiotics (usually ampicillin and gentamycin) to all patients with clinical or radiological evidence of duct obstruction, and whenever therapy seemed probable (which meant about 90% of all cases). The infection rate was < 1%. We gradually reduced the indications for prophylaxis, and changed to oral ciprofloxacin, without any increase in infection [264]. Our current practice is to give oral ciprofloxacin (two doses) before ERCP when failure of complete drainage is predictable (e.g. complex hilar tumors, sclerosing cholangitis, and pseudocysts), and to give it intravenously immediately after any procedure in which we fail to provide drainage. With this policy, the incidence of clinical infection in our unit remains well below 1% (Table 13.6). Some have advocated mixing antibiotics with the contrast media, but this practice has never been validated.

Delayed infection

The commonest cause of delayed biliary sepsis is a blocked stent. Patients can become seriously ill quickly with septic cholangitis. For this reason, patients and their caregivers must be fully informed about this risk and instructed to make contact as soon as symptoms develop. For the same reason, it is common practice to change plastic stents routinely (at 3–4 months), especially in patients with benign biliary strictures. The need to do so in patients with malignant disease (as opposed to waiting for obstructive symptoms) has not been validated in controlled studies, but is still common practice.

Bleeding after ERCP

Clinically significant bleeding has occurred rarely after diagnostic ERCP (due to retching, or after biopsy in patients with tumors or coagulopathy, or after cannulation in patients with biliary varices). However, the main cause of bleeding is sphincterotomy (or other cutting procedure such as papillectomy and pseudocyst drainage). It is common to see a small amount of 'endoscopic' bleeding (Fig. 13.6) (i.e. oozing immediately after sphincterotomy), but clinically relevant bleeding is much rarer.

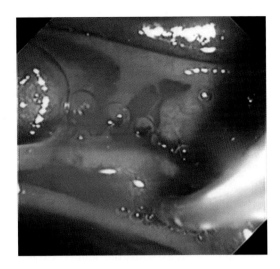

Fig. 13.6 Bleeding immediately after starting sphincterotomy.

Bleeding can occur immediately, but is often delayed for up to 2 weeks.

Whilst significant bleeding is usually manifested by hematemesis and/or melena, occasional patients can present with biliary pain and cholangitis if bleeding fills the bile duct.

Definition of bleeding, and incidence

The consensus conference on complications defined bleeding in clinical terms. Even impressive immediate bleeding is not counted as a complication if it can be stopped by endoscopic manipulation during the procedure. The severity of the bleeding is stratified as follows:

- mild: clinical (not just endoscopic) evidence of bleeding, with a hemoglobin drop of less than 3 g/dl and no transfusion;
- moderate: transfusion (4 units or less), but no angiographic interventional surgery;
- severe: transfusion of 5 units of more, or intervention (angiographic or surgical);
- fatal: death attributable to bleeding.

Memory and some early publications [15,17,19,20,265] indicate that bleeding was the commonest complication of sphincterotomy in the first 10–15 years after its introduction, with an average rate of 2.5% in over 20 000 reported sphincterotomies [15], and a high of 11% [265]. More recent series, using the consensus definitions, report a lower incidence of 0.8–2% [24,25,44]. One series suggested that the true incidence is higher if hematological parameters are followed routinely [266]. More than half the reported episodes of bleeding are delayed for up to 2 weeks.

The rate of bleeding after biliary sphincterotomy was 0.7%; most were delayed.

Risk factors for bleeding, and avoidance

Bleeding is certainly more likely to occur in patients with coagulopathy and/or portal hypertension [267,268], renal failure [268], and apparently also when a sphincterotomy is repeated [93]. There is no evidence that the risk is greater in patients taking aspirin and other agents affecting platelet function [268–270], although it is still common practice to ask patients to discontinue their use. Delayed clinical bleeding may [268] or may not [271] be more common when there has been some immediate oozing.

Prevention

Sphincterotomy should always be performed in a controlled manner, with blended current, avoiding the 'zipper' cut. Coagulopathies should be corrected wherever possible. Anticoagulants should be discontinued, but the need for temporary heparin coverage, and the duration, are controversial. The effect of newer antiplatelet agents has yet to be clearly established, but most endoscopists prefer these to be stopped for 10 days if possible. The type of current used may be relevant. One study showed that the ERBE generator reduced bleeding visible at the time of endoscopy, but not the risk of clinically defined bleeding [272]. Another study utilizing initial cutting current (to reduce the risk of pancreatitis) did show a slightly increased risk of bleeding [273].

Balloon dilatation of the sphincter can be used instead of sphincterotomy for extracting some stones in patients with irreversible coagulopathy or severe portal hypertension [151,274,275].

Management of sphincterotomy bleeding

Bleeding immediately after sphincterotomy usually stops spontaneously, and (unless there is a pumping vessel) it is usually not necessary to take any dramatic action. There are varying opinions about management when treatment is needed [271,276–286]. Some have advocated monopolar cautery [283], local injection of contrast agent [284], even hemoclips [285]. However, it appears that epinephrine injection is the most popular and effective technique [271,286].

My practice (with unimpressive bleeding) is first to spray the site with about 10 ml of a dilute (1 : 100 000) solution of epinephrine. This often stops oozing temporarily, at least enough to see exactly where the bleeding is coming from. If bleeding is impressive, or if oozing persists, balloon tamponade is the next step. A retrieval balloon is overinflated in the bile duct, and then pulled down forcefully to compress the bleeding site between the balloon and the endoscope tip for 5 min. If that fails, we inject epinephrine (diluted 1 : 10 000) using a standard sclerotherapy needle. Up to 5 ml can be injected in aliquots of 1 ml, taking care not to compromise the pancreatic orifice. For this reason, it is my practice to inject just outside the top edges of the sphincterotomy, rather than within it. If there has been much manipulation, it may be wise to place a small protective pancreatic stent (if possible).

Very rarely, bleeding is profuse, and endoscopic vision is quickly lost. Expert angiographic management can be effective [287]. Surgical oversewing would seem logical when all else fails, but re-bleeding may occur [265].

Delayed bleeding

This can occur up to 2 weeks after sphincterotomy, and should be treated like any other episode of bleeding. It is important to confirm the source of bleeding, since patients occasionally bleed from other lesions.

Complications of stents

Biliary and pancreatic stents can cause problems through local trauma, blockage, and migration. Much depends on their size, nature, and position. Sphincterotomy (when placing biliary stents) appears not to affect the rate of blockage [102,288], but may reduce the risk of pancreatitis, at least with hilar tumors [103].

Blockage of (plastic) biliary stents

This is inevitable after a few months, and can cause serious cholangitis. A host of ingenious attempts to prevent this phenomenon over two decades has so far been unavailing (Chapter 3) [289]. It is common practice to reduce the risk by recommending the routine exchange of biliary stents at about 3 months. This is mandatory in patients with benign strictures. It is perhaps legitimate to await events in patients with malignant disease if they (and their caregivers) are well informed about the first symptoms (usually shaking chills), and the need for urgent action. Expandable metal stents usually last much longer, but the consequences of blockage are equally serious.

Stent migration

Stents which migrate outwards may cause damage to the duodenum [235] or distal intestine [236]. Stents which migrate inwards can be difficult to retrieve, especially in the pancreatic duct [290]. Most migrated stents can be teased out of the papilla with a retrieval balloon, or grasped with foreign body forceps, snare, or basket. Rarely, surgery is needed to rectify these situations.

Duct damage due to stents

The presence of a stent in the bile duct for many months may cause some wall irregularity and thickening. This can be seen radiologically (and can cause diagnostic difficulty at EUS), but has no clinical relevance. However, stent-induced duct damage is a serious problem in the pancreas [291–295], especially when the duct initially is normal. Irritation by the tip of the stent (especially at a duct bend), or by internal flaps, often causes wall irregularity, and clinically significant narrowing. Some early descriptions suggested that most of these lesions resolved after stent removal, but we have seen many tight fibrotic strictures, which are very difficult to manage. Relatively stiff pancreatic stents of 7 and even 10 Fr can be used legitimately in some patients with established chronic pancreatitis for the management of stones or strictures. However, when stenting seems indicated in relatively normal ducts, it seems wise to use smaller (3 or 5 Fr) and softer stents, and for only a few weeks [295]. The length of a pancreatic stent should be chosen so that the inner tip is in a straight part of the duct.

Cholecystitis

This has been reported after biliary stenting for malignancy [296–298].

Basket impaction

Baskets may become impacted during attempts to remove large stones from the bile duct [299]. Usually, this situation can be rectified quickly by disengaging the stone, or by crushing it with a 'rescue' lithotripsy sleeve (Chapter 3). To prevent this problem, it is wise to use a mechanical lithotripsy system initially when approaching stones > 1 cm in diameter. Baskets should be used sparingly and with great caution in the pancreatic duct. They are effective for the removal of soft stones (protein plugs) and mucus, but calcified pancreatic stones are very resistant to mechanical lithotripsy. There is a risk that the basket will break inside the duct and remain impacted.

Cardiopulmonary complications and sedation issues

Adverse cardiopulmonary events can occur during any endoscopic procedure [300,301], and myocardial ischemia has been studied specifically during ERCP [302,303].

Transient hypoxia and cardiac dysrhythmias occur occasionally during ERCP procedures, but are usually recognized and managed appropriately without clinical consequences. Very rarely, they may result in severe decompensation during or after procedures, and are a significant cause of the rare fatalities attributable to ERCP.

Risk factors for cardiopulmonary complications include known or unsuspected premorbid conditions, and problems related to sedation and analgesia. Oversedation can be a serious problem, especially in the elderly and frail, and particularly if monitoring is inadequate (in a darkened room).

Cardiopulmonary complications can be largely avoided by careful pre-procedure evaluation, appropriate collaboration with anesthesiologists (and cardiologists) when dealing with high-risk patients, formal training of endoscopists and nurses in sedation and resuscitation, and careful monitoring [304].

Aspiration pneumonia has been described after all types of endoscopic procedures; the incidence is unknown, but it is probably more common than recognized, since the onset may be delayed.

Rare complications

Many other untoward events have followed ERCP. These include:
- **Gallstone ileus** after removing large stones [305,306].
- **Musculo-skeletal injuries** (e.g. dislocation of the temporomandibular joint [307] or shoulder, dental trauma).
- **Opacification of blood vessels.** The portal venous system and lymphatics have been seen [308,309] whilst injecting contrast through tapered tip catheters. The contrast moves rapidly on fluoroscopy. If air is injected as well, the appearances on CT scan are alarming [310], but no sequelae have been reported.
- **Antral sinus infection** after prolonged nasobiliary drainage.
- **Renal dysfunction** [311] with the use of nephrotoxic medications (such as gentamycin).
- **Impaction or fracturing of nasobiliary and nasopancreatic drains.**
- **Allergic reactions to iodine-containing contrast agents.** Allergic reactions have happened, even with the very small doses which enter the bloodstream during ERCP. Endoscopy units should have policies in place to deal with patients who claim to be allergic [312].
- **Increased cholestasis** in patients with sclerosing cholangitis [313].
- **Splenic injury** has been reported several times during ERCP [314–316].
- **Distant abscesses** have occurred in the spleen and kidney [314,317], and no doubt elsewhere.

- **Hemolysis** due to G6PD deficiency and hemolytic–uremic syndrome has been reported [318,319].
- **Dissemination of pancreatic cancer** was reported after sphincterotomy [320].
- **A false aneurysm** of a branch of the pancreatico-duodenal artery developed after needle-knife sphincterotomy [321].

Deaths after ERCP

The literature reporting deaths after ERCP is difficult to analyze as the series contain different spectra of patients and procedures, and some do not distinguish between 30 day mortality and events attributable to the procedure itself. One paper illustrates the difficulty in attributing mortality between concurrent illness, active complications, and complications due to other procedures required after ERCP failure [26]. Data collected for the consensus conference in 1991 reported 103 deaths after 7729 sphincterotomies (1.3%). Most subsequent series report mortality figures of less than 0.5% [24,27,37,44,65,322], with two higher figures of 0.8% [29] and 1% [323].

The causes of death in all of the reported series cover the spectrum of the commonest complications, with approximately equal numbers resulting from pancreatitis, bleeding, perforation, infection, and cardiopulmonary events. Delay in diagnosis of perforation is mentioned as a contributing cause in several publications [217,224,324]. Of nine fatalities resulting in claims to insurance in Denmark, seven were attributable to pancreatitis (two of which had undergone precutting) [325].

Late complications

There are a number of adverse events attributable to ERCP that may not be apparent for months or even years afterwards.

Diagnostic error

Failure to make the correct diagnosis is an under-reported and greatly under-appreciated complication of ERCP. It can be due to poor technique (both endoscopic and radiological), as well as incorrect interpretation of adequate images, or both. Bile duct stones are missed with inadequate duct filling, especially in less obvious sites such as the cystic duct stump and the dependent right intrahepatic duct, or when over-dense contrast is used in a dilated system. Conversely, air bubbles introduced into the system may be misinterpreted as stones (with the potential serious consequences of an unnecessary sphincterotomy).

Poor opacification and ignorance of anatomy may lead to missed or erroneous diagnoses in patients with bile duct injuries. Congenital variations of biliopancreatic drainage are under-recognized. Early stages of chronic pancreatitis and intraductal mucinous tumors are easily missed with inadequate filling. Pancreas divisum may be missed when the ventral duct is rudimentary, and the pancreatic pathology unassessed if dorsal cannulation is not achieved.

Few endoscopists have a radiologist on hand to help with fluoroscopy, film recording, or the immediate interpretation which is needed to formulate therapeutic tactics. It is common practice for radiologists to report the available films after the event, and major discrepancies have been noted [326], a fact which raises complex issues. Providing the reporting radiologist with a detailed copy of the endoscopic report is helpful, and allows radiologists to communicate any differences of opinion.

Late infection

There is a possibility of transmitting non-bacterial infections at ERCP, with an incubation period long enough to hide the relationship, but there are no proven and reported cases. There is a definite risk of sepsis developing when biliary stents become occluded. Patients present with fevers and shaking chills, and can deteriorate rapidly. Any stented patient (and caregivers) must be warned about the possibility, and the need for speedy medical contact and resolution. Patients receiving plastic stents for benign biliary strictures should be advised to undergo a routine stent service at 3–4 months; practice varies with malignant strictures (Chapter 6). Endoscopists placing stents have a continuing responsibility to contact patients with reminders. Occasionally, patients may willfully or accidentally avoid the repeat procedure, with considerable potential for serious complications. The concept of long-term stenting for 'difficult' stones has been discredited because of the risk of delayed cholangitis [327].

Late effects of sphincterotomy

There has been much interest in the possible long-term adverse consequences of biliary sphincterotomy [328–339]. When performed for 'papillary stenosis', there is a significant risk of further biliary-type symptoms, whether due to restenosis or an incorrect diagnosis (Chapter 8).

Sphincterotomy leads almost inevitably to bacterial contamination of the bile [340–344], which may be a potent promoter of pigment stone formation. One study showed a significant increase in the incidence of cholangiocarcinoma after surgical sphincteroplasty [345], but a cohort study in Scandinavia found no such association after endoscopic sphincterotomy [346]. Many patients have been followed for periods of 10 years or more after sphincterotomy for stones [332,334–336,338–340]. The chance of further biliary problems in these studies ranges from 5 to 24%, with an average of about 10% [347]. The Amsterdam study had the highest figure (24%) and all but one of the patients had recurrent stones [330]. In other series, some patients had episodes of cholangitis without stones, even cholangitis without stenosis of the sphincterotomy [332].

Most of these long-term complications of sphincterotomy are easily managed endoscopically, remembering that repeat incisions do carry a slightly greater risk. A few patients continue to reform stones every 6–12 months despite apparently adequate drainage, and may need to be scheduled for repeated endoscopic 'biliary laundry' [348].

Sphincterotomy with the gallbladder in place

Most patients having their ducts cleared of stones endoscopically have undergone cholecystectomy soon afterwards. However, some have not, usually because the risk has been judged to be too great (and especially before the days of laparoscopic cholecystectomy). Several series have examined the long-term risks of leaving the gallbladder in place [349–354]. The reported need for cholecystectomy has ranged from 5 to 33% [337], but most of the follow-up periods are short. Two trials have addressed this issue recently. Thirty-four patients treated endoscopically for acute biliary pancreatitis (and without cholecystectomy) were followed for a mean of 34 months; only 11.6% developed further biliary complications [354]. However, the Amsterdam group performed a randomized trial of 120 patients with the gallbladder in place after biliary sphincterotomy. No fewer than 47% of those treated expectantly developed further biliary symptoms, compared with 2% of those who underwent early cholecystectomy [353]. The suggestion that non-filling of the gallbladder at the index ERCP (indicating cystic duct obstruction) was a predictor of future trouble has not been substantiated [352]. However, it seems clear that the risk is negligible in patients who have no stones remaining in the gallbladder, which is sometimes the case in the context of gallstone pancreatitis [350].

Pancreatic sphincterotomy

The main risk of pancreatic sphincterotomy appears to be restenosis, which occurs in at least 20% of reported cases (Chapters 6, 7 and 8).

It is usually treated endoscopically, but strictures that occur beneath the papilla can be challenging even for surgical repair. Hopefully, better techniques (and new stents) may reduce this risk in the future.

Stenosis of the pancreatic orifice causing recurrent pancreatitis has been reported as a late complication of biliary sphincterotomy [355].

Managing adverse events

All ERCP endoscopists experience complications. Each event requires specific skillful recognition and management (as detailed above), but there are several very important general guidelines.

Prompt recognition and action

The keys to effective management of all complications are early recognition and prompt focused action. Delay is dangerous both medically and legally. Patients in pain and distress after procedures should always be examined carefully, and never simply 'reassured' without careful evaluation. If you are not personally on call on the night after your ERCP procedures, it is helpful to make sure that the person covering is aware of what you have done. Get appropriate laboratory studies and radiographs, consult the extensive literature, and do not hesitate to seek advice from other experts in the relevant fields. It is wise to consult an (informed) surgeon early on for anything that might remotely require surgical intervention. Sometimes it may be appropriate to offer transfer of care of the patient to a specialty colleague, or to a larger medical center, but, if this happens, try to keep in touch, and to show continuing interest and concern. Apparent abandonment alienates patients and their relatives, and may lead to initiation of legal action.

Professionalism and communication

Endoscopists often feel devastated when serious complications occur. Your distress is understandable and worthy, and it is important to be sympathetic, but it is equally important to be composed and matter of fact. Excessive apologies may give an unfortunate impression. Never, never, attempt to cover up the facts. Poor communication is the basis for much unhappiness, and many lawsuits. Remember that the truly informed patient and any accompanying persons have been told already that complications can happen. This is an integral important part of the consent process. So it is appropriate and correct to address suspected complications in that spirit. 'It looks as if we have a perforation here. We discussed that as a remote possibility beforehand, and I am sorry that it has occurred. Here is what I think we should do.' It is also wise to contact and inform other interested relatives, referring physicians, supervisors, and your Risk Management advisors.

Documentation

Document what has happened carefully and honestly in real time. Don't even think of adding notes retrospectively. The results of many lawsuits hang on the quality of the documentation, or lack of it.

Learning from lawsuits

Fortunately, most complications do not result in legal action. Despite the fact that ERCP is the most dangerous of the routine endoscopic procedures, there are far more claims after colonoscopy and upper endoscopy [356]. There are several reasons why patients (or their survivors) may initiate a claim.

Communication

Communication, or lack of it, is often a major complaint. Too often we hear that 'we would never have consented to the procedure if we had known that this might happen'. Sometimes this is simply because patients don't want to hear, but often the consent process is quite inadequate. A hurried conversation immediately before the procedure is not sufficient. Taking time to provide the information (face to face and in writing), making sure that it has been understood, and writing down that you have done it, is simply good medical practice [105].

Good communication after an adverse event is equally important. Show that you care. Litigants are sometimes simply (and justifiably) angry if they get the impression that you do not.

Financial concerns

These are also often prominent, even if not stated. Hospital bills and loss of earnings can be crippling.

Standard of care practice

Once a lawsuit has been filed, the key issue is whether the endoscopist (and others involved) practiced within the 'standard of care'. This is defined in various ways, but comes down to what reasonable colleagues would do (and is expressed in court by what expert witnesses opine). The report from the NIH Consensus Conference is a crucial resource [57], and is particularly forceful in recommending caution when considering ERCP in patients with little or no objective evidence for pathology (i.e. 'suspected sphincter dysfunction').

The key standard of care issues are given below.

Indications

Was the ERCP procedure really indicated in the first place? The task clearly is to balance the possible benefits against the potential risks [357]. Although professional societies publish guidelines for the use of ERCP [358], the devil is in the details, e.g. how much elevation of liver tests or increased duct size constitutes 'objective evidence of pathology'. In practice, the validity of the decision to proceed will be judged by the severity of the symptoms, by the thoroughness of prior treatment and investigations, and the process of communication. Were the symptoms (or other signs of pathology) really that pressing? Had less invasive approaches (nowadays including MRCP) been exhausted, or at least considered and discussed [359]? There are some circumstances (such as postcholecystectomy pain with some abnormality of liver tests) which may justify ERCP even if imaging is negative, but where it may be unwise to strive too hard (e.g. by prolonged attempts or precutting) when cannulation proves difficult.

For less experienced endoscopists, consideration of alternatives (especially for higher risk procedures) should include possible referral to an expert center.

The procedure

Was there an obvious deviation from customary practice, like placing a 10 Fr stent in a normal pancreatic duct, or trying to extract a stone from the bile duct without sphincterotomy (or papillary balloon dilatation)? Did the level of suspicion of pathology really justify a precut? Was there radiological evidence for over-manipulation of the pancreas, over-injection (e.g. acinarization), or injection into a branch duct? The notes of the procedure nurse may contain important evidence, like excessive sedation or contrast, or documentation of patient distress. Pretty endoscopic photographs may also be incriminating, e.g. if they show sphincterotomy in an unusual direction.

Postprocedure care

Was the patient appropriately monitored, discharged in good condition, and properly advised? Was action taken promptly when unexpected symptoms developed? Was the endoscopist available to advise? Among the most common errors are delay in action (particularly in considering and managing perforation) and inadequate fluid resuscitation in patients with pancreatitis.

Conclusion

After more than 30 years, the risks of ERCP and its therapeutic procedures are now well documented. Pancreatitis and sedation-related events are the commonest, but bleeding and perforation still occur. There are a host of rare complications. Understanding and managing the main risk factors can keep these events to a minimum, but cannot eliminate them. For this reason, making sure that patients understand what they are accepting is of crucial importance. Inexperience and over-confidence are dangerous partners.

Outstanding issues and future trends

The two biggest issues for ERCP at the present time are the quality of practice and how to minimize or eliminate postprocedure pancreatitis. These are not unrelated, for we know that experts have lower complication rates, even while dealing with higher risk clientele. Thus, we are forced to focus on how to maximize expertise.

Many experts for a long time have been advocating that fewer endoscopists should be trained in ERCP, so that their skills can be maximized before and after entering practice. This trend is perhaps evident at long last, driven by several forces. Firstly, diagnostic ERCP is becoming obsolescent as non-invasive methods (especially MRCP) improve. This means that would-be ERCP practitioners can often now see the suspected therapeutic issue beforehand. They must be prepared for the challenge, but also have the option of referring problematic cases (e.g. hilar tumors and 'suspected sphincter dysfunction'). Secondly, the seminal studies of Freeman and colleagues, and a few others, have made endoscopists (and lawyers) much more aware of certain high-risk behaviors, such as casual precutting. Thirdly, most gastroenterologists have no shortage of other activities (not least screening colonoscopy) to keep them interested and busy. The final driver is the increasing sophistication of our patients, who are learning that not all interventionists are equal—as is well documented in surgery [8]—and are demanding the data with which to make informed choices [360].

All interventions carry some risks, which are acceptable if the indications are appropriate, i.e. when there are substantial potential benefits. To do a better job of predicting benefit will require many more major prospective outcome studies. We need careful objective and structured cohort studies of ERCP in various clinical contexts, and some randomized studies in comparison with other approaches, such as surgery.

Thus, in the future, we hope that there will be fewer but very well trained and experienced ERCP practitioners, and that both they and their patients will have a better understanding of the risk/benefit ratio in each case.

References

1 Cotton PB. Outcomes of endoscopic procedures: struggling towards definitions. *Gastrointest Endosc* 1994; 40: 514–18.
2 Fleischer DE. Better definition of endoscopic complications and other negative outcomes. *Gastrointest Endosc* 1994; 40 (4): 511–13.
3 Fleischer DE, Van de Mierop F, Eisen GM, Al-Kawas FH, Benjamin SB, Lewis JH *et al.* A new system for defining endoscopic complications emphasizing the measure of importance. *Gastrointest Endosc* 1997; 45 (2): 128–33.
4 Cotton PB. Income and outcome metrics for the objective evaluation of ERCP and alternative methods. *Gastrointest Endosc* 2002; 56 (6): S283–90.
5 Campbell N, Sparrow K, Fortier M, Ponich T. Practical radiation safety and protection for the endoscopist during ERCP. *Gastrointest Endosc* 2002; 55 (4): 552–7.
6 O'Sullivan S, Bridge G, Ponich T. Musculoskeletal injuries among ERCP endoscopists in Canada. *Can J Gastroenterol* 2002; 16 (6): 369–74.
7 Petersen BT. ERCP outcomes: defining the operators, experience, and environments. *Gastrointest Endosc* 2002; 55 (7): 953–8.
8 Birkmeyer JD, Stukel TA, Siewers AE, Goodney PP, Wennberg DE, Lucas FL. Surgeon volume and operative mortality in the United States. *N Engl J Med* 2003; 349: 2117–27.
9 Schutz SM, Abbott RM. Grading ERCPs by degree of difficulty: a new concept to produce more meaningful outcome data. *Gastrointest Endosc* 2000; 51 (5): 535–9.
10 Lambert ME, Betts CD, Hill J, Faragher EB, Martin DF, Tweedle DE. Endoscopic sphincterotomy: the whole truth. *Br J Surg* 1991; 78 (4): 473–6.
11 Cotton PB. Endoscopic management of bile duct stones (apples and oranges). *Gut* 1984; 25: 587–97.
12 Perdue DG, Freeman ML, ERCOST Study Group. Failed biliary ERCP: a prospective multi-center study of risk factors, complications and resource utilization. *Gastrointest Endosc* 2004; 59 (5): AB192.
13 Cotton PB. Randomization is not the (only) answer: a plea for structured objective evaluation of endoscopic therapy. *Endoscopy* 2000; 32 (5): 402–5.
14 Hebert RL, Palesch YY, Tarnasky PR, Aabakken I, Mauldin PD, Cotton PB. DDQ-15 health-related quality of life instrument for patients with digestive disorders. *Health Services Outcomes Res Methodology* 2001; 2: 137–56.
15 Cotton PB, Lehman G, Vennes J, Geenen JE, Russell RC, Meyers WC *et al.* Endoscopic sphincterotomy complications and their management: an attempt at consensus. *Gastrointest Endosc* 1991; 37: 383–93.
16 Bilbao MK, Dotter CT, Lee TG, Katon RM. Complications of endoscopic retrograde cholangiography (ERCP): a study of 10 000 cases. *Gastroenterology* 1976; 70: 314–20.
17 Geenen JE, Vennes JA, Silvis SE. Resume of a seminar on endoscopic retrograde sphincterotomy (ERS). *Gastrointest Endosc* 1981; 27: 31–8.
18 Cotton PB, Progress Report ERCP. *Gut* 1977; 18: 316–41.
19 Neuhaus B, Safrany L. Complications of endoscopic sphincterotomy and their treatment. *Endoscopy* 1981; 13: 197–9.
20 Vaira D, D'Anna L, Ainley C, Dowsett J, Williams S, Baillie J *et al.* Endoscopic sphincterotomy in 1000 consecutive patients. *Lancet* 1989; 2: 431–4.
21 American Society for Gastrointestinal Endoscopy. Standards of Practice Committee. Complications of ERCP. *Gastrointest Endosc* 2003; 57 (6): 633–8.
22 Barthet M, Lesavre N, Desjeux A, Gasml M, Berthezene P, Berdah S *et al.* Complications of endoscopic sphincterotomy: results from a single tertiary referral center. *Endoscopy* 2002; 34 (12): 991–7.
23 Freeman ML. Adverse outcomes of endoscopic retrograde cholangiopancreatography. *Rev Gastroenterol Disord* 2002; 2 (4): 147–67.

24 Loperfido S, Angelini G, Benedetti G, Chilovi F, Costan F, De Berardinis F et al. Major early complications from diagnostic and therapeutic ERCP: a prospective multicenter study. *Gastrointest Endosc* 1998; 48: 1–10.

25 Masci E, Toti G, Mariani A, Curioni S, Lomazzi A, Dinelli M et al. Complications of diagnostic and therapeutic ERCP: a prospective multicenter study. *Am J Gastroenterol* 2001; 96: 417–23.

26 Tzovaras G, Shukla P, Kow L, Mounkley D, Wilson T, Toouli J. What are the risks of diagnostic and therapeutic endoscopic retrograde cholangiopancreatography? *Aust N Z J Surg* 2000; 70: 778–82.

27 Vandervoort J, Soetikno RM, Tham TC, Wong RC, Ferrari AP Jr, Montes H et al. Risk factors for complications after performance of ERCP. *Gastrointest Endosc* 2002; 56: 652–6.

28 Freeman ML. Adverse outcomes of endoscopic retrograde cholangiopancreatography: avoidance and management. *Gastrointest Endosc Clin N Am* 2003; 13 (4): 775–98.

29 Garcia-Cano Lizcano J, Conzalez Martin JA, Morillas Arino J, Perez Sola A. Complications of endoscopic retrograde cholangiopancreatography: a study in a small ERCP unit. *Rev Esp Enferm Dig* 2004; 96 (3): 155–62.

30 Freeman ML. Understanding risk factors and avoiding complications with endoscopic retrograde cholangiopancreatography. *Curr Gastroenterol Rep* 2003; 5 (2): 145–53.

31 Landoni N, Chopita N, Jmelnitzky A. Endoscopic sphincterotomy: its complications and their followup. *Acta Gastroenterol Latinoam* 1992; 22 (3): 155–9.

32 Sherman S, Ruffolo TA, Hawes RH, Glehman GA. Complications of endoscopic sphincterotomy. *Gastroenterology* 1991; 101: 1068–75.

33 Tanner A. ERCP: present practice in a single region. *Eur J Gastroenterol Hepatol* 1996; 8: 145–8.

34 Mallery JS, Baron TH, Dominitz JA, Goldstein JL, Hirota WK, Jacobson BC et al. Complications of ERCP. *Gastrointest Endosc* 2003; 57: 633–8.

35 Aliperti G. Complications related to diagnostic and therapeutic endoscopic retrograde cholangiopancreatography. *Gastrointest Endosc Clin N Am* 1996; 6: 379–40.

36 Freeman ML. Adverse outcomes of ERCP. *Gastrointest Endosc* 2002; 56 (6): S273–82.

37 Farrell RJ, Mahmud N, Noonan N, Kellcher D, Keeling PW. Diagnostic and therapeutic ERCP: a large single centre's experience. *Ir J Med Sci* 2001; 170 (3): 176–80.

38 Munoz SR. Towards safer ERCP: selection, experience and prophylaxis. *Rev Esp Enferm Dig (Madrid)* 2004; 96 (3): 155–62.

39 Misra SP, Dwivedi M. Complications of endoscopic retrograde cholangiopancreatography and endoscopic sphincterotomy: diagnosis, management and prevention. *Natl Med J India* 2002; 15: 27–31.

40 Halme L, Doepel M, von Numers H, Edgren J, Ahonen J. Complications of diagnostic and therapeutic ERCP. *Ann Chir Gynaecol* 1999; 88: 127–31.

41 Rabenstein T, Schneider HT, Nicklas M, Ruppert T, Katalinic A, Hahn EG et al. Impact of skill and experience of the endoscopist on the outcome of endoscopic sphincterotomy techniques. *Gastrointest Endosc* 1999; 50: 628–36.

42 Davis WZ, Cotton PB, Arias R, Williams D, Onken JE. ERCP and sphincterotomy in the context of laparoscopic cholecystectomy: academic and community practice patients and results. *Am J Gastroenterol* 1997; 92: 597–601.

43 Escourrou J, Delvaux M, Busail L et al. Clinical results of endoscopic sphincterotomy: comparison of two activity periods in the same endoscopy units. *Gastrointest Endosc* 1990; 36: 205–6.

44 Freeman ML, Nelson DB, Sherman S, Haber GB, Herman ME, Dorsher PJ et al. Complications of endoscopic biliary sphincterotomy. *N Engl J Med* 1996; 335: 909–18.

45 Newcomer MK, Jowell PS, Cotton PB. Underestimation of adverse events following ERCP: a prospective 30 day follow up study [Abstract]. *Gastrointest Endosc* 1995; 41: 408.

46 Zubarik R, Fleischer DE, Mastropietro C, Lopez J et al. Prospective analysis of complications 30 days after outpatient colonoscopy. *Gastrointest Endosc* 1999; 50 (3): 322–8.

47 Zubarik R, Eisen G, Mastropietro C, Lopez J, Carroll J, Benjamin S et al. Prospective analysis of complications 30 days after outpatient upper endoscopy. *Am J Gastroenterol* 1999; 94 (6): 1539–45.

48 Arenson N, Flamm CR, Bohn RI, Mark DH, Speroff T. Evidence-based assessment: patient procedure, or operator factors associated with ERCP complications. *Gastrointest Endosc* 2002; 56: s294–s301.

49 Deans GT, Sedman P, Martin DF, Royston CMS, Leow CK, Thomas WEG *et al*. Are complications of endoscopic sphincterotomy age related? *Gut* 1997; 41: 545–8.

50 Derkx HHF, Huibregtse K, Taminiau JAJM. The role of endoscopic retrograde cholangiopancreatography in cholestatic infants. *Endoscopy* 1994; 26: 724–8.

51 Guelrud M, Mujica C, Jaen D, Plaz J, Arias J. The role of ERCP in the diagnosis and treatment of idiopathic recurrent pancreatitis in children and adolescents. *Gastrointest Endosc* 1994; 40 (4): 428–33.

52 Mitchell RM, O'Connor F, Dickey W. Endoscopic retrograde cholangiopancreatography is safe and effective in patients 90 years of age and older. *J Clin Gastroenterol* 2003; 36 (1): 72–4.

53 Hui CK, Liu CL, Lai KC, Chan SC, Hu WH, Wong WM *et al*. Outcome of emergency ERCP for acute cholangitis in patients 90 years of age and older. *Aliment Pharmacol Ther* 2004; 19 (11): 1153–8.

54 Leung JW, Chung SC, Sung JJ, Banez VP, Li AK. Urgent endoscopic drainage for acute suppurative cholangitis. *Lancet* 1989; 1 (8650): 1307–9.

55 Cotton PB, Jowell PS, Baillie J, Leung J, Affronti J, Branch MS *et al*. Spectrum of complications after diagnostic ERCP and effect of comorbidities. *Gastrointest Endosc* 1994; 40 (2): P18.

56 Jamidar PA, Beck GJ, Hoffman BJ, Lehman GA, Hawes RH, Agrawal RM *et al*. Endoscopic retrograde cholangiopancreatography in pregnancy. *Am J Gastroenterol* 1995; 98 (8): 1263–7.

57 Cohen S, Bacon BR, Berlin JA, Fleischer D, Hecht GA, Loehrer PJ Sr *et al*. National Institutes of Health State-of-the-Science Conference Statement: ERCP for diagnosis and therapy, January 14–16, 2002. *Gastrointest Endosc* 2002; 56: 803–9.

58 Cotton PB. ERCP is most dangerous for people who need it least. *Gastrointest Endosc* 2001; 54 (4): 535–6.

59 Shemesh E, Klein E, Czerniak A, Coret A, Bat L. Endoscopic sphincterotomy in patients with gallbladder in situ: the influence of periampullary duodenal diverticula. *Surgery* 1990; 107: 163–6.

60 Vaira D, Dowsett JF, Hatfield ARW *et al*. Is duodenal diverticulum a risk factor for sphincterotomy? *Gut* 1989; 30: 939–42.

61 Veitch A, Fairclough P. Endoscopic diathermy in patients with cardiac pacemakers. *Endoscopy* 1998; 30 (6): 544–7.

62 Sherman S, Ruffolo TA, Hawes RH, Lehman GA. Complications of endoscopic sphincterotomy: a prospective series with emphasis on the increased risk associated with sphincter of Oddi dysfunction and nondilated bile duct. *Gastroenterology* 1991; 101: 1068–75.

63 Chen YK, Foliente RL, Santoro MJ, Walter MH, Collen MJ. Endoscopic sphincterotomy-induced pancreatitis: increased risk associated with nondilated bile ducts and sphincter of Oddi dysfunction. *Am J Gastroenterol* 1994; 89 (3): 327–33.

64 Cotton PB, Geenen JE, Sherman S, Cunningham JT, Howell DA, Carr-Locke DL *et al*. Endoscopic sphincterotomy for stones by experts is safe, even in younger patients with normal ducts. *Ann Surg* 1998; 227: 201–4.

65 Wilson MS, Tweedle DEF, Martin DF. Common bile duct diameter and complications of endoscopic sphincterotomy. *Br J Surg* 1992; 79: 1345–7.

66 Huibregtse K. Complications of endoscopic sphincterotomy and their prevention. *N Engl J Med* 1996; 335: 961–2.

67 Boender J, Nix GA, de Ridder MA, van Blankenstein M, Schutte HE, Dees J *et al*. Endoscopic papillotomy for common bile duct stones: factors influencing the complication rate. *Endoscopy* 1994; 26: 209–16.

68 Mehta SN, Pavone E, Barkun JS, Bouchard S, Barkun AN. Predictors of post-ERCP complications in patients with suspected choledocholithiasis. *Endoscopy* 1998; 30: 457–63.

69 Elfant AB, Bourke MJ, Alhalel R, Kortan PP, Haber GB. A prospective study of the safety of endoscopic therapy for choledocholithiasis in an outpatient population. *Am J Gastroenterol* 1996; 91 (8): 1499–502.

70 Alsolaiman M, Cotton P, Hawes R, Aliperti G, Carr-Locke DL, Fogel EL *et al.* Techniques for pancreatic sphincterotomy: lack of expert consensus. *Gastrointest Endosc* 2004; 59 (5): AB210.

71 Elton E, Howell DA, Parsons WG, Qaseem T, Hanson BL. Endoscopic pancreatic sphincterotomy: indications, outcome, and a safe stentless technique. *Gastrointest Endosc* 1998; 47: 240–9.

72 Berkes J, Bernklau S, Halline A, Venu R, Brown R. Minor papillotomy in pancreas divisum: do complications and restenosis rates differ between use of the needle knife papillotome (NKS) vs. ultratapered traction sphincterotome (UTS)? *Gastrointest Endosc* 2004; 59 (5): AB207.

73 Delhaye M, Matos C, Deviere J. Endoscopic technique for the management of pancreatitis and its complications. *Best Pract Res Clin Gastroenterol* 2004; 18 (1): 155–81.

74 Leung JW, Banez VP, Chung SC. Precut (needle knife) papillotomy for impacted common bile duct stone at the ampulla. *Am J Gastroenterol* 1990; 85: 991–3.

75 Cotton PB. Precut papillotomy: a risky technique for experts only. *Gastrointest Endosc* 1989; 35: 578.

76 Cotton PB. Needleknife precut sphincterotomy: the devil is in the indications. *Endoscopy* 1997; 29: 888.

77 Dowsett JF, Polydorou AA, Vaira D *et al.* Needle knife papillotomy: how safe and how effective? *Gastrointest Endosc* 1990; 36 (6): 645–6.

78 Vandervoort J, Carr-Locke DL. Needle-knife access papillotomy: an unfairly maligned technique? *Endoscopy* 1996; 28: 365–6.

79 Rabenstein T, Ruppert T, Schneider HT, Hahn EG, Ell C. Benefits and risks of needle-knife papillotomy. *Gastrointest Endosc* 1997; 46: 207–11.

80 Baillie J. Needle-knife papillotomy revisited [editorial; comment]. *Gastrointest Endosc* 1997; 46: 282.

81 Bruins SW, Schoeman MN, DiSario JA, Wolters F, Tytgat GN, Huibregtse K. Needle-knife sphincterotomy as a precut procedure: a retrospective evaluation of efficacy and complications. *Endoscopy* 1996; 28: 334–9.

82 Dhir V, Swaroop VS, Mohandas KM, Jagannath P, Desouza LJ. Precut papillotomy using a needle knife: experience in 100 patients with malignant obstructive jaundice. *Indian J Gastroenterol* 1997; 16: 52–3.

83 Foutch PG. A prospective assessment of results for needle-knife papillotomy and standard endoscopic sphincterotomy. *Gastrointest Endosc* 1995; 41: 25–32.

84 Gholson CF, Favrot D. Needle knife papillotomy in a University referral practice: safety and efficacy of a modified technique. *J Clin Gastroenterol* 1996; 23: 177–80.

85 Kasmin FE, Cohen D, Batra S, Cohen SA, Siegel JH. Needle-knife sphincterotomy in a tertiary referral center: efficacy and complications. *Gastrointest Endosc* 1996; 44: 48–53.

86 Rollhauser C, Johnson M, Al Kawas FH. Needle-knife papillotomy: a helpful and safe adjunct to endoscopic retrograde cholangiopancreatography in a selected population. *Endoscopy* 1998; 30: 691–6.

87 Harewood GC, Baron TH. An assessment of the learning curve for precut biliary sphincterotomy. *Am J Gastroenterol* 2002; 97: 1708–12.

88 Freeman ML. Precut (access) sphincterotomy: Techniques. *Gastrointest Endosc* 1999; 1: 40–8.

89 Binmoeller KF, Seifert H, Gerke H, Seitz U, Portis M, Soehendra N. Papillary roof incision using the Erlangen-type pre-cut papillotome to achieve selective bile duct cannulation. *Gastrointest Endosc* 1996; 44: 689–95.

90 Goff JS. Long-term experience with the transpancreatic sphincter pre-cut approach to biliary sphincterotomy. *Gastrointest Endosc* 1999; 50: 642–5.

91 Mavrogiannis C, Liatsos C, Papanikolaou IS, Psilopoulos DI, Goulas SS *et al.* Safety of extension of a previous endoscopic sphincterotomy: a prospective study. *Am J Gastroenterol* 2003; 98 (1): 72–6.

92 Choudari CP, Sherman S, Fogel EL, Phillips S, Kochell A, Flueckiger J *et al.* Success of ERCP at a referral center after a previously unsuccessful attempt. *Gastrointest Endosc* 2000; 52 (4): 478–83.

93 Raijman I, Escalante-Glorsky S. Is the complication rate the same for index versus repeat biliary sphincterotomy? *Gastrointest Endosc* 2004; 59 (5): AB193.

94 May GR, Cotton PB, Edmunds EJ, Chong W. Removal of stones from the bile duct at ERCP without sphincterotomy. *Gastrointest Endosc* 1993; 39 (6): 749–54.

95 MacMathuna P. Endoscopic treatment of bile duct stones: should we cut or dilate the sphincter? *Am J Gastroenterol* 1997; 92 (9): 1411–12.

96 Norton ID, Gostout CJ, Baron TH, Geller A, Petersen BT, Wiersema MJ. Safety and outcome of endoscopic snare excision of the major duodenal papilla. *Gastrointest Endosc* 2002; 56: 239–43.

97 Desilets DJ, Dy RM, Ku PM, Hanson BL, Elton E, Mattia A et al. Endoscopic management of tumors of the major duodenal papilla: refined techniques to improve outcome and avoid complications. *Gastrointest Endosc* 2001; 54: 202–8.

98 Zadorova Z, Dvofak M, Hajer J. Endoscopic therapy of benign tumors of the papilla of Vater. *Endoscopy* 2001; 33: 345–7.

99 Catalano MF, Linder JD, Chak A, Sivak MV Jr, Raijman I, Geenen JE et al. Endoscopic management of adenoma of the major duodenal papilla. *Gastrointest Endosc* 2004; 59: 225–32.

100 Fujita N, Noda Y, Kobayashi G, Kimura K, Ito K. Endoscopic papillectomy: is there room for this procedure in clinical practice? *Digestive Endoscopy* 2003; 15: 253–5.

101 Cheng C, Sherman S, Fogel EL, McHenry L, Watkins JL et al. Endoscopic snare papillectomy of ampullary tumors: 10-year review of 55 cases at Indiana University Medical Center. *Gastrointest Endosc* 2004; 59 (5): AB193.

102 Giorgio PD, Luca LD. Comparison of treatment outcomes between biliary plastic stent placements with and without endoscopic sphincterotomy for inoperable malignant common bile duct obstruction. *World J Gastroenterol* 2004; 10 (8): 1212–14.

103 Tarnasky PR, Cunningham JT, Hawes RH, Hoffman BJ et al. Transpapillary stenting of proximal biliary strictures: does biliary sphincterotomy reduce the risk of post-procedure pancreatitis? *Gastrointest Endosc* 1997; 45: 46–51.

104 Baron TH. Endoscopic drainage of pancreatic fluid collections and pancreatic necrosis. *Gastrointest Endosc Clin N Am* 2003; 13 (4): 743–64.

105 Plumeri PA. Informed consent for upper gastrointestinal endoscopy. *Gastroenterol Clin N Am* 1994; 4 (2): 455–61.

106 Duncan HD, Hodgkinson L, Deakin M, Green JR. The safety of diagnostic and therapeutic ERCP as a daycase procedure with a selective admission policy. *Eur J Gastroenterol Hepatol* 1997; 9 (9): 905–8.

107 Ho KY, Montes H, Sossenheimer MJ, Tham TC, Ruymann F, Van Dam J et al. Features that may predict hospital admission following outpatient therapeutic ERCP. *Gastrointest Endosc* 1999; 49: 587–92.

108 Freeman ML, Nelson DB, Sherman S, Haber GB, Fennerty MB, DiSario JA et al. Same-day discharge after endoscopic biliary sphincterotomy: observations from a prospective multicenter complication study. *Gastrointest Endosc* 1999; 49: 580–6.

109 Cvetkovski B, Gerdes H, Kurtz RC. Outpatient therapeutic ERCP with endobiliary stent placement for malignant common bile duct obstruction. *Gastrointest Endosc* 1999; 50: 63–6.

110 Linder JD, Tarnasky P. There are benefits of overnight observation after outpatient ERCP. *Gastrointest Endosc* 2004; 59 (5): AB208.

111 Testoni PA, Bagnolo F, Caporuscio S, Lella F. Serum amylase measured four hours after endoscopic sphincterotomy is a reliable predictor of postprocedure pancreatitis. *Am J Gastroenterol* 1999; 94: 1235–41.

112 Friedland S, Soetikno RM, Vandervoort J, Montes H, Tham T, Carr-Locke DL. Bedside scoring system to predict the risk of developing pancreatitis following ERCP. *Endoscopy* 2002; 34: 483–8.

113 Barthet M, Desjeux A, Gasmi M, Bellon P, Hoi MT, Salducci J et al. Early refeeding after endoscopic biliary or pancreatic sphincterotomy: a randomized prospective study. *Endoscopy* 2002; 34 (7): 546–50.

114 Freeman ML, Guda NM. Prevention of post-ERCP pancreatitis: a comprehensive review. *Gastrointest Endosc* 2004; 59 (7): 845–64.

115 Freeman ML, DiSario JA, Nelson DB, Fennerty MB, Lee JG, Bjorkman DJ *et al.* Risk factors for post-ERCP pancreatitis: a prospective, multicenter study. *Gastrointest Endosc* 2001; 54 (4): 535–6.

116 Testoni PA. Why the incidence of post-ERCP pancreatitis varies considerably? Factors affecting the diagnosis and the incidence of this complication. *JOP* 2002; 3 (6): 195–201.

117 Johnson GK, Geenen JE, Johanson JF, Sherman S, Hogan WJ, Cass O *et al.* Evaluation of post-ERCP pancreatitis: potential causes noted during controlled study of differing contrast media. *Gastrointest Endosc* 1997; 46 (3): 217–22.

118 Rabenstein T, Hahn EG. Post-ERCP pancreatitis: new momentum. *Endoscopy* 2002; 34 (4): 325–9.

119 Sherman S, Lehman GA. ERCP- and endoscopic sphincterotomy-induced pancreatitis. *Pancreas* 1991; 6 (3): 350–67.

120 Gottlieb K, Sherman S. ERCP and biliary endoscopic sphincterotomy-induced pancreatitis. *Gastrointest Endosc Clin N Am* 1998; 8: 87–114.

121 Cotton PB, Baillie J, Leung J, Jowell PS, Affronti J, Branch MS *et al.* Correlations with post-ERCP pancreatitis [Abstract]. *Gastrointest Endosc* 1994; 40: P29.

122 Christoforidis E, Goulimaris I, Kanellos I, Tsalis K, Demetriades C, Betsis D. Post-ERCP pancreatitis and hyperamylasemia: patient-related and operative risk factors. *Endoscopy* 2002; 34: 286–92.

123 Masci E, Mariani A, Curioni S, Testoni PA. Risk factors for pancreatitis following endoscopic retrograde cholangiopancreatography: a meta-analysis. *Endoscopy* 2003; 35: 830–4.

124 Urbach DR, Rabeneck L. Population-based study of the risk of acute pancreatitis following ERCP. *Gastrointest Endosc* 2003; 57 (5): AB116.

125 Roszler MH, Campbell WL. Post-ERCP pancreatitis: association with urographic visualization during ERCP. *Radiology* 1985; 157: 595–8.

126 Haber GB. Prevention of post ERCP pancreatitis. *Gastrointest Endosc* 2000; 51: 100–3.

127 Cortas GA, Mehta SN, Abraham NS, Barkun AN. Selective cannulation of the common bile duct: a prospective randomized trial comparing standard catheters with sphincterotomes. *Gastrointest Endosc* 1999; 50: 775–9.

128 Schwacha H, Allgaier HP, Deibert P, Olschewski M, Allgaier U, Blum HE. A sphincterotome-based technique for selective transpapillary common bile duct cannulation. *Gastrointest Endosc* 2000; 5: 387–91.

129 Laasch HU, Tringali A, Wilbraham L, Marriott A, England RE, Mutignani M *et al.* Comparison of standard and steerable catheters for bile duct cannulation in ERCP. *Endoscopy* 2003; 35: 669–74.

130 Maeda S, Hayashi H, Hosokawa O, Dohden K, Hattori M, Morita M *et al.* Prospective randomized pilot trial of selective biliary cannulation using pancreatic guide-wire placement. *Endoscopy* 2003; 35: 721–4.

131 Maldonado ME, Brady PG, Mamel JJ, Robinson B. Incidence of pancreatitis in patients undergoing sphincter of Oddi manometry (SOM). *Am J Gastroenterol* 1999; 94: 387–90.

132 Singh P, Gurudu SR, Davidoff S, Sivak MV Jr, Indaram A, Kasmin FE *et al.* Sphincter of Oddi manometry does not predispose to post-ERCP acute pancreatitis. *Gastrointest Endosc* 2004; 59 (4): 499–505.

133 Tarnasky P, Cunningham J, Cotton P, Hoffman B, Palesch Y, Freeman J *et al.* Pancreatic sphincter hypertension increases the risk of post-ERCP pancreatitis. *Endoscopy* 1997; 29: 252–7.

134 Lee SJ, Song KS, Chung JP, Lee DY, Jeong YS, Ji SW *et al.* Type of electric currents used for standard endoscopic sphincterotomy does not determine the type of complications. *Korean J Gastroenterol* 2004; 43 (3): 204–10.

135 MacIntosh D, Love J, Abraham N. Endoscopic sphincterotomy using pure-cut current does not reduce the risk of post-ERCP pancreatitis: a prospective randomized trial. *Gastrointest Endosc* 2003; 57: AB189.

136 Elta GH, Barnett JL, Wille RT, Brown KA, Chey WD, Scheiman JM. Pure cut electrocautery current for sphincterotomy causes less post-procedure pancreatitis than blended current. *Gastrointest Endosc* 1998; 47: 149–53.

137 Stefanidis G, Karamanolis G, Viazis N, Sgouros S, Papadopoulou E *et al.* A comparative study of postendoscopic sphincterotomy complications with various types of electrosurgical current in patients with choledocholithiasis. *Gastrointest Endosc* 2003; 57 (2): 192–7.

138 Kohler A, Maier M, Benz C, Martin WR, Farin G, Riemann JF. A new HF current generator with automatically controlled system (Endocut mode) for endoscopic sphincterotomy—preliminary experience. *Endoscopy* 1998; 30: 351–5.

139 Norton I, Bosco J, Meier P, Baron T, Lange S, Nelson D *et al.* A randomized trial of endoscopic sphincterotomy using pure cut versus Endocut electrical waveforms [Abstract]. *Gastrointest Endosc* 2002; 55: AB175.

140 Katsinelos P, Mimidis K, Paroutoglou G, Christodoulou K, Pilpilidis I, Katsiba D *et al.* Needle-knife papillotomy: a safe and effective technique in experienced hands. *Hepatogastroenterology* 2004; 51 (56): 349–52.

141 Komatsu Y, Kawabe T, Toda N, Ohashi M, Isayama M, Tateishi K *et al.* Endoscopic papillary balloon dilation for the management of common bile duct stones: experience of 226 cases. *Endoscopy* 1998; 30: 12–7.

142 MacMathuna PM, White P, Clarke E, Merriman R, Lennon JR, Crowe J. Endoscopic balloon sphincteroplasty (papillary dilation) for bile duct stones: efficacy, safety, and follow-up in 100 patients. *Gastrointest Endosc* 1995; 42: 468–74.

143 Ueno N, Ozawa Y. Pancreatitis induced by endoscopic balloon sphincter dilation and changes in serum amylase levels after the procedure. *Gastrointest Endosc* 1999; 49: 472–6.

144 Bergman JJ, Rauws EA, Fockens P, van Berkel AM, Bossuyt PM, Tijssen JG *et al.* Randomised trial of endoscopic balloon dilation versus endoscopic sphincterotomy for removal of bile duct stones. *Lancet* 1997; 349: 1124–9.

145 Fujita N, Maguchi H, Komatsu Y, Yasuda I, Hasebe O, Igarashi Y *et al.* Endoscopic sphincterotomy and endoscopic papillary balloon dilatation for bile duct stones: a prospective randomized controlled multicenter trial. *Gastrointest Endosc* 2003; 57: 151–5.

146 Minami A, Nakatsu T, Uchida N, Hirabayashi S, Fukuma H, Morshed SA *et al.* Papillary dilation vs. sphincterotomy in endoscopic removal of bile duct stones: a randomized trial with manometric function. *Dig Dis Sci* 1995; 40: 2550–4.

147 Ochi Y, Mukawa K, Kiyosawa K, Akamatsu T. Comparing the treatment outcomes of endoscopic papillary dilation and endoscopic sphincterotomy for removal of bile duct stones. *J Gastroenterol Hepatol* 1999; 14: 90–6.

148 Arnold JC, Benz C, Martin WR, Adamek HE, Riemann JF. Endoscopic papillary balloon dilation vs. sphincterotomy for removal of common bile duct stones: a prospective randomized pilot study. *Endoscopy* 2001; 33: 563–7.

149 Vlavianos P, Chopra K, Mandalia S, Anderson M, Thompson J, Westaby D. Endoscopic balloon dilatation versus endoscopic sphincterotomy for the removal of bile duct stones: a prospective randomised trial. *Gut* 2003; 52: 1165–9.

150 DiSario JA, Freeman ML, Bjorkman DJ, MacMathuna P, Petersen BT, Jaffe PE *et al.* Endoscopic balloon dilation compared with sphincterotomy for extraction of bile duct stones. *Gastroenterology* 2004; 127: 1291–9.

151 Kawabe T, Komatsu Y, Tada M, Toda N, Ohashi M, Shiratori Y *et al.* Endoscopic papillary balloon dilation in cirrhotic patients: removal of common bile duct stones without sphincterotomy. *Endoscopy* 1996; 28: 694–8.

152 Prat F, Fritsch J, Choury AD, Meduri B, Pelletier G, Buffet C. Endoscopic sphincteroclasy: a useful therapeutic tool for biliary endoscopy in Billroth II gastrectomy patients. *Endoscopy* 1997; 29: 79–81.

153 Bergman JJGHM, van Berkel A-M, Bruno MJ, Fockens P, Rauws EAJ *et al.* A randomized trial of endoscopic balloon dilation and endoscopic sphincterotomy for removal of bile duct stones in patients with a prior Billroth II gastrectomy. *Gastrointest Endosc* 2001; 53 (1): 19–26.

154 Goff JS. Common bile duct sphincter of Oddi stenting in patients with suspected sphincter dysfunction. *Am J Gastroenterol* 1995; 90: 586–9.

155 Freeman ML. Prevention of post-ERCP pancreatitis: pharmacologic solution or patient selection and pancreatic stents. *Gastroenterology* 2003; 124 (7): 1977–80.

156 Sherman S, Hawes RH, Troiano FP, Lehman GA. Pancreatitis following bile duct sphincter of Oddi manometry: utility of the aspirating catheter. *Gastrointest Endosc* 1992; 38: 347–50.

157 Wehrmann T, Stergiou N, Schmitt T, Dietrich CF, Seifert H. Reduced risk for pancreatitis after endoscopic microtransducer manometry of the sphincter of Oddi: a randomized comparison with the perfusion manometry technique. *Endoscopy* 2003; 35: 472–7.

158 Cunliffe WJ, Cobden I, Lavelle MI, Lendrum R, Tait NP, Venables CW. A randomised, prospective study comparing two contrast media in ERCP. *Endoscopy* 1987; 19: 201–2.

159 Hannigan BF, Keeling PW, Slavin B, Thompson RP. Hyperamylasemia after ERCP with ionic and non-ionic contrast media. *Gastrointest Endosc* 1985; 31: 109–10.

160 Johnson GK, Geenen JE, Bedford RA, Johanson J, Cass O, Sherman S et al. A comparison of nonionic versus ionic contrast media: results of a prospective, multicenter study. *Gastrointest Endosc* 1995; 42: 312–16.

161 O'Connor HJ, Ellis WR, Manning AP, Lintott DJ, McMahon MJ, Axon AT. Iopamidol as contrast medium in endoscopic retrograde pancreatography: a prospective randomised comparison with diatrizoate. *Endoscopy* 1988; 20: 244–7.

162 Sherman S, Hawes RH, Rathgaber SW, Uzer MF, Smith MT, Khusro QE et al. Post-ERCP pancreatitis: randomized, prospective study comparing a low- and high-osmolality contrast agent. *Gastrointest Endosc* 1994; 40 (4): 422–7.

163 Goebel C, Hardt P, Doppl W, Temme H, Hackstein N, Klor HU. Frequency of pancreatitis after endoscopic retrograde cholangiopancreatography with iopromid or iotrolan: a randomized trial. *Eur Radiol* 2000; 10 (4): 677–80.

164 Andriulli A, Caruso N, Quitadamo M, Forlano R, Leandro G, Spirito F et al. Antisecretory vs. antiproteasic drugs in the prevention of post-ERCP pancreatitis: the evidence-based medicine derived from a meta-analysis study. *JOP* 2003; 4: 41–8.

165 Andriulli A, Leandro G, Niro G, Mangia A, Festa V, Gambassi G et al. Pharmacologic treatment can prevent pancreatic injury after ERCP: a meta-analysis. *Gastrointest Endosc* 2000; 51: 1–7.

166 Raty S, Sand J, Pulkkinen M, Matikainen M, Nordback I. Post-ERCP pancreatitis: reduction by routine antibiotics. *J Gastrointest Surg* 2001; 5: 339–45.

167 Rabenstein T, Roggenbuck S, Framke B, Martus P, Fischer B, Nusko G et al. Complications of endoscopic sphincterotomy: can heparin prevent acute pancreatitis after ERCP? *Gastrointest Endosc* 2002; 55 (4): 476–83.

168 Weiner GR, Geenen JE, Hogan WJ, Catalano MF. Use of corticosteroids in the prevention of post-ERCP pancreatitis. *Gastrointest Endosc* 1995; 42: 579–83.

169 Dumot JA, Conwell DL, O'Connor JB, Ferguson DR, Vargo JJ, Barnes DS et al. Pretreatment with methylprednisolone to prevent ERCP-induced pancreatitis: a randomized, multicenter, placebo-controlled clinical trial. *Am J Gastroenterol* 1998; 93: 61–5.

170 Sherman S, Blaut U, Watkins JL, Barnett J, Freeman M, Geenen J et al. Does prophylactic steroid administration reduce the risk and severity of post-ERCP pancreatitis: a randomized prospective multicenter study. *Gastrointest Endosc* 2003; 58: 23–9.

171 Manolakopoulos S, Avgerinos A, Vlachogiannakos J, Armonis A, Viazis N, Papadimitriou N et al. Octreotide versus hydrocortisone versus placebo in the prevention of post-ERCP pancreatitis: a multicenter randomized controlled trial. *Gastrointest Endosc* 2002; 55: 470–5.

172 Budzynska A, Marek T, Nowak A, Kaczor R, Nowakowska-Dulawa E. A prospective, randomized, placebo-controlled trial of prednisone and allopurinol in the prevention of ERCP-induced pancreatitis. *Endoscopy* 2001; 33: 766–72.

173 De Palma GD, Catanzano C. Use of corticosteroids in the prevention of post-ERCP pancreatitis: results of a controlled prospective study. *Am J Gastroenterol* 1999; 94: 982–5.

174 Prat F, Amaris J, Ducot B, Bocquentin M, Fritsch J, Choury AD et al. Nifedipine for prevention of post-ERCP pancreatitis: a prospective, double-blind randomized study. *Gastrointest Endosc* 2002; 56: 202–8.

175 Sand J, Nordback I. Prospective randomized trial of the effect of nifedipine on pancreatic irritation after endoscopic retrograde cholangiopancreatography. *Digestion* 1993; 54: 105–11.

176 Binmoeller KF, Harris AG, Dumas R, Grimaldi C, Delmont JP. Does the somatostatin analog octreotide protect against ERCP induced pancreatitis? *Gut* 1992; 33: 1129–33.

177 Arvanitidis D, Anagnostopoulos GK, Giannopoulos D, Pantes A, Agaritsi R, Margantinis G *et al.* Can somatostatin prevent post-ERCP pancreatitis? Results of a randomized controlled trial. *J Gastroenterol Hepatol* 2004; 19: 278–82.

178 Bordas JM, Toledo V, Mondelo F, Rodes J. Prevention of pancreatic reactions by bolus somatostatin administration in patients undergoing endoscopic retrograde cholangio-pancreatography and endoscopic sphincterotomy. *Horm Res* 1988; 29: 106–8.

179 Bordas JM, Toledo-Pimentel V, Llach J, Elena M, Mondelo F, Gines A *et al.* Effects of bolus somatostatin in preventing pancreatitis after endoscopic pancreatography: results of a randomized study. *Gastrointest Endosc* 1998; 47: 230–4.

180 Guelrud M, Mendoza S, Viera L, Gelrud D. Somatostatin prevents acute pancreatitis after pancreatic duct sphincter hydrostatic balloon dilation in patients with idiopathic recurrent pancreatitis. *Gastrointest Endosc* 1991; 37: 44–7.

181 Persson B, Slezak P, Efendic S, Haggmark A. Can somatostatin prevent injection pancreatitis after ERCP? *Hepatogastroenterology* 1992; 39: 259–61.

182 Poon RT, Yeung C, Lo CM, Yuen WK, Liu CL, Fan ST. Prophylactic effect of somatostatin on post-ERCP pancreatitis: a randomized controlled trial. *Gastrointest Endosc* 1999; 49: 593–8.

183 Saari A, Kivilaakso E, Schroeder P. The influence of somatostatin on pancreatic irritation after pancreatography: an experimental and clinical study. *Surg Res Comm* 1988; 2: 271–8.

184 Testoni PA, Masci E, Bagnolo F, Tittobello A. Endoscopic papillo-sphincterotomy: prevention of pancreatic reaction by somatostatin. *Ital J Gastroenterol* 1988; 20: 70–3.

185 Arcidiacono R, Gambitta P, Rossi A, Grosso C, Bini M, Zanasi G. The use of a long-acting somatostatin analog (octreotide) for prophylaxis of acute pancreatitis after endoscopic sphincterotomy. *Endoscopy* 1994; 26: 715–18.

186 Arvanitidis D, Hatzipanayiotis J, Koutsounopoulos G, Frangou E. The effect of octreotide on the prevention of acute pancreatitis and hyperamylasemia after diagnostic and therapeutic ERCP. *Hepatogastroenterology* 1998; 45: 248–52.

187 Sternlieb JM, Aronchick CA, Retig JN, Dabezies M, Saunders F, Goosenberg E *et al.* A multicenter, randomized, controlled trial to evaluate the effect of prophylactic octreotide on ERCP-induced pancreatitis. *Am J Gastroenterol* 1992; 87: 1561–6.

188 Testoni PA, Lella F, Bagnolo F, Caporuscio S, Cattani L, Colombo E *et al.* Long-term prophylactic administration of octreotide reduces the rise in serum amylase after endoscopic procedures on Vater's papilla. *Pancreas* 1996; 13: 61–5.

189 Testoni PA, Bagnolo F, Andriulli A, Bernasconi G, Crotta S, Lella F *et al.* Octreotide 24-h prophylaxis in patients at high risk for post-ERCP pancreatitis: results of a multicenter, randomized, controlled trial. *Aliment Pharmacol Ther* 2001; 15: 965–72.

190 Tulassay Z, Papp J. The effect of long-acting somatostatin analog on enzyme changes after endoscopic pancreatography. *Gastrointest Endosc* 1991; 37: 48–50.

191 Tulassay Z, Dobronte Z, Pronai L, Zagoni T, Juhasz L. Octreotide in the prevention of pancreatic injury associated with endoscopic cholangiopancreatography. *Aliment Pharmacol Ther* 1998; 12: 1109–12.

192 Testoni PA, Lella F, Bagnolo F, Buizza M, Colombo E. Controlled trial of different dosages of octreotide in the prevention of hyperamylasemia induced by endoscopic papillosphincterotomy. *Ital J Gastroenterol* 1994; 26: 431–6.

193 Binmoeller KF, Dumas R, Harris AG, Delmont JP. Effect of somatostatin analog octreotide on human sphincter of Oddi. *Dig Dis Sci* 1992; 37: 773–7.

194 Sudhindran S, Bromwich E, Edwards PR. Prospective randomized double-blind placebo-controlled trial of glyceryl trinitrate in endoscopic retrograde cholangiopancreatography-induced pancreatitis. *Br J Surg* 2001; 88: 1178–82.

195 Kaffes A, Alrubaie A, Ding S *et al.* A prospective, randomized, double-blind, placebo-controlled trial of transdermal glyceryl trinitrate in technical success of ERCP and the prevention of post-ERCP pancreatitis: preliminary results. *Gastrointest Endosc* 2003; 57: AB191.

196 Moreto M, Zaballa M, Casado I, Merino O, Rueda M, Ramirez K *et al.* Transdermal glyceryl trinitrate for prevention of post-ERCP pancreatitis: a randomized double-blind trial. *Gastrointest Endosc* 2003; 57: 1–7.

197 Schwartz JJ, Lew RJ, Ahmad NA, Shah JN, Ginsberg GG, Kochman ML *et al.* The effect of lidocaine sprayed on the major duodenal papilla on the frequency of post-ERCP pancreatitis. *Gastrointest Endosc* 2004; 59: 179–84.

198 Cavallini G, Tittobello A, Frulloni L, Masci E, Mariana A, Di Francesco V. Gabexate for the prevention of pancreatic damage related to endoscopic retrograde cholangiopancreatography: gabexate in digestive endoscopy—Italian Group. *N Engl J Med* 1996; 335: 919–23.

199 Masci E, Cavallini G, Mariani A, Frulloni L, Testoni PA, Curioni S *et al.* Comparison of two dosing regimens of gabexate in the prophylaxis of post-ERCP pancreatitis. *Am J Gastroenterol* 2003; 98: 2182–6.

200 Van Laethem JL, Marchant A, Delvaux A, Goldman M, Robberecht P, Velu T *et al.* Interleukin 10 prevents necrosis in murine experimental acute pancreatitis. *Gastroenterology* 1995; 108: 1917–22.

201 Deviere J, Le Moine O, Van Laethem JL, Eisendrath P, Ghilain A, Severs N *et al.* Interleukin 10 reduces the incidence of pancreatitis after therapeutic endoscopic retrograde cholangiopancreatography. *Gastroenterology* 2001; 120: 498–505.

202 Dumot JA, Conwell DL, Zuccaro G Jr, Vargo JJ, Shay SS, Easley KA *et al.* A randomized, double blind study of interleukin 10 for the prevention of ERCP-induced pancreatitis. *Am J Gastroenterol* 2001; 96: 2098–102.

203 Singh P, Lee T, Davidoff S, Bank S. Efficacy of Interleukin 10 (IL10) in the prevention of post-ERCP pancreatitis: a meta-analysis [Abstract]. *Gastrointest Endosc* 2002; 55: AB150.

204 Murray B, Carter R, Imrie C, Evans S, O'Suilleabhain C. Diclofenac reduces the incidence of acute pancreatitis after endoscopic retrograde cholangiopancreatography. *Gastroenterology* 2003; 124: 1786–91.

205 Jowell PS, Branch S, Robuck-Mangum G, Fein S, Purich ED, Stiffler H *et al.* Synthetic secretin administered at the start of the procedure significantly reduces the risk of post-ERCP pancreatitis: a randomized, double-blind, placebo controlled trial (presented at *DDW* 2003). In press.

206 Smithline A, Silverman W, Rogers D, Nisi R, Wiersema M, Jamidar P *et al.* Effect of prophylactic main pancreatic duct stenting on the incidence of biliary endoscopic sphincterotomy-induced pancreatitis in high-risk patients. *Gastrointest Endosc* 1993; 39: 652–7.

207 Tarnasky PR, Palesch YY, Cunningham JT, Mauldin PD, Cotton PB, Hawes RH. Pancreatic stenting prevents pancreatitis after biliary sphincterotomy in patients with sphincter of Oddi dysfunction. *Gastroenterology* 1998; 115: 1518–24.

208 Fogel EL, Eversman D, Jamidar P, Sherman S, Lehman GA. Sphincter of Oddi dysfunction: pancreaticobiliary sphincterotomy with pancreatic stent placement has a lower rate of pancreatitis than biliary sphincterotomy alone. *Endoscopy* 2002; 34: 280–5.

209 Aizawa T, Ueno N. Stent placement in the pancreatic duct prevents pancreatitis after endoscopic sphincter dilation for removal of bile duct stones. *Gastrointest Endosc* 2001; 54: 209–13.

210 Fazel A, Quadri A, Catalano MF, Meyerson SM, Geenen JE. Does a pancreatic duct stent prevent post-ERCP pancreatitis? A prospective randomized study. *Gastrointest Endosc* 2003; 57: 291–4.

211 Sherman S, Earle DT, Bucksot L, Baute P, Gottlieb K, Lehman G. Does leaving a main pancreatic duct stent in place reduce the incidence of precut biliary sphincterotomy (ES)-induced pancreatitis? A final analysis of a randomized prospective study. (Abstract). *Gastrointest Endosc* 1996; 43: A489.

212 Freeman ML, Overby C, Qi D. Pancreatic stent insertion: consequences of failure and results of a modified technique to maximize success. *Gastrointest Endosc* 2004; 5: 8–14.

213 Tarnasky PR. Mechanical prevention of post-ERCP pancreatitis by pancreatic stents: results, techniques, and indications. *JOP* 2003; 4 (1): 58–67.

214 Vege SS, Chari ST, Petersen BT, Baron TH, Jones JR, Munukuti PN *et al.* Morbidity and mortality of ERCP-induced severe acute pancreatitis. *Gastrointest Endosc* 2004; 49 (5): AB207.

215 Enns R, Eloubeidi MA, Mergener K, Jowell PS, Branch MS, Pappas TM *et al.* ERCP-related perforations: risk factors and management. *Endoscopy* 2002; 34 (4): 293–8.

216 Jayaprakash B, Wright R. Common bile duct perforation: an unusual complication of ERCP. *Gastrointest Endosc* 1986; 32: 246–7.

217 Howard TJ, Tan T, Lehman GA, Sherman S, Madura JA, Fogel E *et al.* Classification and management of perforations complicating endoscopic sphincterotomy. *Surgery* 1999; 126 (4): 658–65.

218 Zissin R, Shapiro-Feinberg M, Oscadchy A, Pomeraz I, Leichtmann G, Novis B. Retroperitoneal perforation during endoscopic sphincterotomy: imaging findings. *Abdom Imaging* 2000; 25 (3): 279–82.

219 Genzlinger JL, McPhee MS, Fisher JK, Jacob KM, Helzberg JH. Significance of retroperitoneal air after endoscopic retrograde cholangiopancreatography with sphincterotomy. *Am J Gastroenterol* 1999; 94 (5): 1267–70.

220 Sezgin O, Tezel A, Sahin B. Limited duodenal pneumatosis during needle-knife sphincterotomy. *Endoscopy* 1999; 31: 554.

221 Savides T, Sherman S, Kadell B *et al.* Bilateral pneumothoraces and subcutaneous emphysema after endoscopic sphincterotomy. *Gastrointest Endosc* 1993; 39: 814.

222 Ciaccia D, Branch MS, Baillie J. Pneumomediastinum after endoscopic sphincterotomy. *Am J Gastroenterol* 1995; 90: 475–7.

223 Byrne P, Leung JWC, Cotton PB. Retroperitoneal perforation during duodenoscopic sphincterotomy. *Radiology* 1984; 150: 383–4.

224 Martin DF, Tweedle DE. Retroperitoneal perforation during ERCP and endoscopic sphincterotomy: causes, clinical features and management. *Endoscopy* 1990; 22 (4): 174–5.

225 Dunham F, Bourgeois N, Gelin M *et al.* Retroperitoneal perforations following endoscopic sphincterotomy; clinical course and management. *Endoscopy* 1982; 14: 92–6.

226 Stapfer M, Selby RR, Stain SC, Katkhouda N, Parekh D *et al.* Management of duodenal perforation after endoscopic retrograde cholangiopancreatography and sphincterotomy. *Ann Surg* 2000; 232 (2): 191–8.

227 Scarlett PY, Falk GL. The management of perforation of the duodenum following endoscopic sphincterotomy: a proposal for selective therapy [Review]. *Aust N Z J Surg* 1994; 64: 843–6.

228 Baron TH, Gostout CJ, Herman L. Hemoclip repair of a sphincterotomy-induced duodenal perforation. *Gastrointest Endosc* 2000; 52 (4): 566–8.

229 Tezel A, Sahin T, Kosar Y, Oguz D, Sahin B, Cumhur T. Esophageal perforation due to endoscopic retrograde cholangiopancreatography. *Endoscopy* 1998; 30: 52.

230 Lee DW, Chan AC. Visualization of the peritoneum during endoscopic retrograde cholangiopancreatography. *Hong Kong Med J* 2001; 7 (4): 445–6.

231 Cotton PB. Take care with the tip of your video duodenoscope. *Gastrointest Endosc* 1989; 35: 582–3.

232 Costamagna G. ERCP and endoscopic sphincterotomy in Billroth II patients: a demanding technique for experts only? *Ital J Gastroenterol Hepatol* 1998; 30: 306–9.

233 Faylona JM, Qadir A, Chan AC, Lau JY, Chung SC. Small-bowel perforations related to endoscopic retrograde cholangiopancreatography (ERCP) in patients with Billroth II gastrectomy. *Endoscopy* 1999; 31 (7): 546–9.

234 Kim MH, Lee SK, Lee MH, Myung SJ, Yoo BM, Seo DW *et al.* Endoscopic retrograde cholangiopancreatography and needle knife sphincterotomy in patients with Billroth II gastrectomy: a comparative study of the forward-viewing endoscope and the side-viewing duodenoscope. *Endoscopy* 1997; 29: 82–5.

235 Gould J, Train JS, Dan SL *et al.* Duodenal perforations as a delayed complication of placement of a biliary endoprosthesis. *Radiology* 1988; 157: 467–90.

236 Ruffolo TA, Lehman GA, Sherman S *et al.* Biliary stent migration with colonic diverticular impaction. *Gastrointest Endosc* 1991; 38: 81–3.

237 Nelson DB. Infectious disease complications of GI Endoscopy: Part I, endogenous infections. *Gastrointest Endosc* 2003; 57 (4): 546–56.

238 Benchimol D, Bernard JL, Mouroux J, Dumas R, Elkaim D, Chazal M *et al.* Infectious complications of endoscopic retrograde cholangio-pancreatography managed in a surgical unit. *Int Surg* 1992; 77: 270–3.

239 Motte S, Deviere J, Dumonceau J-M, Serruys E, Thus J-P, Cremer M. Risk factors for septicemia following endoscopic biliary stenting. *Gastroenterology* 1991; 101: 1274–81.

240 YuJ-L, Luungh A. Review. Infections associated with biliary drains. *Scand J Gastroenterol* 1996; 31: 625–30.

241 Deviere J, Motte S, Dumonceau JM *et al*. Septicemia after endoscopic retrograde cholangiopancreatography. *Endoscopy* 1990; 22: 72–5.

242 Mollison LC, Desmond PV, Stockman KA *et al*. A prospective study of septic complications of endoscopic retrograde cholangiopancreatography. *J Gastroenterol Hepatol* 1994; 9: 55–9.

243 Novello P, Hagege H, Ducreux M *et al*. Septicemias after endoscopic retrograde cholangiopancreatography. Risk factors and antibiotic prophylaxis. *Gastroenterol Clin Biol* 1993; 17: 897–902.

244 Kullman E, Borch K, Lindstrom E, Ansehn S, Ihse I, Anderberg B. Bacteremia following diagnostic and therapeutic ERCP. *Gastrointest Endosc* 1992; 38 (4): 444–9.

245 Axon ATR, Cotton PB, Phillips I, Avery SA. Disinfection of gastrointestinal fiber endoscopes. *Lancet* 1974; 1: 656–8.

246 Katsinelos P, Dimiropoulos S, Katsiba D, Arvaniti M, Tsolkas P *et al*. Pseudomonas aeruginosa liver abscesses after diagnostic endoscopic retrograde cholangiography in two patients with sphincter of Oddi dysfunction type 2. *Surg Endosc* 2002; 16 (11): 1638.

247 Bass DH, Oliver S, Bornman PC. Pseudomonas septicaemia after endoscopic retrograde cholangiopancreatography—an unresolved problem [Review]. *S Afr Med J* 1990; 77: 509–11.

248 Struelens MJ, Rost F, Deplano A *et al*. Pseudomonas aeruginosa and enterobacteriaceae bacteremia after biliary endoscopy: an outbreak investigation using DNA macrorestriction analysis. *Am J Med* 1993; 95: 489–98.

249 Allen JI, Allen MO, Olson MM *et al*. Pseudomonas infection of the biliary system resulting from the use of a contaminated endoscope. *Gastroenterology* 1987; 192: 759–63.

250 Novello P, Hagege H, Buffet C, Fritsch J, Choury A, Etienne JP. Septicemia after endoscopic retrograde cholangiopancreatography. *Gastroenterology* 1992; 103: 1367.

251 Baker JP, Haber GB, Gray RR, Handy S. Emphysematous cholecystitis complicating endoscopic retrograde cholangiography. *Gastrointest Endosc* 1982; 28 (3): 184–6.

252 Alvarez C, Hunt K, Ashley SW, Reber HA. Emphysematous cholecystitis after ERCP. *Dig Dis Sci* 1994; 39: 1719–23.

253 Tseng A, Sales DJ, Simonowitz DA, Enker WE. Pancreas abscess: a fatal complication of endoscopic cholangiopancreatography (ERCP). *Endoscopy* 1977; 9: 250–3.

254 Finkelstein R, Yassin K, Suissa A, Lavy A, Eidelman S. Failure of cefonicid prophylaxis for infectious complications related to endoscopic retrograde cholangiopancreatography. *Clin Infect Dis* 1996; 23: 378–9.

255 Byl B, Deviere J. Antibiotic prophylaxis before endoscopic retrograde cholangiopancreatography. *Ann Intern Med* 1997; 126 (12): 1001.

256 Sauter G, Grabein B, Huber G, Mannes GA, Ruckdeschel G, Sauerbruch T. Antibiotic prophylaxis of infectious complications with endoscopic retrograde cholangiopancreatography: a randomized controlled study. *Endoscopy* 1990; 22: 164–7.

257 Subbani JM, Kibbler C, Dooley JS. Review article: antibiotic prophylaxis for endoscopic retrograde cholangiopancreatography (ERCP). *Aliment Pharmacol Ther* 1999; 13 (2): 103–16.

258 Niederau C, Pohlmann U, Lubke H, Thomas L. Prophylactic antibiotic treatment in therapeutic or complicated diagnostic ERCP: results of a randomized controlled clinical study. *Gastrointest Endosc* 1994; 40 (5): 533–7.

259 Van den Hazel SJ, Speelman P, Tytgat GNJ, Dankert J, van Leeuwen DJ. Role of antibiotics in the treatment and prevention of acute and recurrent cholangitis. *Clin Infect Dis* 1994; 19: 279–86.

260 Byl B, Deviere J, Struelens MJ, Roucloux I, De Conick A, Thys J-P *et al*. Antibiotic prophylaxis for infectious complications after therapeutic endoscopic retrograde cholangiopancreatography: a randomized, double-blind, placebo-controlled study. *Clin Infect Dis* 1995; 20: 1236–40.

261 Alveyn CG, Robertson DAF, Wright R, Lowes JA, Tillotson G. Prevention of sepsis following endoscopic retrograde cholangiopancreatography. *J Hosp Infect* 1991; 19 (Suppl. C): 65–70.

262 Van de Meeberg PC, van Berge Henegouwen GP. No routine antibiotic prophylaxis necessary in endoscopic retrograde cholangiopancreatography. *Ned Tijdschr Geneeskd* 1997; 141 (9): 412–3.

263 Alveyn CG. Antimicrobial prophylaxis during biliary endoscopic procedures. *Antimicrob Chemother* 1993; 31 (Suppl B): 101–5.

264 Connor P, Hawes RH, Cunningham JT, Cotton PB. Antibiotics before ERCP; a sequential quality improvement approach. *Gastrointest Endosc* 2002; 55: AB97.

265 Goodall RJR. Bleeding after endoscopic sphincterotomy. *Ann R Coll Surg* 1985; 67: 87–8.

266 Mellinger JD, Ponsky JL. Bleeding after endoscopic sphincterotomy as an underestimated entity. *Surgery* 1991; 172: 465–9.

267 Moreira VF, Arribas R, Sanroman AL *et al*. Choledocholithiasis in cirrhotic patients: is endoscopic sphincterotomy the safest choice? *Am J Gastroenterol* 1991; 86: 1006–9.

268 Nelson DB, Freeman ML. Major hemorrhage from endoscopic sphincterotomy: risk factor analysis. *J Clin Gastroenterol* 1994; 19 (4): 283–7.

269 www.asge.org

270 Hussain N, Toubouti Y, Jean-Francois B. Are medications that affect platelet function associated with bleeding following therapeutic endoscopy: a case–control study. *Am J Gastroenterol* 2003; 98 (9): S220.

271 Wilcox CM, Canakis J, Monkemuller KE, Bondora AW, Geels W. Patterns of bleeding after endoscopic sphincterotomy, the subsequent risk of bleeding, and the role of epinephrine injection. *Am J Gastroenterol* 2004; 99: 244–8.

272 Perini RF, Sadurski R, Cotton PB, Patel RS, Hawes RH, Cunningham JT. Post-sphincterotomy bleeding after the introduction of a microprocessor-controlled electrocautery. Does the new technology make the difference? *Gastrointest Endosc* 2005; 61: 53–7.

273 Gorelick A, Cannon M, Barnett J, Chey W, Scheiman J, Elta G. First cut, then blend: an electrocautery technique affecting bleeding at sphincterotomy. *Endoscopy* 2001; 33: 976–80.

274 Park DH, Kim M-H, Lee SK, Lee SS, Song MH, Choi JS *et al*. Endoscopic sphincterotomy versus endoscopic papillary balloon dilatation for choledocholithiasis in liver cirrhosis with coagulopathy. *Gastrointest Endosc* 2004; 59 (5): AB192.

275 Moneira VF, Morono E, Larraon JL *et al*. Choledocholithiasis in cirrhotic patients: is endoscopic sphincterotomy the safest choice? *Am J Gastroenterol* 1991; 86: 1006–9.

276 Mosca S, Galasso G. Immediate and late bleeding after endoscopic sphincterotomy. *Endoscopy* 1999; 31 (3): 278–9.

277 Ooujaoude J, Pelletier G, Fritsch J, Choury A, Lefebvre JF, Roche A *et al*. Management of clinically relevant bleeding following endoscopic sphincterotomy. *Endoscopy* 1994; 26: 217–21.

278 Matsushita M, Hajiro K, Takakuwa H *et al*. Effective hemostatic injection above the bleeding site for uncontrolled bleeding after endoscopic sphincterotomy. *Gastrointest Endosc* 2000; 51: 221–3.

279 Vasconez C, Llach J, Bordas L *et al*. Injection treatment of hemorrhage induced by endoscopic sphincterotomy. *Endoscopy* 1998; 1: 37–9.

280 Petersen S, Henke G, Freitag M, Ludwig K. Management of hemorrhage and perforation following endoscopic sphincterotomy. *Zentralbl Chir* 2001; 126 (10): 805–9.

281 Costamagna G. What to do when the papilla bleeds after endoscopic sphincterotomy. *Endoscopy* 1998; 30: 40–2.

282 Petersen S, Henke G, Freitag M, Ludwig K. Management of hemorrhage and perforation following endoscopic sphincterotomy. *Zentralbl Chir* 2001; 125 (10): 805–9.

283 Sherman S, Hawes RH, Nisi R, Lehman GA. Endoscopic sphincterotomy-induced hemorrhage: treatment with multipolar electrocoagulation. *Gastrointest Endosc* 1992; 38: 123–6.

284 Lo SK, Patel A. Treatment of endoscopic sphincterotomy-induced hemorrhage: injection of bleeding site with ERCP contrast solution using a minor papilla diagnostic catheter. *Gastrointest Endosc* 1993; 39: 346–9.

285 Baron TH, Norton ID, Herman L. Endoscopic hemoclip for post-sphincterotomy bleeding. *Gastrointest Endosc* 2000; 52: 662.

286 Leung JWC, Chan FK, Sung JJ, Chung S. Endoscopic sphincterotomy-induced hemorrhage: a study of risk factors and the role of epinephrine injection. *Gastrointest Endosc* 1995; 52: 550–4.

287 Saeed M, Kadir S, Kaufman SL, Murray RR *et al*. Bleeding following endoscopic sphincterotomy: angiographic management by transcatheter embolization. *Gastrointest Endosc* 1989; 35: 300–3.

288 Margulies C, Siqueira ES, Silverman WB, Lin XS, Martin JA, Rabinovitz M *et al.* The effect of endoscopic sphincterotomy on acute and chronic complications of biliary endoprostheses. *Gastrointest Endosc* 1999; 49: 716–9.

289 Speer AG, Cotton PB, Rode J *et al.* Biliary stent blockage with bacterial biofilm: a light and electron microscopy study. *Ann Intern Med* 1988; 108: 546–33.

290 Johanson JF, Schmalz MJ, Geenen JE. Incidence and risk factors for biliary and pancreatic stent migration. *Gastrointest Endosc* 1992; 38: 341–6.

291 Kozarek RA. Pancreatic stents can induce ductal changes consistent with chronic pancreatitis. *Gastrointest Endosc* 1990; 36: 93–5.

292 Sherman S, Hawes RH, Savides TJ, Gress FG, Ikenberry SO, Smith MT *et al.* Stent-induced pancreatic ductal and parenchymal changes: correlation of endoscopic ultrasound with ERCP. *Gastrointest Endosc* 1996; 44: 276–82.

293 Siegel J, Veerappan A. Endoscopic management of pancreatic disorders: potential risks of pancreatic prostheses. *Endoscopy* 1991; 23: 177–80.

294 Smith MT, Sherman S, Ikenberry SO, Hawes RH, Lehman GA. Alterations in pancreatic ductal morphology following polyethylene pancreatic stent therapy. *Gastrointest Endosc* 1996; 44: 268–75.

295 Rashdan A, Fogel E, McHenry L, Sherman S, Schmidt S, Lazzell L *et al.* Pancreatic ductal changes following small diameter long length unflanged pancreatic stent placement [Abstract]. *Gastrointest Endosc* 2003; 57: AB213.

296 Dolan R, Pinkas H, Brady PG. Acute cholecystitis after palliative stenting for malignant obstruction of the biliary tree. *Gastrointest Endosc* 1993; 39: 447–9.

297 Ainly CC, Williams SJ, Smith AC, Hatfield ARW, Russel RCG, Lees WR. Gallbladder sepsis after stent insertion for bile duct obstruction: management by percutaneous cholecystostomy. *Br J Surg* 1991; 78: 961–3.

298 Leung JWC, Chung SCS, Sung YJ, Li MKW. Acute cholecystitis after stenting of the common bile duct for obstruction secondary to pancreatic cancer. *Gastrointest Endosc* 1989; 35: 109–10.

299 Payne WG, Norman JG, Pinkas H. Endoscopic basket impaction [Review]. *Ann Surg* 1995; 61: 464–7.

300 Lee JF, Leung JWC, Cotton PB. Acute cardiovascular complications of endoscopy: prevalence and clinical characteristics. *Dig Dis* 1995; 13 (2): 130–5.

301 Lieberman DA, Wuerker CK, Katon RM. Cardiopulmonary risk of esophagogastroduodenoscopy: role of endoscope diameter and systemic sedation. *Gastroenterology* 1985; 88: 468–72.

302 Rosenberg J, Jorgensen LN, Rasmussen V *et al.* Hypoxaemia and myocardial ischaemia during and after endoscopic cholangiopancreatography: Call for further studies. *Scand J Gastroenterol* 1992; 27: 717–20.

303 Johnston SD, McKenna A, Tham TC. Silent myocardial ischaemia during endoscopic retrograde cholangiopancreatography. *Endoscopy* 2003; 35 (12): 1039–42.

304 Freeman ML. Sedation and monitoring for gastrointestinal endoscopy. *Gastrointest Endosc Clin N Am* 1994; 4 (3): 475–98.

305 Despland M, Calvein PA, Mentha G, Rohner A. Gallstone ileus and bowel perforation after endoscopic sphincterotomy. *Am J Gastroenterol* 1992; 87: 886–7.

306 Prackup GM, Baborjee B, Piorkowski RJ, Rossan RS. Gallstone ileus following endoscopic sphincterotomy. *J Clin Gastroenterol* 1990; 12: 230–2.

307 To EW, Pang PC, Lee DW. Temporomandibular joint dislocation during endoscopic retrograde cholangiopancreatography examination. *Endoscopy* 2000; 32 (6): S36–7.

308 Blind PJ, Oberg L, Hedberg B. Hepatic portal vein gas following ERCP with sphincterotomy. *Eur J Surg* 1991; 157: 299–300.

309 Dickey W, Huibregtse K, Rauws EAJ *et al.* Direct pancreatic lymphangiography during ERCP. *Gastrointest Endosc* 1995; 41: 528.

310 Herman JB, Levine MS, Long WB. Portal venous gas as a complication of ERCP and endoscopic sphincterotomy. *Am J Gastroenterol* 1995; 90: 828–9.

311 Seibert DG, Al-Kawas FH, Graves J, Gaskins RD. Prospective evaluation of renal function following ERCP. *Endoscopy* 1991; 23: 355–6.

312 Draganov P, Cotton PB. Iodinated contrast sensitivity in ERCP. *Am J Gastroenterol* 2000; 95 (6): 1398–401.

313 Beuers U, Spengler U, Sackmann M, Paumgartner G, Sauerbruch T. Deterioration of cholestasis after endoscopic retrograde cholangiography in advanced primary sclerosing cholangitis. *J Hepatol* 1992; 15: 140–3.

314 Furman G, Morgenstern L. Splenic injury and abscess complicating endoscopic retrograde cholangiopancreatography. *Surg Endosc* 1993; 39: 343–4.

315 Lewis FW, Moloo N, Steigmann GV, Goff JS. Splenic injury complicating therapeutic upper gastrointestinal endoscopy and ERCP. *Gastrointest Endosc* 1991; 37: 632–3.

316 Tronsden E, Rosseland AR, Moer A, Solheim K. Rupture of the spleen following endoscopic retrograde cholangiopancreatography. *Acta Chir Scand* 1989; 155: 75–6.

317 Gilad J, David A, Hertzanu Y, Flusser D, Wolak T, Levi I *et al.* Endoscopic biliary sphincterotomy complicated by abscess formation in a simple renal cyst. *Endoscopy* 1999; 31 (2): S5–6.

318 Katsinelos P, Eugenidis N, Vasilliadis T, Tsoukalas I, Xiarchos P, Triantopoulos I. Hemolysis due to G-6-PD deficiency induced by endoscopic sphincterotomy. *Endoscopy* 1998; 30 (6): 581.

319 Nguyen NQ, Maddern GJ, Berry DP. Endoscopic retrograde cholangiopancreatography-induced hemolytic uraemic syndrome. *Aust N Z J Surg* 2000; 70: 235–6.

320 Studley JGN, Sami AR, Williamson RCN. Dissemination of pancreatic carcinoma following endoscopic sphincterotomy. *Endoscopy* 1993; 25: 301–2.

321 Al-Jeroudi A, Belli AM, Shorvon PJ. False aneurysm of the pancreaticoduodenal artery complicating therapeutic endoscopic retrograde cholangiopancreatography. *Br J Radiol* 2001; 74 (880): 375–7.

322 Male R, Lehman G, Sherman S, Cotton P, Hawes R, Gottlieb K, *et al.* Severe and fatal complications from diagnostic and therapeutic ERCPs. *Gastrointest Endosc* 1994; 40 (2): P29.

323 Klimczak J, Markert R. Retrospective analysis of post-endoscopic retrograde cholangiopancreatography mortalities. *Pol Merkuriusz Lek* 2003; 15 (86): 199–201.

324 Thompson AM, Wright DJ, Murray W, Ritchie GL, Burton HD, Stonebridge PA. Analysis of 153 deaths after upper gastrointestinal endoscopy: room for improvement? *Surg Endosc* 2004; 18: 22–5.

325 Trap R, Adamsen S, Hart-Hansen O, Henriksen M. Severe and fatal complications after diagnostic and therapeutic ERCP: a prospective series of claims to insurance covering public hospitals. *Endoscopy* 1999; 31 (2): 125–30.

326 Khanna N, May G, Cole M, Bass S, Romagnuolo J. Post-ERCP radiology interpretation of cholangio-pancreatograms appears to be of limited benefit and may be inaccurate. *Gastrointest Endosc* 2004; 59 (5): AB186.

327 Cotton PB. Stents for stones: short-term good, long-term uncertain. *Gastrointest Endosc* 1995; 42: 272–3.

328 Prat F. The long term consequences of endoscopic sphincterotomy. *Acta Gastro Enterologica Belgica* 2000; LXIII: 395–6.

329 Sheth SG, Howell DA. What are really the true late complications of endoscopic biliary sphincterotomy? *Am J Gastroenterol* 2002; 97 (11): 2699–701.

330 Bergman JJGHM, van der Mey S, Rauws EAJ, Tijssen JGP, Gouma D-J, Tytgat GNJ *et al.* Long-term follow-up after endoscopic sphincterotomy for bile duct stones in patients younger than 60 years of age. *Gastrointest Endosc* 1996; 44 (6): 643–9.

331 Prat F, Malak NA, Pelletier G, Buffet C, Fritsch J, Choury AD *et al.* Biliary symptoms and complications more than 8 years after endoscopic sphincterotomy for choledocholithiasis. *Gastroenterology* 1996; 110: 894–9.

332 Hawes RH, Cotton PB, Vallon AG. Follow-up at 6–11 years after duodenoscopic sphincterotomy for stones in patients with prior cholecystectomy. *Gastroenterology* 1990; 98: 1008–12.

333 Sugiyama M, Atomi Y. Risk factors predictive of late complications after endoscopic sphincterotomy for bile duct stones: long-term (more than 10 years) follow-up study. *Am J Gastroenterol* 2002; 97 (11): 2763–7.

334 Costamagna G, Tringali A, Shah SK, Mutignani M, Zuccala G, Perri V. Long-term follow-up of patients after endoscopic sphincterotomy for choledocholithiasis, and risk factors for recurrence. *Endoscopy* 2002; 34 (4): 273–9.

335 Pereira-Lima JC, Jakobs R, Winter UH, Benz C, Martin WR *et al.* Long-term results (7–10 years) of endoscopic papillotomy for choledocholithiasis: multivariate analysis of prognostic factors for the recurrence of biliary symptoms. *Gastrointest Endosc* 1998; 48: 457–64.

336 Tanaka M, Takahata S, Konomi H, Matsunaga H, Yokohata K *et al.* Long-term consequences of endoscopic sphincterotomy for bile duct stones. *Gastrointest Endosc* 1996; 44: 465–9.

337 Frimberger E. Long-term sequelae of endoscopic papillotomy. *Endoscopy* 1998; 30 (9): A221–7.

338 Kullman E, Borch K, Liedberg G. Long-term follow-up after endoscopic management of retained and recurrent common duct stones. *Acta Chir Scand* 1989; 155: 395–9.

339 Park SH, Watkins JL, Fogel EL, Sherman S, Lazzell L, Bucksot L *et al.* Long-term outcome of endoscopic dual pancreatobiliary sphincterotomy in patients with manometry-documented sphincter of Oddi dysfunction and normal pancreatogram. *Gastrointest Endosc* 2003; 57 (4): 483–91.

340 Sugiyama M, Atomi Y. Does endoscopic sphincterotomy cause prolonged pancreatobiliary reflux? *Am J Gastroenterol* 1999; 94 (3): 795–8.

341 Cetta F. The possible role of sphincteroplasty and surgical sphincterotomy in the pathogenesis of recurrent common duct brown stones. *HPB Surg* 1991; 4: 261–70.

342 Sand J, Airo I, Hiltunen K-M, Mattila J, Nordback I. Changes in biliary bacteria after endoscopic cholangiography and sphincterotomy. *Am Surg* 1992; 5: 324–8.

343 Bordas JM, Elizalde I, Llach J, Mondelo F, Bataller R, Teres J. Biliary reflux due to sphincter of Oddi ablation: a new pathogenetic explanation for long-term major biliary symptoms after endoscopic-sphincterotomy. *Endoscopy* 1996; 28 (7): 642.

344 Johnston GW. Iatrogenic chymobilia—A disease of the nineties? *HPB Surg* 1991; 4: 187–90.

345 Hakamada K, Sasaki M, Endoh M, Itoh T, Morita T, Konn M. Does sphincteroplasty predispose to bile duct cancer? *Surgery* 1997; 121: 488–92.

346 Karlson BM, Ekbom A, Arvidsson D, Yuen J, Krusemo UB. Population-based study of cancer risk and relative survival following sphincterotomy for stones in the common bile ducts. *Br J Surg* 1997; 84: 1235–8.

347 Tham TCK, Carr-Locke DL, Collins JSA. Endoscopic sphincterotomy in the young patient: is there cause for concern? *Gut* 1997; 40: 697–700.

348 Geenen DJ, Geenen JE, Jafri FM, Hogan WJ, Catalano MF, Johnson GK *et al.* The role of surveillance endoscopic retrograde cholangiopancreatography in preventing episodic cholangitis in patients with recurrent common bile duct stones. *Endoscopy* 1998; 30: 18–20.

349 Escourrou J, Cordova JA, Lazorthes F, Frexinos J. Early and late complications after endoscopic sphincterotomy for biliary lithiasis with and without the gallbladder 'in situ'. *Gut* 1984; 25: 598–602.

350 Tanaka M, Ikeda S, Yoshimoto H *et al.* The long-term fate of the gallbladder after endoscopic sphincterotomy: complete follow-up study of 122 patients. *Am J Surg* 1987; 154: 505.

351 Ingoldby CJH, El-Saadi J, Hall RI *et al.* Late results of endoscopic sphincterotomy for bile duct stones in the elderly patient with gallbladders in situ. *Gut* 1989; 30: 1129.

352 Hill J, Martin DE, Tweedle DEF. Risks of leaving the gallbladder in situ after endoscopic sphincterotomy for bile duct stones. *Br J Surg* 1991; 78: 554.

353 Boerma D, Rauws EA, Keulemans YC, Janssen IM, Bolwerk CJ, Timmer R *et al.* Wait-and-see policy or laparoscopic cholecystectomy after endoscopic sphincterotomy for bile-duct stones: a randomized trial. *Lancet* 2002; 360 (9335): 761–5.

354 Kaw M, Al-Antably Y, Kaw P. Management of gallstone pancreatitis: cholecystectomy or ERCP and endoscopic sphincterotomy. *Gastrointest Endosc* 2002; 56 (1): 61–5.

355 Asbun HJ, Rossi RL, Heiss FW, Shea JA. Acute relapsing pancreatitis as a complication of papillary stenosis after endoscopic sphincterotomy. *Gastroenterology* 1993; 104: 1814–17.

356 Gerstenberger PD, Plumeri PA. Malpractice claims in gastrointestinal endoscopy: analysis of an insurance industry data base. *Gastrointest Endosc* 1993; 39 (2): 132–8.

357 Cotton PB. Is your sphincterotomy really safe—and necessary? *Gastrointest Endosc* 1996; 44 (6): 752–5.

358 www.asge.org

359 Martin DF. Endoscopic retrograde cholangiopancreatography should no longer be used as a diagnostic test: an independent verdict. *Digest Liv Dis* 2002; 34: 381–2.

360 Cotton PB. How many times have you done this procedure, Doctor? *Am J Gastroenterol* 2002; 97: 522–3.

INDEX

Note: page numbers in *italics* refer to figures, those in **bold** refer to tables.

405